Bio-inspired Algorithms in Machine Learning and Deep Learning for Disease Detection

Editors:

Balasubramaniam S
School of Computer Science and Engineering
Kerala University of Digital Sciences, Innovation and
Technology (Formerly IIITM-K), Digital University Kerala
Thiruvananthapuram, Kerala, India

Seifedine Kadry
Department of Applied Data Science
Noroff University College, Kristiansand, Norway
or
Department of Computer Science and Mathematics
Lebanese American University, Beirut, Lebanon

Manoj Kumar T K
School of Digital Sciences
Kerala University of Digital Sciences, Innovation and Technology
Thiruvananthapuram, Kerala, India

K. Satheesh Kumar
School of Digital Sciences
Kerala University of Digital Sciences, Innovation and Technology
Thiruvananthapuram, Kerala, India

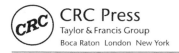

CRC Press is an imprint of the
Taylor & Francis Group, an **informa** business

A SCIENCE PUBLISHERS BOOK

First edition published 2025
by CRC Press
2385 NW Executive Center Drive, Suite 320, Boca Raton FL 33431

and by CRC Press
4 Park Square, Milton Park, Abingdon, Oxon, OX14 4RN

© 2025 Balasubramaniam S, Seifedine Kadry, Manoj Kumar T K and K. Satheesh Kumar

CRC Press is an imprint of Taylor & Francis Group, LLC

Reasonable efforts have been made to publish reliable data and information, but the author and publisher cannot assume responsibility for the validity of all materials or the consequences of their use. The authors and publishers have attempted to trace the copyright holders of all material reproduced in this publication and apologize to copyright holders if permission to publish in this form has not been obtained. If any copyright material has not been acknowledged please write and let us know so we may rectify in any future reprint.

Except as permitted under U.S. Copyright Law, no part of this book may be reprinted, reproduced, transmitted, or utilized in any form by any electronic, mechanical, or other means, now known or hereafter invented, including photocopying, microfilming, and recording, or in any information storage or retrieval system, without written permission from the publishers.

For permission to photocopy or use material electronically from this work, access www.copyright.com or contact the Copyright Clearance Center, Inc. (CCC), 222 Rosewood Drive, Danvers, MA 01923, 978-750-8400. For works that are not available on CCC please contact mpkbookspermissions@tandf.co.uk

Trademark notice: Product or corporate names may be trademarks or registered trademarks and are used only for identification and explanation without intent to infringe.

Library of Congress Cataloging-in-Publication Data (applied for)

ISBN: 978-1-032-86548-5 (hbk)
ISBN: 978-1-032-88509-4 (pbk)
ISBN: 978-1-003-53815-8 (ebk)

DOI: 10.1201/9781003538158

Typeset in Times New Roman
by Prime Publishing Services

Preface

Currently, computational intelligence approaches are utilised in various science and engineering applications to analyse information, make decisions, and achieve optimisation goals. Over the past few decades, various techniques and algorithms have been created in disciplines such as genetic algorithms, artificial neural networks, evolutionary algorithms, and fuzzy algorithms. In the coming years, intelligent optimisation algorithms are anticipated to become more efficient in addressing various issues in engineering, scientific, medical, space, and artificial satellite fields, particularly in early disease diagnosis. A metaheuristic in computer science is designed to discover optimisation algorithms capable of solving intricate issues. Metaheuristics are optimisation algorithms that mimic biological behaviours of animals or birds and are utilised to discover the best solution for a certain problem. A meta-heuristic is an advanced approach used by heuristics to tackle intricate optimisation problems. A metaheuristic in mathematical programming is a method that seeks a solution to an optimisation problem. Metaheuristics utilise a heuristic function to assist in the search process. Heuristic search can be categorised as a blind or informed search. Metaheuristic optimisation algorithms are gaining popularity in various applications due to their simplicity, independence from data trends, ability to find optimal solutions, and versatility across different fields.

Recently, many nature-inspired computation algorithms have been utilised to diagnose people with different diseases. Nature-inspired methodologies are now widely utilised across several fields for tasks such as data analysis, decision-making, and optimisation. Techniques inspired by nature are categorised as either biology-based or natural phenomena-based. Bio-inspired computing encompasses various topics in computer science, mathematics, and biology in recent years. Bio-inspired computer optimisation algorithms are a developing method that utilises concepts and inspiration from biological development to create new and resilient competitive strategies. Bio-inspired optimisation algorithms have gained recognition in machine learning and deep learning for solving complicated issues in science and engineering. Utilising BIAs learning methods with machine learning and deep learning shows great promise for accurately classifying medical conditions.

This book explores the potential benefits of bio-inspired algorithms (BIAs) and their application in machine learning and deep learning models for disease diagnosis, including COVID-19, heart diseases, cancer, diabetes, and some other diseases. It discusses the advantages of using bio-inspired algorithms in disease diagnosis and concludes with research directions and future prospects in this field.

Contents

Preface	*iii*
About the Editors	*vii*
List of Contributors	*ix*

1. Potential Benefits of BIAs-based ML/DL Models   **1**
*Gopirajan P.V., Hariharan B., Wilfred Blessing N.R. and
Anupama C.G.*

2. BIAs-based Deep Learning (DL) Models   **23**
N. Sanjana, R. Immanual, K.M. Kirthika, S. Sangeetha, and
K. Maharaja

**3. Evaluation of Bio-Inspired Algorithm-based Machine
Learning and Deep Learning Models**   **48**
Selvam Durairaj, Malik Mohamed Umar and *Natarajan B.*

**4. Disease Diagnosis: Traditional vs. Bio-Inspired
Algorithm Approaches**   **70**
Varun Saagar Saravanan, Dawn Sivan, K. Satheesh Kumar
and *Rajan Jose*

**5. Algorithmic Heartbeat with Bio-Inspired Algorithms in
Cardiac Health Monitoring**   **89**
Ashwini A., Kavitha V., Balasubramaniam S. and *Seifedine Kadry*

**6. Bio-Inspired Algorithms-based Machine Learning and
Deep Learning Models for COVID-19 Diagnosis**   **107**
S. Sheik Asraf, M. Subash, P. Nagaraj V. Muneeswaran and
Christopher Samuel Raj Balraj

**7. Bio-Inspired Intelligence in Early Cancer Detection:
A Machine Learning Approach**   **122**
Ashwini A., Balasubramaniam S. and *Sundaravadivazhagan B.*

**8. Bio-Inspired Algorithms in Machine Learning and
Deep Learning for Diabetes Diagnosis**   **141**
S. Aathilakshmi, Balasubramaniam S. and *Ayodeji Olalekan Salau*

vi | Contents

9. **A Multi-objective Optimized Bio-inspired Deep Learning Framework for Autism Spectrum Disorder Diagnosis in Toddlers**   **158**
K. Vijayalakshmi and *Venkatesh Naganathan*

10. **Bio-Inspired Algorithms using Machine Learning and Deep Learning for Social Phobia Treatment**   **183**
Abinaya M., Vadivu G., Balasubramaniam S. and *Sundaravadivazhagan B.*

11. **Bio-Inspired Algorithms-based Machine Learning Models for Neural Disorders Prediction: A Focus on Depression Detection**   **203**
Tekulapally Shriya Reddy, Kishor Kumar Reddy C., Manoj Kumar Reddy D. and *Srinath Doss*

12. **Research Directions and Challenges in Bio-Inspired Algorithms for Machine Learning and Deep Learning Models in Healthcare**   **230**
Mani Deepak Choudhry, Sundarrajan M., Akshya Jothi and *Seifedine Kadry*

Index   **249**

About the Editors

Dr. Balasubramaniam S (IEEE Senior Member) is working as an Assistant Professor in School of Computer Science and Engineering, Kerala University of Digital Sciences, Innovation and Technology (Formerly IIITM-K), Digital University Kerala, Thiruvananthapuram, Kerala, India. He has totally around 15+ years of experience in teaching, research and industry. He has completed his Post Doctoral Research in Department of Applied Data Science, Noroff University College, Kristiansand, Norway. He holds a Ph.D degree in Computer Science and Engineering from Anna University, Chennai, India in 2015. He has published nearly 25+ research papers in reputed SCI/WoS/Scopus indexed Journals. He has also granted with 1 Australian patent and 2 Indian Patents and published 2 Indian patents. He has presented papers at conferences, contributed chapters to the edited books and editor in few books published by international publishers. His research and publication interests include machine learning and deep learning-based disease diagnosis, cloud computing security, Generative AI and Electric Vehicles.

Prof. Seifedine Kadry has a bachelor's degree in 1999 from Lebanese University, MS degree in 2002 from Reims University (France) and EPFL (Lausanne), PhD in 2007 from Blaise Pascal University (France), HDR degree in 2017 from Rouen University (France). At present his research focuses on Data Science, education using technology, system prognostics, stochastic systems, and applied mathematics. He is an ABET program evaluator for computing, and ABET program evaluator for Engineering Tech. he is a full professor of data science at Noroff University College, Norway and Department of Computer Science, Lebanese American University, Beirut, Lebanon.

Prof.T K Manojkumar, currently serving as Dean (Research) and Professor at Kerala University of Digital Sciences, Innovation and Technology, Thiruvananthapuram, Kerala, India. He is having 5 years of post-doctoral research experience in prestigious institutions like IIT-Madras and Pohang University of Science & Technology, Korea. With an impressive 17-year track record in post-graduate teaching, Dr Manoj has imparted knowledge across a diverse range of subjects including Data Analytics, Deep Learning, Computational Sciences, Predictive Analytics, Big data technologies and Cloud computing, Discrete mathematics, Ordinary differential Equations, Automata, Data Structure and Algorithm, Artificial Intelligence, and Quantum Chemistry. Their scholarly contributions extend to 80 publications in international journals of high impact, marking a significant impact in their respective fields. Previously, he has holding key administrative roles such as Chair of the School of Digital Sciences; Registrar, Digital University Kerala; Registrar, Indian Institute of Information Technology and Management – Kerala and Director of the International Centre for Free and Open-Source Systems, Kerala, India.

Prof. K. Satheesh Kumar presently holds the role of Visiting Professor at the Kerala University of Digital Sciences, Innovation, and Technology, Thiruvananthapuram Kerala, India. Previously, he served as Professor and Head of the Department of Futures Studies at the University of Kerala, Kerala, India. Dr. Kumar's academic journey began with a degree in mathematics, followed by doctoral research in suspension rheology and chaotic dynamics at the CSIR Lab in Thiruvananthapuram. He subsequently pursued post-doctoral research positions at Monash University, Australia, and POSTECH, South Korea. Dr. Kumar's research interests span suspension and polymer rheology, chaotic dynamics, nonlinear time series analysis, geophysics, complex network analysis, and wind energy modeling and forecasting.

List of Contributors

Abinaya M.
Department of Data Science and Business Systems SRM Institute of Science and Technology, Kattankulathur, Chennai, India.

Akshya Jothi
Department of Computational Intelligence, SRM Institute of Science and Technology, Kattankalathur, Chengalpattu, Tamil Nadu, India.

Anupama C.G.
Department of Computational Intelligence, School of Computing, SRM Institute of Science and Technology, Kattankulathur, Chennai, India.

Ashwini A.
Department of Electronics and Communication Engineering, Vel Tech Rangarajan Dr. Sagunthala R&D Institute of Science and Technology, Avadi, Chennai, Tamilnadu, India.

Ayodeji Olalekan Salau
Department of Electrical and Computer Engineering, Afe Babalola University, Nigeria.

Balasubramaniam S.
School of Computer Science and Engineering, Kerala University of Digital Sciences, Innovation and Technology (Formerly IIITM-K), Digital University Kerala, Thiruvananthapuram, Kerala, India.

Christopher Samuel Raj Balraj
International College of the Cayman Islands, Grand Cayman, Cayman Islands.

Dawn Sivan
Center for Advanced Intelligent Materials and Faculty of Industrial Sciences and Technology, Universiti Malaysia Pahang Al-Sultan Abdullah, 26300, Kuantan, Pahang, Malaysia.

Gopirajan P.V.
Department of Computational Intelligence, School of Computing, SRM Institute of Science and Technology, Kattankulathur, Chennai, India.

List of Contributors

Hariharan B.
Department of Computational Intelligence, School of Computing, SRM Institute of Science and Technology, Kattankulathur, Chennai, India.

K. Maharaja
Department of Electrical and Electronics Engineering, AI Musanna College of Oman, Oman.

K. Satheesh Kumar
School of Digital Sciences, Kerala University of Digital Sciences, Innovation and Technology, Thiruvananthapuram, Kerala, India

K. Vijayalakshmi
School of Computer Science and Applications, REVA University, Bangalore, Karnataka, India.

K.M. Kirthika
Department of Computer Science and Engineering, Sri Ramakrishna Institute of Technology. Coimbatore, India.

Kavitha V.
University College of Engineering, Kancheepuram, Tamilnadu, India.

Kishor Kumar Reddy C.
Department of Computer Science & Engineering, Stanley College of Engineering and Technology for Women, India.

M. Subash
Department of Biotechnology, School of Bio, Chemical and Processing Engineering, Kalasalingam Academy of Research and Education (Deemed to be University), Anand Nagar, Krishnankoil, Tamil Nadu, India.

Malik Mohamed Umar
National Space Science & Technology Center (NSSTC), United Arab Emirates University (UAEU), Al Ain, 15551, Abu Dhabi, UAE.

Mani Deepak Choudhry
Department of Computing Technologies, SRM Institute of Science and Technology, Kattankalathur, Chengalpattu, Tamil Nadu, India.

Manoj Kumar Reddy D.
Department of Electrical and Electronics Engineering, Vardhaman College of Engineering, Hyderabad, India.

N. Sanjana
Department of Computer Science and Engineering, Sri Ramakrishna Institute of Technology. Coimbatore, India.

Natarajan B.
School of Computer Science and Engineering (SCOPE), Vellore Institute of Technology, Chennai Campus, 600127, Tamil Nadu, India.

P. Nagaraj
Department of Computer Science and Engineering, School of Computing, Kalasalingam Academy of Research and Education (Deemed to be University), Anand Nagar, Krishnankoil, Tamil Nadu, India.

R. Immanual
Department of Mechanical Engineering, Sri Ramakrishna Institute of Technology. Coimbatore,India.

Rajan Jose
Center for Advanced Intelligent Materials and Faculty of Industrial Sciences and Technology, Universiti Malaysia Pahang Al-Sultan Abdullah, 26300, Kuantan, Pahang, Malaysia.

S. Sangeetha
Department of Electrical and Electronics Engineering, Sri Ramakrishna Institute of Technology. Coimbatore, India.

S. Sheik Asraf
Department of Biotechnology, School of Bio, Chemical and Processing Engineering, Kalasalingam Academy of Research and Education (Deemed to be University), Anand Nagar, Krishnankoil, Tamil Nadu, India.

Seifedine Kadry
Department of Applied Data Science, Noroff University College, Norway.

Selvam Durairaj
School of Computer Science and Engineering (SCOPE), Vellore Institute of Technology, Chennai Campus, 600127, Tamil Nadu, India.

Srinath Doss
Faculty of Engineering & Technology, Botho University, Botswana.

Sundaravadivazhagan B.
Department of Information Technology, University of Technology and Applied Science-AL Mussanah, Oman.

Sundarrajan M
Department of Networking and Communications, SRM Institute of Science and Technology, Kattankalathur, Chengalpattu, Tamil Nadu, India.

Tekulapally Shriya Reddy
Department of Computer Science & Engineering, Stanley College of Engineering and Technology for Women, India.

V. Muneeswaran
Department of Electronics and Communication Engineering, School of Electronics, Electrical and Biomedical Technology, Kalasalingam Academy of Research and Education (Deemed to be University), Anand Nagar, Krishnankoil, Tamil Nadu, India.

List of Contributors

Vadivu G.

Department of Data Science and Business Systems SRM Institute of Science and Technology, Kattankulathur, Chennai, India.

Varunsaagar Saravanan

Lead AI ML, Asianet News Media and Entertainment Pvt. Ltd., Crescent Road, Gandhi Nagar, Bangalore, India.

Venkatesh Naganathan

Senior Consultant cum Professor, Amity Global Institute, Singapore.

Wilfred Blessing N.R.

IT Department, College of Computing and Information Sciences, University of Technology and Applied Sciences-Ibri, Sultanate of Oman.

1 Potential Benefits of BIAs-based ML/DL Models

Gopirajan P.V.,[1] Hariharan B.,[1*] Wilfred Blessing N.R.[2] and Anupama C.G.[1]

Integrating bio-inspired algorithms with machine learning (ML) and deep learning (DL) models enhances computational intelligence. These algorithms, like neural networks modeling the human brain, ant colony optimization, and particle swarm optimization, offer robust, efficient, and flexible models. Their inherent parallelism, adaptability, and self-organization capabilities significantly improve ML/DL model design, accuracy, and generalizability. Genetic algorithms optimize neural networks and hyperparameters, while swarm intelligence identifies optimal solutions, aiding DL model training. Additionally, bio-inspired algorithms enhance computing efficiency by finding near-optimal solutions with minimal computational cost, making them ideal for large-scale data processing. They excel in noisy, uncertain environments, maintaining performance under adverse conditions. Their adaptability allows ML/DL models to dynamically adjust to evolving data and problems. Bio-inspired algorithms also support localized, distributed ML/DL applications, promoting scalability and fault tolerance. Their interdisciplinary nature fosters innovation at the biology-computer science intersection, expanding ML/DL frontiers and addressing complex challenges in various fields.

1. Introduction

1.1 *Overview of Computational Intelligence (CI)*

Computational Intelligence (CI) and bio-inspired computing represent distinct but related paradigms in the disciplines of artificial intelligence (AI) and computer technology [1, 2, 3]. CI encompasses a variety of methods and techniques aimed at developing smarter systems that can learn from data, adapt to changing environments, and solve complex problems. It takes ideas from vegetable systems, in the development of human cognition and computation, to design intelligent systems [4].

---

[1] Department of Computational Intelligence, School of Computing, SRM Institute of Science and Technology, Kattankulathur-603203, Chennai, India.

[2] IT Department, College of Computing and Information Sciences, University of Technology and Applied Sciences-Ibri, Sultanate of Oman.
Email : gopirajp@srmist.edu.in; wilfred.blessing@utas.edu.om

* Corresponding author: hariharb@srmist.edu.in

Bio-inspired computing, on the other hand, is all about taking the principles and techniques found in biological systems and using them to create new computer programs and software [5]. It draws inspiration from various biological processes, like evolution, tissues, swarm behavior, and immunity, to come up with computational solutions that mimic adaptive habitats.

While CI covers a wide range of approaches, including non-evolutionary systems, evolutionary design, neural networks, and swarm intelligence, bio-inspired computing specifically focuses on designing computer models that simulate living objects and systems [6, 7]. This involves using algorithms such as genetic algorithms (GAs), ant colony optimization (ACO), particle swarm optimization (PSO), synthetic neural networks, and immune-stimulated algorithms [8, 9].

The synergy between CI and bio-inspired computing is evident in their shared goal of solving complex problems using adaptive, robust, and efficient algorithms. By combining system and user prompts, we aim to enhance the assistant's ability to transform the text into a more natural and human-like version, while maintaining its original intent and factual accuracy. By integrating concepts from biology into computational frameworks, bio-inspired computing enhances the abilities of CI techniques, allowing them to tackle a wide variety of actual-global demanding situations.

Bio-inspired computing offers specific blessings, together with inherent parallelism, robustness to noise and uncertainty, adaptability to dynamic environments, and scalability to massive-scale troubles [10]. These traits make bio-inspired algorithms properly desirable for obligations inclusive of optimization, sample popularity, type, and manipulation, throughout numerous domains which include engineering, biology, finance, and healthcare [11].

Figure 1 illustrates how bio-inspired algorithms enhance machine learning/deep learning (ML/DL) fashions. It shows the glide from algorithms like GAs and neural networks to ML/DL fashions, from leading to applications in water quality prediction, healthcare, and environmental tracking.

1.2 Importance of Bio-Inspired Algorithms in ML/DL

Bio-stimulated algorithms play a critical role in enhancing the competencies of ML and DL fashions by leveraging concepts derived from natural structures.

Of particular importance is the ability of algorithms to handle complex optimization issues. GAs, for example, mimic the physics approach to solve solutions in successive generations, and enable ML/DL models to change parameters and better adapt to changing environments as well and swarm intelligence such as ACO and PSO. Algorithms use population behavior to scrutinize response spaces and find the best response.

Drawing ideas from immune systems, those algorithms can discover and adapt to modifications in information distributions or environments, mainly to greater resilient fashions. Additionally, their parallelism and scalability lead them to appropriate for huge-scale and disbursed computing duties, improving the overall performance and scalability of ML/DL structures.

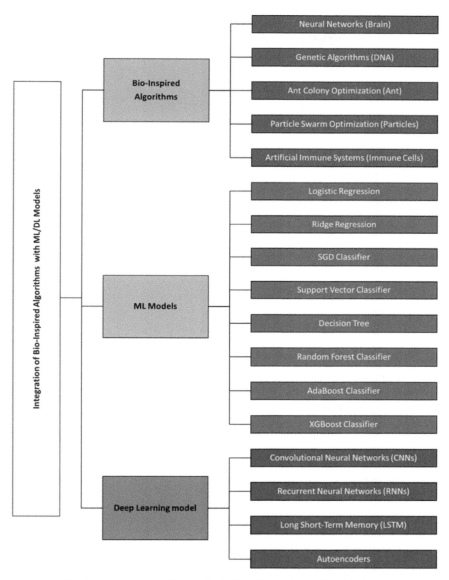

Fig. 1 Integration of Bio-inspired Algorithms with ML/DL Models.

1.3 Objectives of Integrating Bio-inspired Algorithms with ML/DL

The integration of bio-inspired algorithms with ML and DL serves several key objectives, every contribution to the advancement and improvement of sensible structures is given in Figure 2.

Bio-inspired algorithms can improve how ML/DL models find optimal solutions.
This can be applied to tasks like parameter tuning, feature selection, and model architecture optimization.

Enhanced Optimization

- Bio-inspired algorithms can improve how ML/DL models find optimal solutions.
- This can be applied to tasks like parameter tuning, feature selection, and model architecture optimization.

Improved Robustness and Adaptability

- By learning from biological systems, ML/DL models can become more resilient to changes and uncertainties.
- This can involve anomaly detection, adapting to new data, and maintaining performance in dynamic environments.

Exploration of Novel Problem-Solving Approaches

- Bio-inspired algorithms offer unique ways to solve problems compared to traditional methods.
- Integration with ML/DL encourages exploration of these approaches, potentially leading to breakthroughs in challenging domains.

Scalability and Efficiency

- Bio-inspired algorithms often work well with parallel computing.
- Integrating them with ML/DL can improve how these models handle large datasets and complex computations.

Interdisciplinary Innovation

- This combination fosters collaboration between different fields, leading to a richer exchange of ideas and the development of more diverse and innovative intelligent systems with broad applications.

Fig. 2 Objectives of Integrating Bio-inspired Algorithms with ML/DL.

2 Understanding Bio-Inspired Algorithms

2.1 Definition and Concept of Bio-Inspired Algorithms

Bio-inspired algorithms are computational strategies that draw concepts from standards observed in biological structures to clear up complicated troubles. They mimic the behavior, strategies, and mechanisms found in nature, which includes evolution, neural networks, swarm intelligence, and immune structures. The idea behind bio-stimulated algorithms is to emulate the adaptive, self-organizing, and green nature of organic structures in computational fashions [12].

These algorithms embody a huge range of methodologies, which includes GAs, ACO, PSO, artificial neural networks (ANNs), and immune-stimulated algorithms. By harnessing ideas from biology, bio-inspired algorithms offer modern tactics to optimize, sample popularity, type, and manage duties. They showcase residences which includes robustness, adaptability, scalability, and efficiency, making them suitable for addressing complex actual-world problems throughout diverse domain names, together with engineering, healthcare, finance, and environmental technological know-how. The essence of bio-inspired algorithms lies in their ability to translate biological principles into computational frameworks to increase intelligent systems able to solve various demanding situations effectively.

2.2 Types of Bio-Inspired Algorithms

Bio-inspired algorithms encompass a numerous variety of computational techniques, each drawing inspiration from exclusive organic phenomena located in nature. GAs replicate the process of herbal choice and evolution to iteratively optimize solutions via mimicking duplicate, mutation, and choice mechanisms. ACO algorithms simulate ant feeding behavior, placing optimal paths on graphs by pheromone deposition and evaporation; PSO fashions collective behavior of chook swarms or fish faculties, iteratively adjusting particle locations that answers in a search space; Adaptable ANNs are computational models inspired by biological neural network morphology and functions, which are used for tasks such as popular modeling and classification [13, 14, 15, 16]. Immune-inspired algorithms draw attention from the ability of the immune system to detect and remove pathogens, which are used in anomaly detection, optimization, and class issues [17, 18]. Each bio-inspired algorithm offers specific efficiencies and applications in different industries, contributing to the effectiveness of intelligent computing systems.

2.2.1 Neural Networks Modeling the Human Brain

Neural networks that largely mimic the workings of the human mind encourage broader development in AI by reproducing sensory mechanisms These fibers receive emotions from the structure of the mind, with billions of neurons a through synapses that are electrically connected and modulated by synaptic plasticity [19]. ANNs mimic this process with perceptrons—for layered neurons: input, storage, and output. Statistics are applied to the use of weighted combinations and activation functions such as sigmoid and ReLU, enabling the selection and learning of styles [20, 21]. Learning in these networks' parallels Hebbi's principle from biology, which states that "cells that fire together, string together". This is achieved through backpropagation, a technique wherein community weights are adjusted to limit errors using gradient descent. Different types of neural networks emulate various brain features: feedforward networks are effective in sample recognition, Convolutional Neural Networks (CNNs) [22], inspired by using the visible cortex, excel in image processing, and Recurrent Neural Networks (RNNs) [23], together with Long Short-Term Memory (LSTM) networks [24, 25], are adept at modeling temporal sequences for language and time-series analysis. Advances in neuromorphic engineering, which targets to develop hardware that mimics the mind's neural structure and Spiking Neural Networks (SNNs) [26], which use discrete spikes for communication, retain to push the frontiers of AI studies. These mind-stimulated networks have big packages, from improving cognitive computing structures to assisting inside the diagnosis and treatment of neurological disorders.

6 | Bio-inspired Algorithms in Machine Learning and Deep Learning for Disease Detection

However, in addition they increase moral worries, particularly concerning the development of self-sustaining systems and their impact on society. The destiny of NNs lies in the ongoing convergence of neuroscience and AI, with the pursuit of Artificial General Intelligence (AGI) aiming to create incredibly adaptable AI structures with cognitive skills that would at some point surpass human intelligence, marking a new technology of technological and cognitive innovation.

2.2.2 Ant Colony Optimization (ACO)

ACO is an influential algorithm stimulated via the foraging behavior of ants, designed to address complex optimization issues. Developed through Marco Dorigo in the early 1990s, ACO replicates how ants discover shortest paths to meals' sources using pheromones, guiding different ants to most fulfilling routes through a collective intelligence system. In nature, ants deposit pheromones alongside their paths, with shorter routes collecting stronger pheromones trails due to frequent traversal, growing a superb remarks loop that highlights the maximum efficient paths [27]. This natural system is translated into ACO's computational model, where synthetic ants construct answers by using probabilistically choosing steps based on pheromone intensity and heuristic data precise to the hassle. High-great answers bring about stronger pheromone trails, at the same time less favorable paths see pheromone evaporation to hold exploration. ACO excels in solving combinatorial optimization issues including the journeying salesman problem, vehicle routing, community routing, and scheduling, way to its flexibility and adaptability. Despite its robustness and parallelization capability, ACO faces demanding situations like parameter tuning and handling massive-scale problems. Effective balance among exploration and exploitation through pheromone control is crucial to avoid neighborhood optima and reap worldwide solutions. Ongoing studies goals to enhance ACO's efficiency by integrating hybrid algorithms and real-time adaptive mechanisms, promising extra effective answers for dynamic and complicated tasks. ACO stands as a testament to the potential of bio-stimulated algorithms in fixing complex issues throughout numerous domain names.

2.2.3 Particle Swarm Optimization (PSO)

PSO is an evolutionary computation technique stimulated by way of the social behavior of birds flocking and fish training, delivered by means of James Kennedy and Russell Eberhart in 1995 [28]. This set of rules simulates a populace of debris—analogous to male or female birds or fish—that traverse a multidimensional answer space to find ultimate solutions. Each particle adjusts its role based totally on its own level in, and the experience of neighboring particles, guided by using two number one factors: the particle's personal great role and the worldwide first-class role observed through the swarm. These changes permit particles to converge toward optimal answers through an aggregate of exploration and exploitation, balancing the want to search new regions and refine current solutions. PSO is

Potential Benefits of BIAs-based ML/DL Models | 7

distinguished by its simplicity, requiring fewer parameters to tune as compared to different evolutionary algorithms, and its potential to correctly clear up nonlinear, multimodal optimization problems [29].

PSO has been efficiently implemented to a huge variety of traditional optimization demanding situations, consisting of characteristic optimization, NN education, and control systems. However, its novel applications in recent years have validated its versatility and flexibility across various fields [30, 31]. In healthcare, PSO is applied for optimizing remedy plans in radiation therapy, making sure it is concentrated on/of tumors, and at the same time minimizing harm to wholesome tissue. In renewable power, PSO allows in optimizing the location and operation of windmills and solar panels to maximize electricity production and performance. In the realm of finance, it aids in portfolio optimization by way of locating an excellent mixture of property to acquire preferred returns even as minimizing threat. PSO is also making strides in robotics, wherein it is hired for route-making plans and swarm robotics, allowing a couple of robots to navigate and collaborate effectively in complicated environments. Additionally, PSO has discovered programs in the system gaining knowledge of, specifically in hyperparameter tuning for DL models, in which it optimizes the parameters that extensively impact a model's overall performance.

The adaptability of PSO to numerous problem domains, coupled with its truthful implementation, has spurred ongoing research to similarly decorate its talents. Hybrid PSO algorithms, which integrate PSO with other optimization strategies that include GAs or differential evolution, goal to leverage the strengths of multiple strategies for superior overall performance. Furthermore, adaptive editions of PSO dynamically regulate algorithm parameters in response to the optimization procedure, improving convergence quotes and solution satisfactory. As PSO continues to evolve, its packages expand, providing sturdy and green answers to increasingly complicated and dynamic issues across a multitude of disciplines.

2.2.4 Artificial Immune Systems (AIS)

The non-stop evolution of AIS is pushed with the aid of ongoing studies aimed toward enhancing its algorithms and expanding its application domains. Hybrid strategies that integrate AIS with different computational techniques, along with NNs and GAs, are being developed to leverage their complementary strengths, resulting in extra effective and green hassle-solving equipment. As AIS continues to strengthen, its capability to imitate the state-of-the-art adaptive and defensive mechanisms of the biological immune system guarantees to offer innovative answers to an increasing number of complex demanding situations throughout diverse fields.

2.3 Three Key Features of Bio-Inspired Algorithms

Bio-inspired algorithms, drawing concepts from nature, provide specific benefits over conventional techniques. Here's a breakdown of 3 key features:

2.3.1 Inherent Parallelism

Imagine a colony of ants working together to discover food. Individual ants discover distinctive paths, and hit one to leave pheromone trails for others to comply with. This disbursed approach is an indicator of inherent parallelism in bio-inspired algorithms.

2.3.2 Flexibility in Dynamic Environments

The natural worldwide is constantly converting and the ecosystems that inhabit it have developed a fantastic capacity for model. Bio-stimulated algorithms capture this essence via modifications in dynamic environments. Unlike traditional systems, which could resist unexpected adjustments, these systems can fully alter their movements based totally on new information or evolving situations

One example is a set of rules which can be prompted with the assist of an improvement software. Imagine multiple responses (which include a completely unique bridge system) that are continuously changing through mutation and selection. When environmental situations change (e.g., higher wind speeds), selection strain offers the satisfactory advanced method to deal with those forces. Similarly, the bio-inspired algorithm is touchy to unpredictable situations by way of constantly adjusting itself to discover it primarily based on remarks or changes within the goal.

2.3.3 Self-Organization and Learning

Bio-prompted algorithms can also similarly exhibit autonomy, with man or woman creditors working collectively to acquire a non-specific purpose without explicit command. This self-organizing behavior comes from simple regulations carried out to every item.

Another crucial factor is to recognize. Many bio-inspired algorithms comprise inspired mechanisms, the usage of biological getting-to-know techniques. For example, an algorithm stimulated through NNs can alternate its simple inner interactions based totally on experience (records), enhancing its universal overall performance over the years. This self-organizing know-how of competencies presents bio-stimulated algorithms that can continuously boom their effectiveness as they stumble throughout new records or manner new facts.

3. Enhancing ML/DL Models with Bio-Inspired Algorithms

3.1 Improving Accuracy and Generalizability

Another important thing is to know that many bio-stimulated algorithms incorporate stimulated mechanisms using biological learning techniques. For example, an algorithm inspired by NNs can change its basic internal interactions based on experience (data), improving its overall performance over the years. This self-earned knowledge of capabilities provides again-inspired algorithms that can continuously increase their effectiveness as they stumble across new facts or process new information.

3.1.1 Role of Genetic Algorithms in Optimization

Genetic simulations (GAs) are basically optimization methods based on the principles of herbal selection and inheritance (Flux Optimization using GAs in Membrane [32]. They are particularly effective in obtaining large complex areas for high-quality solutions. For ML and DL, GAs can be used to optimize hyperparameters, pick capacities, and design neural network architectures.

3.2 Enhancing Computational Efficiency

3.2.1 Minimizing Computational Costs

Bio-inspired algorithms can significantly reduce computational costs in ML and DL models. Methods such as genetic design and PSO simplify the optimization process and require fewer resources than traditional methods.

3.3 Robustness in Noisy and Uncertain Environments

3.3.1 Handling Noise and Data Variability

Bio-inspired algorithms are mainly adept at fixing noise and statistical variability, which aren't unusual challenges in actual-global programs. As an example, GAs use strategies inclusive of mutation and crossover to discover answers that are greater, increasing their robustness to noisy calculations by considering more than one solution simultaneously, thereby a more reliable method by which errors and insights can be generalized.

3.3.2 Maintaining Performance under Adverse Conditions

Bio-inspired algorithms additionally excel in preserving overall performance under adverse conditions, including environmental fluctuations and sudden disturbances. Evolutionary techniques and techniques such as ACO are inherently adaptive for it enables styles to rethink and remain efficient, even if conditions do not change, for example, GAs can actively change their parameters to meet new demanding conditions, ensuring a more appropriate performance than each in a consistent manner. Similarly, the ACO algorithm can adapt new routes and search for new routes in real time, predicting the adaptation of bee colonies to boundaries. These characteristics are important for applications in dynamic environments with autonomous devices, robotics, and disaster response, where work environments can change rapidly and unpredictably. It is the ability to be robust and useful in situations where required, thus ensuring that bio-inspired models provide reliable performance and choice of materials. Comments increase between the various events.

4. Adaptability and Scalability of Bio-Inspired ML/DL Models

4.1 Dynamic Adaptation to Changing Data Patterns

Bio-inspired ML/DL models are known for their dynamic versioning skills, which makes them appear attractive for dealing with changing reality systems. Algorithms such as GAs and PSO are designed to adapt and change in response to new information, reflecting vegetable evolutionary processes. This adjustment ensures that the fashions are appropriate and correct only when the underlying record distribution changes. For example, in financial markets where conditions often vary, bio-inspired models can constantly adapt to new trends and anomalies.

4.1.1 Real-World Application Scenarios

Bio-stimulated ML/DL models reveal great advantages in various real-world software products. Figure 3 shows a typical real-world application.

1. **Healthcare**
   - Drug discovery and development: GAs and PSO are used to optimize drug structures and to map and analyze molecular interactions for new drug therapies.
   - Medical imaging: Evolutionary algorithms improve the classification and class accuracy of medical images, which help in the early diagnosis of cancerous diseases.

2. **Financial Services**
   - *Algorithmic trading*: Herd intelligence and evolutionary techniques are used to optimize buying and selling strategies by learning market trends to maximize returns and limit opportunities.
   - *Fraud detection*: Bio-stimulated algorithms improve detection of fraudulent activities by identifying unusual patterns in big datasets.

3. **Environmental Monitoring**
   - *Climate prediction*: Evolutionary computing helps model and forecast climate research by supporting complex simulation fashions based on classical climate statistics.
   - *Wildlife conservation*: Biological models examine the population and movement patterns of wildlife, helping to improve powerful conservation strategies.

4. **Industrial Applications**
   - *Predictive maintenance*: GAs and PSO anticipate system screw-ups with the help of read-performance statistics, enabling reduced uptime and renewal costs.
   - *Process optimization*: Bio-stimulated algorithms optimize production processes, improve chain control, and refine the distribution of useful products.

5. Transportation

- **_Traffic management_**: ACO and PSO are hired to optimize traffic glide in smart cities, decreasing congestion and improving journey instances.
- **_Autonomous vehicles_**: Evolutionary algorithms useful resource in developing navigation and choice-making systems for self-riding cars, permitting adaptation to converting environments.

6. Energy

- **_Smart Grid Optimization_**: Bio-stimulated algorithms optimize the distribution and intake of power in smart grids, correctly balancing deliver and call for.
- **_Renewable energy systems_**: Genetic algorithms are used to layout and optimize renewable strength structures, which include wind farms and sun panels, to maximize electricity production.

7. Cybersecurity

- **_Threat detection_**: Swarm intelligence and evolutionary computation decorate the detection of cyber threats with the aid of identifying unusual styles and behaviors in network traffic.
- **_Intrusion prevention_**: Bio-inspired models constantly adapt to new kinds of assaults, improving the effectiveness of intrusion prevention structures.

8. Robotics

- **_Swarm robotics_**: Inspired by means of social bugs, swarm intelligence algorithms coordinate the actions of more than one robot, permitting them to carry out complex duties together.
- **_Adaptive control systems_**: Evolutionary algorithms optimize robot control systems, permitting them to conform to new responsibilities and environments.

9. Agriculture

- **_Precision farming_**: Bio-inspired algorithms examine records from sensors and satellite TV for PC imagery to optimize irrigation, fertilization, and pest manage, thereby improving crop yields and resource performance.
- **_Supply Chain Optimization_**: GAs help optimize the agricultural supply chain from manufacturing to distribution, decreasing waste, and improving performance.

10. Telecommunications

- **_Network optimization_**: Evolutionary algorithms optimize the layout and control of telecommunications networks, improving insurance and reducing latency.
- **_Resource allocation_**: Bio-inspired models correctly allocate bandwidth and different network resources, enhancing the first-rate of provider.

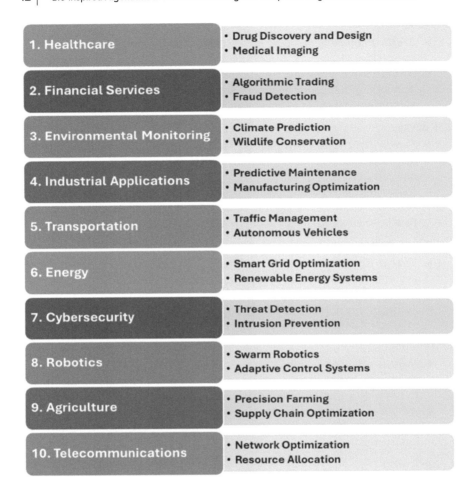

Fig. 3 Real-world applications of Bio-inspired computing.

4.1.2 Continuous Learning without Reprogramming

One of the important thing strengths of bio-stimulated ML/DL fashions is their ability to engage in non-stop gaining knowledge, without the want for reprogramming. Unlike conventional fashions, which may require common updates and guide adjustments, bio-stimulated algorithms along with Evolutionary Strategies (ES) and ACO obviously evolve through the years. This continuous mastering functionality is particularly precious in dynamic environments in which statistics is constantly changing. For instance, in smart town applications, models can constantly adapt to visitors' styles, optimizing routing and decreasing congestion in real-time. In the financial sector, these models can examine from new market statistics, adjusting buying and selling strategies to preserve profitability. This ongoing variation reduces the want for human intervention, decreasing renovation prices and growing performance. Moreover, in industrial settings, non-stop gaining knowledge of guarantees that predictive upkeep structures stay accurate as machinery a long time and working situations trade. By putting off the need for common reprogramming, bio-inspired models offer a scalable and green solution for long-term deployment in diverse industries.

4.2 Development of Localized and Distributed ML/DL Programs

4.2.1 Scalability in Large Systems

Scalability is a crucial issue of growing ML/DL applications, especially in huge structures. Localized and distributed ML/DL programs are designed to address full-size increases in records extent and computational demands without performance degradation. Scalability in these structures is completed through parallel processing, where duties are allotted throughout more than one node or processors. This allows for efficient dealing with of huge datasets and complex models by way of dividing the workload, which significantly reduces training times. Techniques along with information partitioning, version parallelism, and federated mastering allow the machine to control and manner widespread information in real time.

4.2.2 Fault Tolerance in Distributed Environments

Fault tolerance is important for the reliability and robustness of the distributed ML/DL implementation. In distributed environments, the failure of an unmarried node or group can destroy the entire machine, especially information loss and statistical errors. Replication techniques, where information is duplicated between two nodes, ensure that a backup will continue to occur if one node fails. Checkpointing periodically retrieves the state of the device, which upon failure is restarted from the last stored object. Furthermore, strong dialogue protocols and error-correcting rules help keep information consistent during transmission between distributed nodes. The inclusion of these fault-tolerant mechanisms enables delivered ML/DL packages to achieve high levels of scalability and reliability.

5. Interdisciplinary Innovations and Applications

5.1 Intersection of Biology and Computer Science

The intersection of biology and laptop technology has led to groundbreaking innovations especially through the development of bio-stimulated algorithms in ML and DL. Experimental biology methods and systems enable researchers to draw parallels that affect computational design types, increasing their performance and strength. Biological systems that have evolved over thousands and thousands of years to adapt and thrive in different environments provide valuable insights for solving complex computational problems. This synergy no longer simply advances the abilities of ML/DL fashions; however, it additionally gives new gear and methodologies for biological studies, developing a virtuous cycle of innovation and discovery.

5.1.1 Exploring Biological Principles

Exploring biological standards offers a wealth of information that may be translated into innovative algorithmic solutions in computer technology. Biological systems show off extremely good capabilities which includes self-business enterprise, adaptability, and robustness, that are proper in computational models. By analyzing processes like natural choice, neural processing, and collective conduct in organisms, researchers can expand algorithms that mimic those green and adaptive mechanisms. For example, GAs draw idea from the manner of natural choice to remedy optimization troubles, even as swarm intelligence algorithms are based on the collective behavior of social insects like ants and bees. These biologically inspired algorithms can address complex issues in dynamic and uncertain environments, making them appropriate for a huge range of packages, from robotics to facts evaluation. Understanding and leveraging these organic standards allow the advent of greater resilient and green computational structures, bridging the distance among herbal and AI.

5.1.2 New Algorithmic Methods from Biology

New algorithmic techniques derived from organic insights have revolutionized the sphere of laptop technology, particularly in system gaining knowledge of and AI. Algorithms stimulated with the aid of biological procedures, which includes NNs, GAs, and swarm intelligence, have demonstrated to be relatively powerful in solving complicated computational issues. NNs, modeled after the human brain's architecture, have enabled considerable improvements in areas like photo and speech recognition. GAs, based totally at the concepts of herbal selection, provide strong solutions for optimization demanding situations, new frontiers for innovation and alertness.

This listing explores diverse algorithms inspired by organic phenomena, imparting modern solutions to complex computational demanding situations.

1. **Neural Networks**
   - *ANN*: Inspired by the human brain, these networks top in tasks like image and speech recognition via DL [33].
   - *CNN*: Dedicated for processing grid-like records (photographs) by using mirroring the visible cortex's structure [22].
   - *RNNs*: Aimed to address consecutive data like time series or natural language, taking notion from how the mind systems information over time.

2. **Evolutionary Computation**
   - *GAs*: Mimic organic evolution's principles of choice, mutation, and crossover to find finest solutions for diverse issues.

Potential Benefits of BIAs-based ML/DL Models | 15

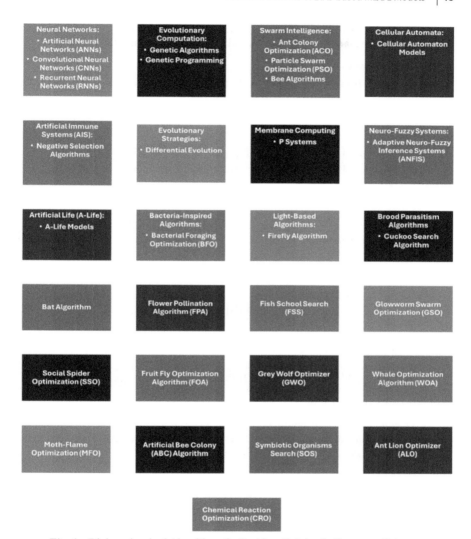

Fig. 4 Biology-inspired Algorithms for Problem-Solving in Computer Science.

- **Genetic Programming**: Grows requests or capabilities by way of repeating herbal genetic strategies, allowing them to solve precise duties [34].

3. **Swarm Intelligence**
   - **ACO**: Inspired by means of ant hunting behavior, this procedure helps find greatest answers via suggesting how ants discover food sources.
   - **PSO**: Based on the combined motion of birds or fish, PSO accelerates discover premier solutions with the aid of mimicking how these swarms traverse and optimize their actions.

- ***Bee Algorithms***: Outstanding by way of bee foraging patterns, these procedures tackle optimization and search troubles correctly.

4. Cellular Automata

- ***Cellular Automaton Models***: Model complex routines the use of simple, discrete units (cells) that interact and evolve based totally on nearby strategies [35].

5. AIS

- Encouraged by means of the human immune machine, AIS algorithms address challenges like anomaly detection, sample reputation, and optimization.
- ***Negative Selection Algorithms***: Model the immune system's ability to differentiate among self and non-self-factors.

6. Evolutionary Strategies

- ***Differential Evolution***: Iteratively improves candidate answers to find most excellent solutions for a given hassle.

7. Membrane Computing

- ***P Systems***: Inspired with the aid of the shape and functions of living cells, these fashions provide parallel computation capabilities [16, 36, 37].

8. Neuro-Fuzzy Systems

- ***Adaptive Neuro-Fuzzy Inference Systems (ANFIS)***: Combine NNs and fuzzy good judgment, creating models that learn and adapt to facts.

9. Artificial Life (A-Life)

- ***A-Life models***: Simulate real looking behaviors and evolution of synthetic organisms, with applications in robotics and complicated machine simulations.

10. Bacteria-Inspired Algorithms

- ***Bacterial Foraging Optimization (BFO)***: Mimics the foraging strategy of E. Coli microorganism to remedy optimization troubles [38, 39].

11. Light-Based Algorithms

- ***Firefly algorithm***: Based at the flashing conduct of fireflies to find greatest answers for optimization and seek duties.

12. Brood Parasitism Algorithms

- ***Cuckoo Search Algorithm***: Inspired via the brood parasitism of a few cuckoo species, this algorithm tackles optimization issues.

13. Bat Algorithm

- ***Bat Algorithm***: Mimics the echolocation behavior of bats, locating most suitable answers for numerous problems.

14. Flower Pollination Algorithm (FPA)

- *Flower Pollination Algorithm*: Inspired with the aid of the pollination system of flowering flowers, FPA addresses optimization troubles.
- *Cross-Disciplinary Collaboration*: The integration of bio-inspired algorithms fosters collaboration among PC science, biology, and different disciplines. This change of thoughts leads to more various and revolutionary smart structures.
- *Biomimicry for AI Advancement*: By gaining knowledge of from the hassle-fixing techniques of nature, AI can evolve into greater robust and adaptable structures able to tackling complicated challenges.
- *The Future of AI*: Bio-stimulated algorithms are a promising avenue for the destiny of AI, probably leading to the improvement of greater clever and autonomous systems with wide programs throughout various fields.
- *Fish School Search Optimization Algorithm*: Inspired by means of the collective conduct of fish faculties, FSS tackles optimization and seek issues.

15. Glow-worm Swarm Optimization (GSO)

- *GSO*: Mimics the conduct of glow worms in finding most desirable solutions.
  By drawing proposal from the herbal global, those bio-inspired algorithms offer effective tools for tackling complicated computational challenges in PC technological know-how. Their inherent robustness, adaptability, and efficiency cause them to precious assets for numerous packages.
- *Social Spider Optimization (SSO)*: Inspired with the aid of the social hunting behavior of spiders, where they collaborate to capture prey. This algorithm can be used for optimization problems involving a couple of retailers working together.
- *Fruit Fly Optimization Algorithm (FOA)*: Mimics the efficient fruit fly olfactory search for locating food resources. This set of rules excels at locating most fulfilling answers in complex seek spaces.
- *Grey Wolf Optimizer (GWO)*: Inspired by the hunting strategies and social hierarchy of grey wolves, GWO can be implemented to various optimization troubles requiring green exploration and exploitation.
- *Whale Optimization Algorithm (WOA)*: Based at the social foraging behavior of humpback whales, WOA utilizes an aggregate of bubble-internet searching and Levy flight seek styles for optimization.
- *Moth-Flame Optimization (MFO)*: Inspired via the navigation behavior of moths around a mild supply, MFO can be used for optimization problems requiring efficient convergence in the direction of most beneficial solutions.
- *Artificial Bee Colony (ABC) Algorithm*: Mimics the foraging conduct of honeybees, consisting of scout bees trying to find food assets and worker bees exploiting the ones assets. ABC algorithms are powerful for numerous optimization problems.

- ***Symbiotic Organisms Search (SOS):*** Inspired by means of the symbiotic relationships determined in nature, along with mutualism and commensalism, SOS algorithms may be used for complex optimization issues related to multiple interacting retailers.
- ***Ant Lion Optimizer (ALO):*** Based on the hunting conduct of antlion larvae, wherein they invent traps to capture prey, ALO algorithms are treasured for optimization responsibilities requiring green seek strategies.
- ***Chemical Reaction Optimization (CRO):*** Inspired via chemical reaction concepts, in which molecules have interaction and react to form new ones, CRO algorithms can be carried out to diverse optimization problems related to complex interactions.

5.2   Cross-Domain Contributions

5.2.1   Enriching ML/DL Fields

Bio-inspired algorithms have considerably enriched the fields of ML and DL via introducing innovative procedures to trouble-fixing.

5.2.2   Addressing Complex Challenges

5.2.2.1   Healthcare Bioinformatics

These advancements allow more unique and early analysis, improving affected person care and remedy efficiency. Bio-stimulated strategies hence play an important position in managing and interpreting the significant and complicated datasets normal in healthcare [40].

5.2.2.2   Policy Independent Species

Bio-stimulated algorithms can address complex demanding situations in ecological and environmental studies, together with managing policy-independent species. These species, which thrive regardless of human interventions, pose widespread threats to biodiversity and environment stability. Algorithms stimulated through natural methods, such as ACO and GAs, assist version and predict the spread of those species, examine impacts, and increase powerful management strategies [41].

6.   Emerging Trends in Bio-Inspired ML/DL

6.1   Potential Research Areas

Bio-inspired computing, drawing concept from nature's problem-fixing strategies, offers a rich landscape for studies. Here are a few promising regions to explore, together with three novel ideas [42]:

1.   Novel Bio-stimulated Algorithms
- ***Explore new organic phenomena for notion:*** Which includes slime mildew foraging patterns or bacterial communique mechanisms. This could result in the improvement of new algorithms with unique strengths.

- *Hybrid processes*: Investigate how to combine distinct BIAs or integrate them with traditional optimization techniques to leverage the blessings of every technique.

2. **Bio-inspired DL Architectures**
   - *Develop neural community architectures*: Inspired by using the shape and feature of the mind. This should involve exploring opportunity activation features, gaining knowledge of policies, or community topologies based totally on biological ideas.
   - *Explore the capacity of neuromorphic computing:* Which pursuits to create hardware that mimics the mind's energy efficiency and parallel processing competencies.

3. **Bio-stimulated Robotics and Control Systems**
   - *Design robots*: That can learn and adapt like animals, using BIAs for managing and selection-making. This ought to result in robots with improved autonomy and flexibility in complicated environments.
   - *Investigate bio-stimulated methods*: To robotic locomotion, drawing proposal from the green movement styles located in nature.

4. **Bio-stimulated Optimization for Complex Problems**
   - *Develop bio-stimulated algorithms*: Particularly tailored for solving complex problems in diverse domain names like logistics, resource allocation, and scheduling.
   - *Bio-inspired algorithms for big-scale records*: Explore the way to scale bio-stimulated algorithms to handle the huge datasets encountered in big data applications.

Conclusion

This review of bio-inspired algorithms in ML/DL has a number of major findings:
- *Bio-inspired algorithms*: Are exceptionally strong in solving complicated optimization problems in ML/DL. Some of such tasks include parameter optimization, function selection, and version architecture optimization.
- *Bio-stimulated algorithms*: Enhance the robustness and flexibility of ML/DL models, by referring to biological systems. Dynamic environments, uncertain situations can be well adapted to these models and perhaps even exhibit their recovery properties.
- *Future AI*: A prospective approach to Destiny of AI is the bio-stimulated algorithms which may lead to development of highly intelligent autonomous systems with multiple configurations across industries.

References

[1] Vamos, T. (Jan. 1980). Artificial Intelligence, Automatic Control and Development. *IFAC Proceedings Volumes, 13*(11), xxxvii–xliii. doi: 10.1016/S1474-6670(17)64407-0.

[2] El Hechi, M., et al. (2021). Artificial Intelligence, Machine Learning, and Surgical Science: Reality Versus Hype. *Journal of Surgical Research, 2021.* doi: https://doi.org/10.1016/j.jss.2021.01.046.

[3] Sadiku, M.N.O., Ajayi-Majebi, A.J. and Adebo, P.O. (2023). Artificial Intelligence in Manufacturing. *In:* M.N.O. Sadiku, A.J. Ajayi-Majebi, and P.O. Adebo (Eds.), *Emerging Technologies in Manufacturing.* Cham: Springer International Publishing, pp. 13–32. doi: 10.1007/978-3-031-23156-8_2.

[4] Petković, D. (2017). Prediction of laser welding quality by computational intelligence approaches. *Optik (Stuttg), 140,* 597–600. doi: 10.1016/j.ijleo.2017.04.088.

[5] I. Rafegas and M. Vanrell, "Color encoding in biologically-inspired convolutional neural networks," *Vision Res,* vol. 151, no. March, pp. 7–17, 2018, doi: 10.1016/j.visres.2018.03.010.

[6] Bracconi, M. and Maestri, M. (2020). Training set design for machine learning techniques applied to the approximation of computationally intensive first-principles kinetic models. *Chemical Engineering Journal, 400*(April), 125469. doi: 10.1016/j.cej.2020.125469.

[7] Mair, C., et al., (2019). Estimation of temporal covariances in pathogen dynamics using Bayesian multivariate autoregressive models. *PLoS Comput. Biol., 15*(12), e1007492. doi: 10.1371/journal.pcbi.1007492.

[8] Aghbashlo, M., Hosseinpour, S., Tabatabaei, M., Younesi, H. and Najafpour, G. (2016). On the exergetic optimization of continuous photobiological hydrogen production using hybrid ANFIS-NSGA-II (adaptive neuro-fuzzy inference system-non-dominated sorting genetic algorithm-II). *Energy, 96,* 507–520. doi: 10.1016/j.energy.2015.12.084.

[9] Mantilla-Gaviria, I A., Díaz-Morcillo, A. and J.V. Balbastre-Tejedor, J.V. (2013). An Ant Colony Optimization Algorithm for Microwave Corrugated Filters Design. *Journal of Computational Engineering, 2013,* 942126. doi: 10.1155/2013/942126.

[10] Martínez-del-Amor, M.A., Pérez-Hurtado, I., Orellana-Martín, D. and Pérez-Jiménez, M.J. (2020). Adaptative parallel simulators for bio-inspired computing models. *Future Generation Computer Systems, 107,* 469–84. doi: https://doi.org/10.1016/j.future.2020.02.012.

[11] Vaiapury, K., et al., (2024). Chapter Nine–Recent trends in human- and bio-inspired computing: Use-case study from a retail perspective. *In:* A. Biswas, A.P. Tonda, R. Patgiri, and K.K. Mishra (Eds.), *Applications of Nature-Inspired Computing and Optimization Techniques,* in *Advances in Computers, 135,* 211–29. Elsevier. doi: https://doi.org/10.1016/bs.adcom.2023.11.013.

[12] K. Meshram, "8 - Bioinspired computing models for civil engineering," in *Machine Learning Applications in Civil Engineering,* K. Meshram, Ed., in Woodhead Publishing Series in Civil and Structural Engineering. Elsevier, 2024, pp. 121–147. doi: https://doi.org/10.1016/B978-0-443-15364-8.00008-1.

[13] dos Santos, C.M., Escobedo, J.F., Teramoto, É.T. and da Silva, S.H.M.G. (2016). Assessment of ANN and SVM models for estimating normal direct irradiation (Hb). *Energy Convers. Manag., 126,* 826–36. doi: 10.1016/j.enconman.2016.08.020.

[14] Shanmugaprakash, M. and Sivakumar, V. (2013). Development of experimental design approach and ANN-based models for determination of Cr(VI) ions uptake rate from aqueous solution onto the solid biodiesel waste residue. *Bioresour Technol, 148,* 550–59. doi: 10.1016/j.biortech.2013.08.149.

[15] Yusuf, Z., Abdul Wahab, N., Abdul Wahab, N., Sahlan, S. and Sahlan, S. (Sep. 2017). Modeling of Filtration Process Using PSO-Neural Network." *Journal of Telecommunication, Electronic, and Computer Engineering (JTEC), 9*(3) SE-Articles, 15–19. [Online]. Available: https://jtec.utem.edu.my/jtec/article/view/1075.

[16] Zhifeng, L., Dan, P., Jianhua, W. and Shuangxi, Y. (2010). Modelling of Membrane Fouling by PCA-PSOBP Neural Network. *In: 2010 International Conference on Computing, Control, and Industrial Engineering,* pp. 34–37. doi: 10.1109/CCIE.2010.16.

[17] Choudhury, H.A., Sinha, N. and Saikia, M. (2020). Nature inspired algorithms (NIA) for efficient video compression: A brief study. *Engineering Science and Technology, An International Journal*, 23(3), 507–526. doi: https://doi.org/10.1016/j.jestch.2019.10.001.

[18] Hemeida, A.M., et al. (2020). Nature-inspired algorithms for feed-forward neural network classifiers: A survey of one decade of research. *Ain Shams Engineering Journal*, 11(3), 659–75. doi: https://doi.org/10.1016/j.asej.2020.01.007.

[19] Mammoli, D., et al. (2020). Kinetic Modeling of Hyperpolarized Carbon-13 Pyruvate Metabolism in the Human Brain. *IEEE Trans. Med. Imaging*, 39(2), 320–27. doi: 10.1109/TMI.2019.2926437.

[20] Sewsynker-Sukai, Y., Faloye, F. and Kana, E.B.G. (2017). Artificial neural networks: An efficient tool for modelling and optimization of biofuel production: A mini review. *Biotechnology and Biotechnological Equipment*, 31(2), 221–35. doi: 10.1080/13102818.2016.1269616.

[21] Ireaneus Anna Rejani, Y. and Thamarai Selvi, S. (2008). Digital Mammogram Segmentation and Tumour Detection using Artificial Neural Networks. *International Journal of Soft Computing*, 112–119. [Online]. Available: https://medwelljournals.com/abstract/?doi=ijscomp.2008.112.119.

[22] H. Tang. (2022). "Image Classification based on CNN: Models and Modules. *In: 2022 International Conference on Big Data, Information, and Computer Network* (*BDICN*), pp. 693–96. doi: 10.1109/BDICN55575.2022.00134.

[23] Zhou, W., Zhu, C. and Ma, J.(Apr. 2024). Single-layer folded RNN for time-series prediction, and classification under a non-Von Neumann architecture. *Digit Signal Process*, 147, 104415. doi: 10.1016/J.DSP.2024.104415.

[24] Lin, H., Zhang, S., Li, Q., Li, Y., Li, J. and Yang, Y. (Feb. 2023). A new method for heart rate prediction based on LSTM-BiLSTM-Att. *Measurement*, 207, 112384. doi: 10.1016/J.MEASUREMENT.2022.112384.

[25] Lu, M., Xiao, X., Pang, Y., Liu, G. and Lu, H. (2022). Detection and Localization of Breast Cancer Using UWB Microwave Technology and CNN-LSTM Framework. *IEEE Trans. Microw. Theory Tech.*, 70(11), 5085–94. doi: 10.1109/TMTT.2022.3209679.

[26] A. Tavanaei, A., Ghodrati, M., Kheradpisheh, S.R., Masquelier, T. and Maida, A. (2019). Deep learning in spiking neural networks." *Neural Networks*, 111, 47–63. doi: https://doi.org/10.1016/j.neunet.2018.12.002.

[27] Triche, A., Maida, A.S. and Kumar, A. (2022). Exploration in neo-Hebbian reinforcement learning: Computational approaches to the exploration–exploitation balance with bio-inspired neural networks. *Neural Networks*, 151, 16–33. doi: https://doi.org/10.1016/j.neunet.2022.03.021.

[28] Luo, T., Xie, J., Zhang, B., Zhang, Y., Li, C. and Zhou, J. (2024). An improved levy chaotic particle swarm optimization algorithm for energy-efficient cluster routing scheme in industrial wireless sensor networks." *Expert Syst. Appl.*, 241, 122780. doi: https://doi.org/10.1016/j.eswa.2023.122780.

[29] Li, Z., et al., (2024). Adaptive fusion of different platform point cloud with improved particle swarm optimization and supervoxels. *International Journal of Applied Earth Observation and Geoinformation*, 130, 103934. doi: https://doi.org/10.1016/j.jag.2024.103934.

[30] Su, B., Lin, Y., Wang, J., Quan, X., Chang, Z. and Rui, C. (2022). Sewage treatment system for improving energy efficiency based on particle swarm optimization algorithm. *Energy Reports*, 8, 8701–08. doi: https://doi.org/10.1016/j.egyr.2022.06.053.

[31] Zhao, F., Ji, F., Xu, T., Zhu, N. and Jonrinaldi. (2024). Hierarchical parallel search with automatic parameter configuration for particle swarm optimization. *Appl. Soft Comput.*, 151, 111126. doi: https://doi.org/10.1016/j.asoc.2023.111126.

[32] Zahmatkesh, S., Gholian-Jouybari, F., Klemeš, J.J., Bokhari, A. and Hajiaghaei-Keshteli, M. (Sep. 2023). Sustainable and optimized values for municipal wastewater: The removal

of biological oxygen demand and chemical oxygen demand by various levels of geranular activated carbon- and genetic algorithm-based simulation. *J. Clean Prod., 417*, 137932. doi: 10.1016/J.JCLEPRO.2023.137932.

[33] Ray, P.P. (Sep. 2022). A survey on cognitive packet networks: Taxonomy, state-of-the-art, recurrent neural networks, and QoS metrics. *Journal of King Saud University - Computer and Information Sciences, 34*, (8), 5663–83. doi: 10.1016/J.JKSUCI.2021.05.017.

[34] Márquez-Vera, C., Cano, A., Romero, C. and Ventura, S. (Apr. 2013). Predicting student failure at school using genetic programming and different data mining approaches with high dimensional and imbalanced data. *Applied Intelligence, 38*, (3), 315–30. doi: 10.1007/s10489-012-0374-8.

[35] Pastor, E., Zárate, L., Planas, E. and Arnaldos, J. (2003). Mathematical models and calculation systems for the study of wildland fire behaviour. *Prog. Energy Combust. Sci., 29*, (2), 139–53. doi: https://doi.org/10.1016/S0360-1285(03)00017-0.

[36] Zhang, X., Liu, X., Ren, Q., Sun, M. and Zhao, Y. (2024). A general neural membrane computing model. *Inf. Sci. (N.Y), 672*, 120686. doi: https://doi.org/10.1016/j.ins.2024.120686.

[37] Visalaxi, G. and Muthukumaravel, A. (2023). IOT monitoring membrane computing based on quantum inspiration to enhance security in cloud network." *Measurement: Sensors, 27*, 100755. doi: https://doi.org/10.1016/j.measen.2023.100755.

[38] Nicolau, D.V., Burrage, K. and Maini, P.K. (2008). 'Extremotaxis': Computing with a bacterial-inspired algorithm. *Biosystems, 94*, (1), 47–54. oi: https://doi.org/10.1016/j.biosystems.2008.05.009.

[39] Swayamsiddha, S. (2020). Chapter 4: Bio-inspired algorithms: Principles, implementation, and applications to wireless communication. *In*: X.-S. Yang (Ed.), *Nature-Inspired Computation and Swarm Intelligence*. Academic Press, pp. 49–63. doi: https://doi.org/10.1016/B978-0-12-819714-1.00013-0.

[40] Shorey, S., Chan, V., Rajendran, P. and Ang, E. (Nov. 2021). Learning styles, preferences, and needs of generation Z healthcare students: Scoping review. *Nurse Educ. Pract., 57*, 103247. doi: 10.1016/J.NEPR.2021.103247.

[41] Balasubramaniam, S., Kadry, S. and Kumar, K.S. (2024). Osprey Gannet optimization enabled CNN based Transfer learning for optic disc detection and cardiovascular risk prediction using retinal fundus images. *Biomedical Signal Processing and Control, 93*, 106177.

[42] Balasubramaniam, S., Arishma, M. and Dhanaraj, R.K. (2024). A Comprehensive Exploration of Artificial Intelligence Methods for COVID-19 Diagnosis. *EAI Endorsed Transactions on Pervasive Health and Technology, 10*.

2 | BIAs-based Deep Learning (DL) Models

N. Sanjana,[1*] R. Immanual,[2] K.M. Kirthika,[1] S. Sangeetha[3] and K. Maharaja[4]

This chapter provides a comprehensive overview of bio-inspired algorithms (BIAs) in optimization models and machine learning. It explores how BIAs, inspired by biological systems, solve complex problems by emulating natural processes. The chapter introduces BIAs and their natural origins, discussing their applications and advantages in optimization and machine learning. It examines both traditional and contemporary BIAs, including Evolutionary Algorithms, Genetic Algorithms, and newer developments like Artificial Immune Systems and Membrane Computing Algorithms, with a focus on Particle Swarm Optimization and Ant Colony Optimization. The integration of BIAs with deep learning techniques is explored, highlighting their role in enhancing optimization strategies and improving deep learning models. Applications of BIAs in deep learning are discussed, covering model tuning, hyperparameter selection, neural architecture search, and regularization. The chapter addresses BIAs' contribution to explainable artificial intelligence (AI) and visualization in deep learning models, and explores their practical applications in disease diagnostics, including computer-aided diagnosis systems, medical imaging, and Omics data analysis. The chapter concludes by examining current challenges and opportunities in the field, such as computational complexity, scalability, epistemological frameworks, convergence analysis, and deep learning integration. This review offers insights into the current state and future directions of BIAs in optimization and machine learning.

1. Introduction to Bio-Inspired Algorithms (BIAs)

At any rate, even if one disregards the technicalities of the evolution mechanism spanning millions of years, nature is a treasure chest filled with different ideas for

---

[1] Department of Computer Science and Engineering, Sri Ramakrishna Institute of Technology. Coimbatore, India.

[2] Department of Mechanical Engineering, Sri Ramakrishna Institute of Technology. Coimbatore, India.

[3] Department of Electrical and Electronics Engineering, Sri Ramakrishna Institute of Technology. Coimbatore, India.

[4] Department of Electrical and Electronics Engineering, Al Musanna College of Oman, Oman.
Email : immangwu@gmail.com; kirthikakmbe@gmail.com; sangeetha.ram02@gmail.com; maharajasrit@gmail.com

[*] Corresponding author: sanjananithykumar06@gmail.com

24 | Bio-inspired Algorithms in Machine Learning and Deep Learning for Disease Detection

mankind in relation to the different issues that they are faced with. Every engineer, scientist, or, at some times, the mere problem solver is bound to find oneself at a point in their careers where what they consider the most challenging of tasks is the order of the day especially when modeling a system or even dealing with paradigms. Trust me or beat me, but actually a huge number of questions people pose, and some responses provided every day, can be provided just by paying attention to the sounds of nature. From this perspective, the reader is brought to a world of the future where swarms are manageable, information can be retrieved from the structure of the evolutions, and bacteria can be cloned to address issues and look for more opportunities. To understand what this knowledge of BIAs permits one to do is invite you to consider the vast range of professions within computer science and engineering, finance, and other business areas where it might be deployed.

Moreover, it is also helpful in giving good practice to learn how bio-inspired methods intend and work out natural-like solutions in order to advance computational methods. This is due to the fact that they are rooted in biology and are thus extraordinarily effective. You'll also find out how it was that the folks came up with the evolutionary algorithms, and (SI), and hoi', bacterial foraging optimization. Explicit, simple, and illustrated by example from a lot of areas, you will soon discover how these high level concepts can be used and how they can be easily tailored towards formulating solutions for any particular need, and with the knowledge of the numerous techniques that are available in your HD Toolbox of approaches for managing practically any issue that may be facing you at a certain or another stage of your further study.

1.1 Overview of BIAs and Their Inspiration from Natural Systems

BIAs, in general, deserve particular attention since it belongs to the group of modern and promising methods of solving complex optimization problems, and which is inspired by the natural world. These algorithms are the subject of some attention as some of the most effective methods of solving various problems in computing, engineering, biology, and even in the field of Finance. The primary subordinate areas of BIAs are EEAs (Extended Euclidean Algorithms), SIAH, and BFAHs, which are relatively more recent forms of the established BIAs [1]. EAs, built using concepts of genetic evolution and natural selection, work on a fitness model which involves the best fit to be the fittest; solutions to optimization problems change over generations through mutation, crossover, and selection. There are several types of this family of algorithms, for example; Genetic Algorithms (GA), Genetic Programming (GP), Evolution Strategies (ES), Differential Evolution (DE), and Particle Swarm Optimization (PSO). These population-adaptive search methods use stochastic items and pick out first-class solutions for difficult issues of population. Contrarily, SI algorithms work with reference to the social insects and animals and show how the complex cooperative behavior of the small components results in the appearance of a collective complex whole behavior. Some of the most popular algorithms are the PSO, the Ant Colony Optimization (ACO), Artificial Bee Colony optimization (ABC), Bacterial Foraging Optimization Algorithm (BFOA), and the Firefly Algorithm (FFA). These algorithms often use the populations of abstract agents that can work in parallel with each other and with the environment to find the best solution based on cooperation. An addition to the BIA family, only a few years ago, is the BFAs which basically work in foraging patterns similar to bacteria and solve optimization issues.

From the BFA (bacteria foraging algorithm) model, current models of BFA have become both population-based BFA and the individual-based BFA which incorporate the individual based modeling-InbM for computational balance. Thus, future work on the development of all kinds of BFAs exhibits the promise of effectiveness in addressing increasingly difficult optimization problems by employing the heuristics of bacteria in the search and optimization processes. More so, increase advancements in the BIAs are expected as researchers continue to explore the depths of analysis of intricate biological units and develop even more elaborate optimizations' algorithms that will be relevant to solve real-life problems. Figure 1 shows that the use of BIA comes with the following sequence of engagements: Initialization of the algorithm involves creating the population of solutions, the number of iterations, and the stop criteria. These are important control parameters for the algorithm execution and can be tweaked quite often by the researchers considering the trial-and-error method. The detailed process of how the field works is as follows: The fitness evaluation stage involves inputting the individual solutions such as feature subsets as used in the feature selection phase into a classifier and the accuracy of the classifier serves as the fitness of the solutions. The central idea of the iterative optimizations is the periodically repeated steps reminiscent to the biological processes. It goes on cycling through these stages until it satisfies some exit condition such as the number of iterations equaling to some fixed upper limit or some predetermined level of error. Specifically, the following basic elements of bio-inspirational designs assist BIAs to function as natural evolutionary and social conduct by seeking for better solutions within the optimization problems [2].

1.2 Principles and Advantages of BIAs in Optimization and Machine Learning

BIAs were indeed found to be rich in principles as well as they offer numerous advantages in the field of optimization and therefore, BIA remains as one of the most useful tools that can be used to solve complex problems with a high level of efficiency. These algorithms aim for their motives from nature-inspired behavior or phenomena like evolution, searching behavior exhibited by animals, and bacterial colony behavior to design efficient optimization approaches. In the light of the above elaborations, it can be inferred that like natural processes, BIAs are well capable of searching the solution space, learning from the environment, and solving even the most complex optimization problems. It should be noted, however,

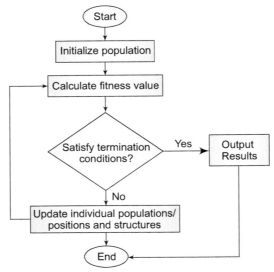

Fig. 1 Common framework of bio-inspired algorithms.

that one of the peculiarities of BIAs by design is the utilization of randomized algorithms, which situates them in a particular category of optimization algorithms. Randomness in decision-making and stochastic movements add to the fact that BIAs avoid solutions located in local optima and explore the various regions of the solution space; and the general ability for search and problem-solving scenarios gives BIAs the potential to perform complex optimization tasks [3].

Some main types of BIAs include the Evolutionary Algorithms (EAs) and SI- based algorithms, which use the population-based search methodologies. These approaches enable BIAs to have a wide range of solutions and enable the exploration of the solution space to the full extent while making the optimization process more reliable. In essence, by replicating some forms of natural processes like mutation, crossover, and selection, BIAs successfully perform solution searches, solutions' identification, environment changes accommodation, and, in particular, solve extremely complex optimization problems effectively. BIAs also have another major benefit in that they can be used in a Global Optimization context, the goal of which is to identify the best solution within the huge and complex problem space. By incorporating the feature of population-based search along with random variation and selection, BIAs are able to surmount the complexities involved in searching through optimization landscapes, even if it is trapped at a local optimum, and this makes BIAs highly efficient search techniques as they are able to look for global optima when required. Furthermore, BIAs are relatively general and flexible, that can be used in a vague number of instances in various fields according to optimization issues. This flexibility makes it possible for BIAs to adjust solutions and the problem-solving process, throughout iterations and over time, so that it remarks a high ability to solve optimization of different types of objectives.

BIAs are currently one of the defining features of the machine learning domain and are characterized by specific principles that provide synergistic benefits when designing new promising learning models. In the current study, it will be established that one of the most useful areas of BIAs when applied to machine learning is feature selection and dimensionality reduction. Natural selection-based algorithms such as GA or PSO can identify the prominent features for learning as they actually mimic nature and help in dimensionality reduction thereby improving the efficiency of the models and reducing the computation load. Furthermore, BIAs are most useful for fine-tuning normal hyperparameters and architectural characteristics of machine learning. Now, by using EAs and SI algorithms, the search space of model configurations is examined and the best settings for better learning performances are determined, itself being a model selection process that results in finding better models. BIAs are more effective when the current model contains a prerequisite workflow of diverse functions and numerous target variables dependent on features for consistent learning in machine learning tasks. GP, based on evolutionary theory and Artificial Neural Networks (ANNs) that mimic neurons in the human brain, can hail complex relationships and predict outcomes by seeking out optimal solutions and flexible strategies in extensive search spaces and discontinuous landscapes. Furthermore, these BIAs can be applied as a part of ensemble learning methodologies where a number of models are used for prediction-making. Ensemble learning enabled by BIAs can utilize various populations of models with different properties and synchronize them into a single improved and less vulnerable learning system. EAs evolve various populations of models, which have different parameters and strengths, and join their predictive capabilities in a way that can make an ensemble learning system more accurate and less sensitive.

Another strength that is apparent when using BIAs in the field of machine learning is the flexibility of learning and the possibility of online learning from the streaming data. ACO and BFO inspired from the behavioral aspects of animals are capable of integrating new knowledge that reflects the ongoing and dynamic learning tasks in the course of improving the algorithms. Additionally, some of the BIAs like Decision Tree-based algorithms and Rule-based systems promising approximations to natural systems can provide interpretability and rank features based on importance. BIA-based algorithms are able to produce human-interpretable rules or decision trees describing the learned-feature-to-target associations; thereby improving the credibility and reliability of machine learning models based on this knowledge assimilation technique.

The benefits of BIAs in machine learning include maximizing model performance, managing of intricate relationships between model variables, and encouraging the concept of diversity, making it easier to adapt to dynamically changing settings and easier interpretation of the model. BIAs assist in designing high performance and efficient progressive models for the analysis and learning from data using the inspiration that is drawn from biological systems and evolutionary processes and are used across different fields of pattern recognition, data mining, and predictive modeling. With the future advancement of research in this field, BIAs combined with machine learning can be very useful in developing solutions for many unpredicted real-world applications and the development of even more intelligent systems [4]. Figure 2 presents the information and the advantages of BIAs in optimization and machine learning.

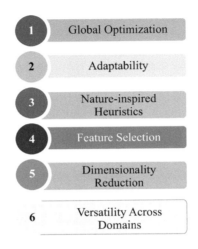

Fig. 2 Advantages of BIAs in optimization and machine learning.

2. Ancient and Classical BIAs

2.1 Evolutionary Algorithms (EAs)

EAs are metaheuristic optimization methods that are based on natural evolution processes where different solutions are adapted in the hope of finding better solutions. They operate by the basis of a generation of a population of solution candidates; selection and variation of the candidates mimicking the process of natural genetic inheritance. It mimics the idea about survival of the fittest, especially regarding the choice of solutions, since the better solution will have a higher chance of being copied or used in the next generation. Mutation operators alter the selected individuals just as the recombination (crossover) operators do; they create variation in the population as in natural selection. This process of selection and variation is repeated and builds up over many generations, groping towards the right solution. Both the exploration by using the variation operators and the exploitation by the selection can optimize the space of search of an EA and adapt it to the problem to finally reach the optimum or near-optimum solutions. GAs are known to solve diverse optimization problems with success and such problems may involve complicated and more difficult features including, nonlinear problems, and multimodal problems making EA a key resource pool for researchers and developers for a variety of disciplines.

2.2 Genetic Algorithms (GAs)

GAs are an important category of the EAs that have been applied in numerous and successful ways with regards to enhancing different aspects of the deep learning (DL) model. In this regard, each member in the GAs population can be viewed as a potential solution, or in other words, a certain neural network architecture, a method for weight initialization, along with some network-related parameters like learning rates and activation functions. The individuals are represented more or less in the form of genomes, which could be of Boolean, Real, or some other data types or even more complex structures [5]. As GAs replicate new generations of individuals, the process of selection, crossover, and mutation operators produce fitter individuals and generate better fit population over the generations. Taking the nature selection step, higher fitness scores are selected, as these may be established using the validation set or other performances related measurements. Crossover incorporate the genotypes of two parent individuals to produce off springs. On the other hand, mutation brings in random changes allowing the algorithm to move to different region in the search space. Over time, more generations of the GA are produced resulting in the overall population of the GA moving towards the optimal deep learning models or configurations that are best suited to the given task. This strong optimization strategy has been successful in the theoretical and empirical contexts of designing and fine-tuning DNNs because of the GA capacity to search through exceedingly intricate solutions as shown in Figure 3.

2.3 Evolutionary Strategies (ES)

ES constitute another important class of Everett algorithms targeted at numerical optimization tasks. The general form of ES algorithms is distinct from most GAs that work on integer or binary representations since they utilize derived mutation and selection methods to evolve species of real-valued prospects. In ES, the mutation operation is defined in order to fast navigate the continuous search space by sampling of new solutions according to predefined probability distributions so that the sample is much more biased and efficient compared to purely random mutations. This makes ES particularly suitable for fine-tuning of the real-valued parameters fields in deep learning models like weights and biases. Furthermore, ES techniques have also been intensified in the field of neuro evolution, where weights and architectures of neural networks are evolved at once through the initiation of a single process. Combining the capability of new ES to search high-dimensional solution spaces and the parallelism, the contributors have managed to reuse these algorithms to identify new neural network topologies and weight assignments that yield optimal performance on the multiple tasks. The valuable properties involving the stability and adaptability of ES along with the ability to search for the best solution of constant and discrete characteristics of deep learning makes it an effective tool for AutoML, architecture search.

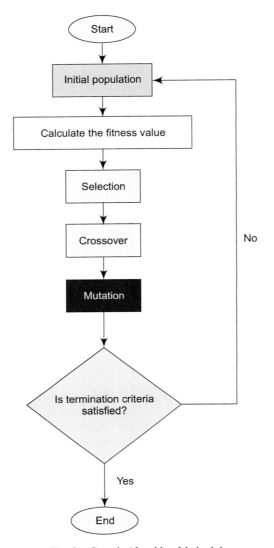

Fig. 3 Genetic Algorithm Methodology.

2.4 Genetic Programming (GP)

GP is one of the most specific techniques within the EAs paradigm that evolves computer programs or models in the form of trees or any other forms of executable sets of rules. Therefore, the GP becomes a popular technique over the other DL methods for the automation of the architectures of the Neural Network (NN). Unlike the typical global optimization paradigm of EAs that insists on their string-mutating counterparts, Differential Evolution, GP is capable of creating search

BIAs-based Deep Learning (DL) Models | 31

space of different sizes and Tree-depths for DL architectures. May be something like mutation, crossover, selection GP repeatedly improves population of NN models, and during that will find out how to assemble right parts into successful complex of subroutines. Moreover, GP has been used at the problem of generating optimized network topologies, interconnections, and feature representations for the given data, especially for the cases when a necessary structure is expected to be hierarchical and complex, and capable of capturing the subtle interrelations inherent to the data [6]. Through that integration, GP allows to set up powerful and very flexible tools for automation of various aspects of DL model construction that in turn leads to the new possibilities for researches and further development of the existing ideas in such field as architecture engineering.

2.5 Swarm Intelligence (SI) Algorithms

SI algorithms means getting inspired from synergistic, self-organizing collective behavior that can be observed in natural world like ants, birds, or bees, etc. These algorithms unveil the emergent intelligence that stems from the transaction that exists between the individual agents that have simple routines to follow. Even though every individual agent is very simple, it is sufficient when taken collectively of sufficient number to solve real problems in the world, explore labyrinthine search spaces, and find near-optimal solutions. Similarly, they employ the principles like positive feedback, negative feedback, and that promote the intelligibility of the swarm collectivity. These algorithms are noted for their flexibility in exploring different environments, their resilience to failures and inherent parallelism, and that makes them relevant to solve a number of optimization problems especially when working with DL where they have successfully exhibited their efficacy in tasks such as neural architecture search and hyperparameter tuning.

2.6 Particle Swarm Optimization (PSO)

SI is a broad family of artificial intelligence (AI) techniques modeled after the behavior of natural systems: flocks of birds, schools of fishes, etc. Movement of these particles is guided by two main principles using PSO. In PSO, "a swarm" refers to a collection of particles where each of them is a candidate solution to the problem being searching, and the particles move in the search space through the adjustment of position and velocity of each particle and through the information exchange between the particles in the swarm. The updating of each swarmed particle is thus made such that each particle is influenced by both its own best solution and the global best solution giving the swarm an exploration-exploitation nature. This coordinated movement of individual particles makes the swarm to search efficiently in the presumed globalization search space and slowly converge to the global optima. For instance, in DL, PSO has been used in several ways in optimizing NN such as the model parameters, the structure of the network, and other parameterized irregularities of neural net models [7]. It is playable in a way of balancing between exploration and exploitation which is particularly useful when dealing with high-dimensional and often non-convex search spaces that are characteristic for DL problems. As a result, the fact that PSO states the particle SI, it has been shown that it cuts across DL configuration space, and has been proven to search better than other optimization routines in some instances as depicted in the Figure 4.

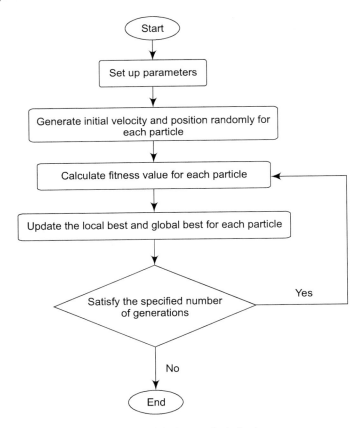

Fig. 4 Particle Swarm Optimization.

2.7 Ant Colony Optimization (ACO)

ACO is a metaheuristic algorithm derived from the stigmergy process observed with ants searching for their food. ACO algorithms mimic the predefined ants' pheromone trail-laying and trail-following to determine the better solution path. ACO has been adopted in feature selection, model pruning, and NAS (network-attached storage) where it has showcased its effectiveness in DL applications. ACO, as such, takes advantage of the collective intelligence realized in artificial ants to search the vast possibility landscape in searching for forms of DL architectures.

Derived from nature and evolution, these BIAs provide tough optimization techniques to unfold the issues of DL. They make it possible to find the best architecture, the right set of parameters, and appropriate feature descriptions that will in one way or another help enhance DL models, and, as a result, expand their applicability to many areas.

3. Modern and Hybrid BIAs

3.1 Artificial Immune Systems (AIS)

AIS refers to a set of computational methods based on the immune system approach to resolve problems in the presence of uncertainties. In line with the features of the immune system, such as self-recognition, learning, adaptation and diversity, AIS algorithms recognize and classify aberrations, categorize patterns, and even optimize the solutions in a similar fashion as how the immune system fights threats to the body. Basic theories of AIS, like Clonal Selection, Immune Networks, and Negative Selection constitute the primary basis for algorithmic modeling derived from the action of the immune system. AIS streams are widespread in various areas, such as data analytics, optimization, security, and robotics, combined with proven solidity and flexibility. AIS has a substantial amount of empirical evidence, and there is a more theory-based approach in AH and AIS development, where researchers investigate more advanced mathematical models and analysis to improve the implementation and knowledge of AIS. Conclusively, AIS implies a brand new powerful computational intelligence methodology that draws on biological understanding to proffer creative solutions to diverse types of problems in multiple fields.

3.2 Membrane Computing Algorithms

Membrane Computing Algorithms are defined as computational algorithms that have conceptual similarity to the biological membranes at some levels of abstraction. These algorithms are based on an area of the study of membranes which are a way of computing inspired by the structure and specific processes of cells. Indeed, in this computational model, the computations occur in parallel and distributed, always involving multisets of symbol-objects contained in the membranes. Of equal importance in Membrane Computing Algorithms is the interaction between these compartments and more specifically with other compartments or the rest of the environment in the system.

Membrane computing is a relatively novel approach, and several models have been proposed with different characteristics and uses. These models are the symbol-object P systems with multiset rewriting rules in which documents are changed, the system using symport/antiport, string-objects, tissue-like P systems, and neural-like P systems. There are some variations in what they represent regarding computation, which still relies on the principles observed in biological systems.

A wide spectrum of fields is benefitted or implemented by Membrane Computing Algorithms; these are Biology, Computer Science, Optimization, and Pattern Recognition; the list is not exhaustive. As most of the biological read and process information through neural network like structures, these algorithms offer a novel way to look at computational problems, quite possibly holding the keys to new solutions.

3.3 Hybrid BIAs for Deep Learning

The bibliometry of the integration of BIAs into DL models examines the ways in which BIAs help to refine and improve DL models. These algorithms comprise multiple aspects of several bio-inspired optimization algorithms in an effort to solve various complicated problems in DL tasks including the selection, optimization, and classification of features.

Hybrid BIA falls within the scope of DL while Meta heuristic optimization algorithm is conceptually used to improve the efficiency and effectiveness of learning in DL, hybrid BIAs conceptually have used different metaheuristic optimization algorithms concurrently. As seen in the combinations of WOA and APSO (adaptive particle swarm optimization) where the integration of the two improves feature selection and optimization in DL.

In this approach, to cooperate with several EAs, the researchers plan to leverage the unique feature of each algorithm for developing a powerful optimization solution for DL problems. The above hybrid methods may help avoid the deficiency of a single algorithm and improve the optimization effect from various fronts, including accuracy, convergence rate, and generalization ability.

3.4 Integrating BIAs with Deep Learning Models

BIAs and DL means that in programming the natural systems and processes are incorporated into the DL structures to make them more performant and more efficient. By mimicking the actions of these particles like bees, ants, or even genetic evolution of DL, these algorithmic strategies present new ways of enhancing these DL models. Integralization process refers to the application of fresh bio-inspired optimization algorithms like PSO, GAs or the ABC optimization to conform to the hyperparameters, or the architectural construction of DL models or their training processes. This integration helps in exploring parts of the solution space systematically and helps in achieving better model fitting, faster rate of convergence, and overcoming the problem of overfitting. Through incorporation of BIAs, despite the adaptive and self-organizing crucial characteristics of DL, it will be possible to obtain even more powerful, open-ended computer systems with increased competency in multiplicity of tasks in many range of applications from image recognition, natural language processing and medical diagnosis.

4. BIAs for Deep Learning Model Optimization

BIAs, as a method, is one of the practices used within structural engineering and DL models with good outcomes. Scientists have amplified the effectiveness in providing engineering the DL prognosis technique related to structural structure and strength by including concepts derived from nature into AI alternative. BIAs, namely, GAs and ANNs methodology are based on the observation of biological systems to tackle complex optimization problems. Such algorithms have very favorable performances in tuning all the parameters of the DL models enabling the models to predict effectively and to perform equally well on different environments [1]. In addition to using BIAs and AI models, both of them are promising in predicting the shear strength capacity of deep beams. Support vector regression (SVR) technique has also been hybridized with GA for enhancement of the proposed framework of estimating the shear strength of reinforced concrete deep beams. Apart from that it also helps to enhance the accuracy of the predictions and at the same time addresses a crucial issue of tuning of parameters in SVR models. Also, it should also be noted that the data handling and structural dependencies among the variables are nonlinear and that BIAs have some significant advantages over other existing methods, which makes their usage crucial for optimizing DL models in structural engineering.

4.1 Hyperparameter Tuning using BIAs

Recently, the BIAs, in combination with DL models for the role of hyperparameter tuning have also evolved and have been adapted in most of the sectors of machine learning. This novel approach is based on the Natural Selection theory and SI principles of which the fundamentals are designed to offer immense performance increase to DL models. Algorithms that apply the principles found in nature to select the hyperparameters for a computationally demanding problem also apply bio-signature. BIAs, therefore, offer the best approach to the optimization of the DL models given that they can search for an immense hyperparameter space for the best combination possible.

The basic mode of searching the hyperparameter space such as the grid search or even entirely random search, which perform very poorly when searching for high dimensions and come with the added disadvantage of improved computational cost. The steps involved in the above BIAs are GAs, PSO, and the ACO which are effective ways of exploring the hyperparameter space and can help find the optimum set of hyperparameters. Besides, these algorithms are characterized by self-improvement traits which enable them to dynamically alter hyperparameters based on the model's evaluation. The flexibility of DL is particularly beneficial in terms of hyperparameter optimization, which depends on dataset complexity as well as NN architecture [8]. Within iterations, BIAs keep adjusting hyperparameters settings, thus improving overall DL models' performance and generalization. Figure 5 shows the General Schema of Hyperparameters Tuning by ABC.

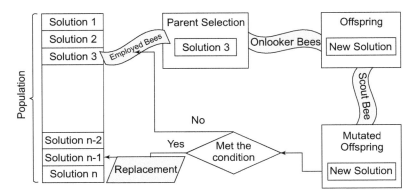

Fig. 5 A General Schema of Hyperparameters Tuning by ABC.

In addition to that, combining the BIAs with DL models makes it not only a good tool for hyperparameter tuning but also provides an entirely new perspective towards solving challenging optimization problems. Using a mix of the two paradigms, harnessing both advantages at once can yield a quicker convergence, greater scalability, and robustness in training complex NNs. Then by utilizing the properties of the features which are inspired from nature, this can increase the success rate in optimizing the hyperparameters in DL.

4.2 Neural Architecture Search (NAS) with BIAs

The field of NAS was only recently transitioning to a reality for creating a new generation of complicated structures for DL using creativity-based algorithms. These algorithms emulate the inherent processing architecture of the natural world; thus, they constitute efficient optimization approaches for countless issues in NAS. In the case of using metaheuristic algorithms, it is possible to refer to EAs, GAs, and RL that have proved effective in automating the formation of neural network structures. These algorithms actually duplicate principles of natural selection, heredity and training based on reinforcement which facilitate powerful search of the seemingly infinite hypothesis space for network configuration.

Biological methods inspired by weight sharing in NSGA-Net include network morphisms, and multi-objective optimization to perform an efficient search for a design space that balances the performance of architectures and the computational requirement [9]. These algorithms learn and optimize network topologies through genetic processes like gene transfers, mutations or crossover, and selection over successive generations. BIAs also help in establishing the right foundation for the discovery of the true trade-off frontier regarding the performance objectives and the resource and architectural constraints in NAS. With the help of using evolutionary methods and Bayesian optimization, meta-modeling and multi-objective selection schemes, these algorithms provide an efficient basis for searching for the optimal deep learning models in NAS.

Another area of research in NAS, which points to the promising future of applying BIAs into complex systems, is the automation of the NN's architecture. With the help of evolutionary principles and molecular biology strategies, reinforcement learning, and reinforcement healing strategies, new possibilities can be opened for improving DL models and artificial intelligence [10].

4.3 BIA-based Regularization Techniques

By focusing on BIA and more broadly on the trends of integrating BIAs in the DLM optimization domain, it is possible to conclude that the general idea of applying bio-inspired approaches to design novel regularization algorithms for enhancing the model performance is a promising research direction in the current state of IT (information technology) development. These algorithms are inspired by biological systems, and their primary objective is to mimic the under-connectivity and the specific firing patterns intrinsic to NNs, in the context of shallow and DL models. Scientists have created crucial bio-inspired procedures, including Deep Feedback Control (DFC) and winner-take-all or sparseness systems, which play a significant role in training deep systems. These algorithms imitate the process that are used by the brain to learn, hence providing faster and better results in learning.

It is noteworthy that through the employment of the BIA-based regularization techniques, DL models benefit from the performance enhancement while being endowed with the features to overcome obstacles such as catastrophic forgetting. Such techniques enhance incremental and dynamic learning which makes the models to update the accumulated knowledge with new knowledge without erasing the previous knowledge. These levels of regularization when incorporated into DL models through BIBA have shown to have great benefits especially through the following applications. This research proves that using nature-inspired techniques can improve reliability and adaptability of models to a noisy environment and their ability to solve intricate problems.

Therefore, the incorporation of BIAs, especially measured in the context of BIA, has become the practical method of selecting optimal DL models through postmodern forms of regularization. Thus, by favoring after processing stints from biological systems and imitating brain type solutions for information processing, these algorithms can contribute to the optimization of the model results, solve some of the issues such as catastrophic forgetting, and create the fundamental groundwork for the advancement of deep learning algorithms in the future.

5. BIAs for Enhancing Deep Learning Interpretability

Machine learning interpretable models have become a distinct possibility due to the application of BIAs in DL models. These algorithms refer to the affairs of biological systems in order to seek to understand the nature of a neuron, by emulating biological procedures. This can, for instance, be done by employing GAs that mimic evolution in the attempt to interpret model results in a more straightforward manner. GAs aid in the selection process of relevant features in improving the performance of the model by going through cycles of feature selection to arrive at the most relevant and informative features thereby giving the Event-driven Stream Processing (ESP) models modulatory and comprehensible characteristics [11]. Another area of improvement based on SMTs is the improvement of interpretability using swarm intelligence techniques that borrowed their ideas from the way ants, bees, and other social organisms behave. Both methods help in the process of selecting relevant features and enable us to fully understand how the model arrives at its conclusions.

The general potential of CI (continuous integration) as the driving force behind the swarm algorithms could help to predict and emphasize the vital characteristics and their interrelations in the model. NN models that are inspired by the structure and function of the human brain are helpful in gaining insights into the process of information flow in DL models. These generated networks resemble the connectivity of the brain and represent the activation dynamics of the data when passed through the various layers of a DL model. This is due to ACO ability, similar to ants' foraging of food source, to trace and predict the flow of data within the network, thus analyzing the important paths traveled by the model. Remote look at the paths of participating 'ants' helps reveal the most important features in the network and their effectiveness in terms of the model's predictions. Based on these, the contribution of BIAs in various fields, including image classification, natural language processing, and healthcare, has been made apparent in terms of improving the reliability and acceptance of AI systems. The application of these algorithms for achieving interpretability improvements has been verified through case studies, as well as Experimental Assessment. In the further development of research in this area, improving the possibilities of linking BIAs is seen for the future, DL models that combine interpretability and ease of understanding by users. It is now only possible to more fully realize the potential of DL concepts for assisting human decision-making in an increasingly complex world, and in so doing, create more trustworthy AI systems.

5.1 Explainable AI through BIAs

The Area of Research known as Explainable AI (XAI) has observed a rising curve in the use of biological mimic algorithms to improve comprehensible AI systems. The process of natural evolution or the structure and function of the human brain has therefore inspired researchers when designing models that will offer high ability as well as a comprehensible manner on how and why the model arrived at that particular ability. NNs, which are inspired by the structures of the human brain, GAs imitating the process of the natural selection of species, and swarm intelligence concepts inspired by interactions of social bees, ants, and other insects are the subclass of the AI that has the potential to enhance the explainability of the AI systems. Thus, such heuristics allow designing the models, which not only are effective, but also can be easily explained to the users, as the principles, supported by the developed algorithms, reflect the patterns observed in nature. In the field of XAI, BIAs have a crucial task of explaining the actions of complex AI schemes to their human counterparts.

It is advantageous for researchers to incorporate elements paraphrased from natural systems to AI models that enable the system to go further than making accurate predictions, it can also explain the basis of its decision. This transparency is especially needed in fields including healthcare, finance, and automobiles where the AI models require clear explanation of how they operate. When applied to Explainable AI, the concepts and methods of BIAs are the essential steps that can lead science to a new level of development and ensure AI's transparency and accountability while retaining its power and effectiveness. By integrating bio-inspired knowledge into creating and developing systems, it will be possible to unleash the complete potential of the AI, while at the same time guaranteeing the ethical, reliable, and explainable nature of these systems to all the parties that are impacted by them. However, as more studies continue to be conducted in the area of XAI, it can be further noted that there is so much potential for the future of the application of AI in industries as they leverage BIAs in solving problems. Thus, by following the inspiration from biological systems, which can be regarded as sophisticated, integrated, and highly perceptible, we can develop AI models of agents that not only solve tasks efficiently and effectively but also make explanations that can be understood and trusted by humans and can contribute to further collaboration of people and artificially intelligent systems.

5.2 Visualizing and Understanding Deep Learning Models with BIAs

For DL, especially for analyzing the models' mechanisms, the model's visualization and interpretation are meaningful. Biologically Inspired Attribution Scores (BIAS) have, therefore, been proposed more recently as a computationally efficient technique of generating visual explanations of a model's predictions especially, but not necessarily only in the genomic sequences context. Saliency maps and feature attribution techniques are actually the kind of models that allow to check how each input feature contributes to the emergence of results. These methods depict the feature visualization as an idea based on real data instead of the hypothetical case, giving some form of explanation of the model's reasoning. It is noteworthy that the researchers have come up with the explanation models that are capable of determining the decision-making process of deep NNs by integrating the additive feature attribution methods and the distillation techniques.

DL algorithm is one of the most popular algorithms in use today, every model designer should consider interpretability. Thus, designing interpretable mechanisms not only improves the predictive qualities of the model but also makes it possible to explain to a wider audience what is happening at the theoretical level but in practice. This emphasis on model interpretability is important, to some extent, to restore people's trust in machine learning systems and to make the algorithmic decisions affecting society comprehensible [12].

Ideally in the context of networks architecture, DL deftly draws its success from a set of model architectures for distinct levels which in turn has the ability to learn a representation of data in terms of hierarchy with other layers able to learn both global and localized features. Hence doing so, in a broader sense, investigating prototypes has made researchers enable the working of DL models on tractable sets, yet their interpretability remains intact. In particular, the above mentioned approach enables obtaining a more flexible view on the representation of features in space and the limitations of the proposed system's performance.

When it comes to analyzing DNA sequences and patterns, the Deep Motif Dashboard is certainly a helpful and ready tool in the field of bioinformatics. The PhyloMotifs rich dashboard sums up a set of graphical approaches to identify motifs and sequence patterns learned by deep NNs, especially for discriminating transcription factor-binding sites. By using such models as convolutional, recurrent, and convolutional-recurrent ones, the researchers receive ideas on how these models determine the signals in DNA sequences and draw the reflections on why the transcription factors function in the specific locations. These saliency maps can be used to analyze the influence that each individual nucleotide within a given DNA sequence has on the final output of a DL NN. The strength of this method is that, apart from identifying which parts of the sequence contribute more to the classification and, therefore, being able to interpret why the model's outputs are what they are, Additionally, it provides a temporal dimension of the output scores showing how recurrent models predict the response through time of sequential inputs and which indicate the fluctuation of the transcription factors binding process. Further, the use of class-specific visualization strategy for the consider transcription factor bind site-positive class helps in determining the right feed-forward input sequence of the considered transcription factor bind site-positive class through stochastic gradient optimization.

This method helps to describe and pinpoint certain periodicity trends that qualify transcription factor binding sites to clearly identify the processes that support the patterns of transcript expression [13]. Hence, the ways that learning models, predominantly about genomic sequences, can be visualized and understood through such tools as saliency maps or a temporal output score, or class-specific visual methodologies are the main focus of the numerous and multiple correspondences concerning DNA sequences and transcription factor binding. Indeed, availing of these solutions in the analysis and visualization aspect puts the researchers in a position to unlock the information hidden within the genomics study and introduce new advancements within the bioinformatics niche. Primarily, the use of biologically inspired attribution scores and interpretable mechanisms embedded within the DL models enhance the performance of the classifier, and secondarily, the usage of such techniques contributes to the formulation of the basic premise of transparency and comprehensibility of any algorithmic decision; altogether, the advancement of more interpretable and reliable AI systems.

6. Applications of BIA-based Deep Learning Models in Disease Detection

BIAs associated with DL Models have become quite popular in the past few years and have strikingly indicated matured outcomes in the disease detection area. This amalgamation of BIA and DL can be revolutionary as it integrates the advantages of both these domains and can revolutionize the medical imaging and diagnosing mechanisms through enhancing the disease-detecting systems. Hence, there are obvious advantages to applying BIA-based DL models in disease detection, one of which is the capacity to deal with extensive and sophisticated medical data. The bio-inspired optimization algorithms help in fine-tuning the DL model to improve the performance specificity on patterns and abnormality detection in medical scan images. The suggested application of BIA in conjunction with DL is highly beneficial in disease detection as it leads to more accurate and dependable results that can then improve the quality of patient care experienced by patients and healthcare professionals. Moreover, when combining BIA and DL, there is a possibility of developing disease detection systems that are innovative and capable of learning from their experiences. These models are able to adapt their techniques to each new set of data that is given to it and its repetitions to enhance precision these features are helpful in the dynamic world of medical images where new diseases and changes are emerging in the market. Moreover, the integration of Biomedical Image Analysis-based DL techniques in disease diagnosis allows the provision of a personalized approach to treatments. This approach allows for a more effective approach and usage of individual patient data to enhance algorithms in delivering high-quality care. The outlined form of treatment can go down in the history of the development of healthcare as the one that brought about a revolution in clinical operations to increase patient satisfaction. To sum up, it is possible to note that incorporating BIAs with DL models as an effective tool for improving disease detection in medical images. Using BIA optimization and the pattern analysis of DL, researchers not only can create new and more accurate diagnosis and detection systems for various diseases but can also make the process faster and smarter that can eventually lead to so-called individualized medicine This symbiosis between BIA and DL is a starting point on the way to the use of highly innovative approaches in the healthcare field [15– 17].

6.1 Computer-Aided Diagnosis (CADx) Systems

The fusion of DL models using BIAs has become the focus of attention in CADx systems, and has demonstrated significant performance levels in the diagnosis of diseases. Employing the CADx systems for a diverse range of diseases, the investigators demonstrated the enhancement of accuracy, speed, and reliability of the systems by applying BIA-based DL models. One of the key areas to focus in the integration is the use of BIA in the feature selection and training of DL libraries. Deeper Learning researchers have succeeded in applying Moth-Flame Optimization, Firefly Optimization, ABC Optimization, as well as ACO algorithms to select some of the best features from the medical imaging data to improve the DL models in disease detection applications. These integrated with Convolutional Neural Networks (CNNs) and Long Short-Term Memory (LSTM), BIA-based feature selection has empowered the capability of automatically classifying complex patterns in medical images contributing to the improvement of diagnostic and predictive accuracy. They were able to classify patterns of emphysema in chest CT scans by using DL model consisting of both CNN and LSTM parts. Furthermore, when CADx systems incorporate BIA algorithms, accuracy of the segmentation of the lung tissues and extraction of ROIs (region of interest) has received a boost. With the application of specialized algorithms like SIFCM, the researchers have improved the ability to spot specific features pertaining to a disease through the images, thus improving the chances of early diagnosis of ailments like bronchiectasis and lung cancer. Therefore, the combination of computer-aided diagnostic tools such as the DL model and BIA-based optimization has enhanced disease diagnosis in medical imaging. Together, these methods have given impetus to developed, precise, and quicker ways toward diagnosing several diseases that can greatly enhance the possibilities of diagnosis and treatment within healthcare.

6.2 Medical Image Analysis and Segmentation

DL models and BIA integrated with DL models have shown incredible advancements in the medical image (MI) analysis and segmentation of diseases. Several researchers have employed and enhanced the performance of DL architectures in terms of the accuracy and complexity of the medical image analysis of a variety of diseases by integrating the optimization aspects of BIAs. The integration of CNNs with BIA is a significant step in this approach and is used to extract the features of medical images. These can help with the automatic recognition and delineation of pathological areas, including tumors or lesions, at a higher efficiency and with increased accuracy. Also, due to the adaptability of BIA, the hyperparameters of DL models involved are tuned correspondingly with enhanced efficiency in disease detection missions. Furthermore, the use of BIA-based DL models in the detection of diseases has demonstrated several benefits whereby feature engineering does not provide adequate solutions [14]. Rather than using the prespecified features, the models can learn from the data and this leads to an important aspect that can be captured through the raw image data which is the patterns and details that are vital in diagnosis. The combination of DL models and BIOT in the fields of MI analysis and segmentation have promising opportunities for the development of better disease diagnosis. Researchers must understand the advantages of using both these methodologies to enhance diagnoses in healthcare structures.

6.3 Omics Data Analysis for Disease Prediction

Precision medicine, as a revolutionary concept that has implications in disease prediction and segmentation, has received massive improvement through Omics data analysis. The involvement of different techniques like genomics, proteomics, metabolomics helps in understanding the root cause of diseases and offers potential biomarkers. This approach benefits a deeper understanding of the disease heterogeneity and helps in the creation of unique approaches to the treatment of the patients. Moreover, the integration of Omics data with bioinformatics and machine learning including the BIA-based DL models, etc., offers newer vistas for early and accurate diagnosis and classification of diseases. These models take advantage by using the self-features of Omics data for identifying the noticeable pattern and features which can help in effective disease modeling and categorization. Omics data analysis, in conjunction with BIA-based DL models, improves the diagnostic capacity and comprehensible variables that are inherent to disease diagnostic tools. This is the prospect of the upcoming book chapter in which we will attempt to discuss the potential of Omics data analysis for the alteration of disease models and their forecasts as well as for the disease categorization using the application of BIA-based DL models. Our work here is to introduce the reader to the major principles, methods, accomplishments, as well as to provide a number of case studies to reveal how these progressive approaches are changing the world of diagnostics and PEM (protein-energy malnutrition). In this context, the intended goal of this chapter is to present state-of-the-art findings and framework that may spearhead progressive innovations in precision healthcare.

7. Challenges and Future Directions

7.1 Computational Complexity and Scalability

Considering the issues of computational comprehensiveness and sustainability of BIAs, the use of these approaches in optimization and, in particular, in machine learning processes is critical. These challenges come about from the high dimensional spaces in the optimization problems and large volume of data available across different fields, which makes the efficiency of the BIAs in handling big data a huge challenge. In addition, there are issues like small-scale infrastructure curtailing the growth of BIAs due to constraints in computational resources required for computation of optimization problems. To overcome such challenges with computer resources, the future direction might involve the use parallel and distributive computing in order to handle the data more efficiently, using advanced optimization techniques and incorporating hybrid methods to increase the scalability of the technique along with cloud computing for the scalable resources, using hardware acceleration to perform the techniques at a faster rate, designing more efficient algorithm and search methods. These challenges and future directions should be observed to enhance the BIAs' performance and thus their usefulness in meeting real-world problems effectively in the future [18–21].

7.2 Theoretical Foundations and Convergence Analysis

The following major bottlenecks in BIA research have been identified: The major bottleneck is the fact that there seem to be only limited attempts at establishing sound theoretical frameworks and systematically and extensively conducting convergence analysis of BIAs. The existence nonlinearity in biological systems and the attempt to model biological systems through algorithms are some of the challenges that orphan BIAs from a robust theoretical framework. Moreover, conformity of convergence properties in BIAs is more complicated to attain because of their stochastic characteristics, heuristic search purposes, and dynamic optima's environment, which makes it quite hard to achieve convergence with definite optimization solutions. To deal with such challenges, the future work involves the propositions of mathematical formulations as well as theoretical models that can be used in the determination of convergence properties as well as the stability of the BIAs together with the convergence rates. Some strategies are suggested to validate them theoretically and empirically such as solving the standard optimization problems, conducting experimentation and comparing the results obtained for different methods. More careful analyses of algorithm behaviors with BIAs, such as comparing theoretical results with real-world data and conducting sensitivity analysis on step size, maximum iterations and convergence criteria, on different BIAs problems and analyzing which kind of problems are more suitable for the algorithm would improve the BIAs in optimization tasks. The present paper raises some of these prospects and suggests further adjustments to the theoretical framework and empirical discoveries relevant to BIAs to enhance the convergence analysis and development of more efficient and robust optimization approaches to tackle multifaceted application problems in reality [22– 23].

7.3 Integration with Emerging Deep Learning Techniques

Combining BIAs with new learning NNs presents a unique problem as there is a vast gap between the two in terms of logical structure and what might be considered 'clean' mathematical principles when compared to traditional BIAs. The training paradigms of DL models, which is the case with NNs, are not in the same category with the evolutionary and swarm-based optimization paradigms of BIAs, thus increasing the problem of their integration to work more effectively. While making existing BIAs compatible with DL architecture, especially CNNs and RNNs (recurrent NNs) as well as dealing with issues of tuning and convergence within the objective function within frameworks of hybrid optimization, smart approaches, methods of attack, and defenses that aim at adversarial training. To overcome these challenges, future directions include the following; future research aims at integrating BIAs with the DL technique; future work also seeks to fine-tune pretrained model using BIAs; metaheuristics optimization is also desirable to be employed for optimizing DL architecture; finally, interdisciplinary researchers should collaborate in the future working on integration of these approaches. To this end, resolving these challenges and discussing their potential developments may lead researchers to new horizons of further development of the optimization algorithms in the context of growth and changes of DL rates.

Conclusion

In conclusion, this book chapter has discussed in detail the modern and hybrid BIAs and their relevance in the field of DL as well as disease detection. BIAs can be described as a method of solving the given problem which is derived from analyzing the various biological systems. The heuristic aspects of the living phenomena have been incorporated in these algorithms where they have been seen to perform very well despite being used in the solution of complex and dynamic models. From the BIAs of historical and classical origins including EAs and Swarm Intelligence Algorithms through to modern and convincingly composite BIAs, including AIS and Membrane Computing Algorithms, a detailed description of these BIAs has been included in the chapter. The now-published synergistic coupling of BIAs with DL models has been explained and general areas such as model selection, hyperparameter, NAS, and (L1/L2) regularizations have been covered in the literature. The chapter has also focused on how BIAs can be used to improve the usability of models derived through DL and AI through explainability techniques and graphical representations. A brief introduction about the potential of BIA-based DL models in the fields of disease detection has been provided as follows: CAD Systems, MI analysis, and segmentation and Disease prediction by analyzing omics data. These applications point out that BIAs can be a game-changer in the area of healthcare because they help diagnose diseases and recommend their treatment quicker and with almost total reliability. Yet it has also highlighted the issues and possibilities in this area of study discussed in the chapter. Some of the challenges that need discussed or to be faced, are as follows: A major challenge relates to the computational complexity and scalability of the algorithms, as well as to fundamental theoretical aspects of the approach; another significant topic concerns the convergence analysis of the current algorithms in the framework of BIAs both in DL and in the context of disease detection; finally, the integration of the present BIAs with state-of-art deep learning methodologies. The suggestions for future work encompass the following: The proposal to pay more attention to designing of effective BIAs and scalable algorithms with good accuracy, the need to set up more refined theoretical backgrounds, more rigorous convergence analysis, and the integration of BIAs with DL. Multidisciplinary cooperation and integration between academic collaborators in computer science, biology, and healthcare is and will continue to be a key factor that can drive the progress of the scientific field and produce usable and beneficial services and products that address current needs. In conclusion, this book chapter enables the reader to garner valuable insights and ideas to continue further research in the fields of DL and disease identification using modern and hybrid BIAs. To reduce the complexity level of various problem domains and to gain a better understanding about the key principles, applications, issues, and future research directions of Fuzzy systems, it is possible to argue that this is an important avenue of research for the researchers.

References

[1] Pham, T.H. and Raahemi, B. (2023). Bio-inspired feature selection algorithms with their applications: A systematic literature review. *IEEE Access*, *11*, 43733–43758.

[2] Bozorg-Haddad, O. (Ed.). (2018). *Advanced Optimization by Nature-inspired Algorithms* (Vol. 720). Singapore: Springer.

[3] Balasaraswathi, V.R., Sugumaran, M. and Hamid, Y. (2017). Feature selection techniques for intrusion detection using non-bio-inspired and bio-inspired optimization algorithms. *Journal of Communications and Information Networks*, *2*, 107–19.

[4] Binitha, S. and Sathya, S.S. (2012). A survey of bio-inspired optimization algorithms. *International Journal of Soft Computing and Engineering*, *2*(2), 137–51.

[5] Whitley, D. (1994). A genetic algorithm tutorial. *Statistics and Computing*, 4(2), 65–85.

[6] Koza, J.R. (1992). *Genetic Programming: On the Programming of Computers by Means of Natural Selection* (Vol. 1). MIT Press.

[7] Kennedy, J. and Eberhart, R. (1995). Particle swarm optimization. *In: Proceedings of ICNN'95-International Conference on Neural Networks*, *4*, 1942–48. IEEE.

[8] Zhang, G., Ali, Z.H., Aldlemy, M.S., Mussa, M.H., Salih, S.Q., Hameed, M. M., ... and Yaseen, Z.M. (2022). Reinforced concrete deep beam shear strength capacity modelling using an integrative bio-inspired algorithm with an artificial intelligence model. *Engineering with Computers*, *38*(Suppl 1), 15–28.

[9] Lu, Z., Whalen, I., Boddeti, V., Dhebar, Y., Deb, K., Goodman, E. and Banzhaf, W. (Jul. 2019). Nsga-net: Neural architecture search using multi-objective genetic algorithm. *In: Proceedings of the Genetic and Evolutionary Computation Conference* (pp. 419–27).

[10] Liu, Y., Sun, Y., Xue, B., Zhang, M., Yen, G.G. and Tan, K.C. (2021). A survey on evolutionary neural architecture search. *IEEE Transactions on Neural Networks and Learning Systems*, *34*(2), 550–70.

[11] Dong, Y., Su, H., Zhu, J. and Zhang, B. (2017). Improving interpretability of deep neural networks with semantic information. *In: Proceedings of the IEEE Conference on Computer Vision and Pattern Recognition* (pp. 4306–14).

[12] Lanchantin, J., Singh, R., Wang, B. and Qi, Y. (2017). Deep motif dashboard: Visualizing and understanding genomic sequences using deep neural networks. *In: Pacific Symposium on Biocomputing*, *2017* (pp. 254–65).

[13] Drumond, T.F., Viéville, T. and Alexandre, F. (2019). Bio-inspired analysis of deep learning on not-so-big data using data-prototypes. *Frontiers in Computational Neuroscience*, *12*, 100.

[14] Ghoniem, R.M. (2020). A novel bio-inspired deep learning approach for liver cancer diagnosis. *Information*, *11*(2), 80.

[15] Fan, X., Sayers, W., Zhang, S., Han, Z., Ren, L. and Chizari, H. (2020). Review and classification of bio-inspired algorithms and their applications. *Journal of Bionic Engineering*, *17*, 611– 31.

[16] Kar, A.K. (2016). Bio-inspired computing: A review of algorithms and scope of applications. *Expert Systems with Applications*, *59*, 20–32.

[17] Meng, X., Liu, Y., Gao, X. and Zhang, H. (2014). A new bio-inspired algorithm: chicken swarm optimization. *In: Advances in Swarm Intelligence: 5th International Conference, ICSI 2014*, Hefei, China, October 17–20. *Proceedings, Part I 5* (pp. 86– 94). Springer International Publishing.

[18] Selvaraj, C., Kumar, R.S. and Karnan, M. (2014). A survey on application of bio-inspired algorithms. *International Journal of Computer Science and Information Technologies*, *5*(1), 366–70.

[19] Dhiman, G. and Kumar, V. (2018). Emperor penguin optimizer: A bio-inspired algorithm for engineering problems. *Knowledge-Based Systems*, *159*, 20–50.

[20] Brabazon, A. and O'Neill, M. (2006). *Biologically iIspired Algorithms for Financial Modelling.* Springer Science & Business Media.

[21] Kadry, S., Dhanaraj, R.K., K, S.K. and Manthiramoorthy, C. (2024). Res-Unet based blood vessel segmentation and cardio vascular disease prediction using chronological chef-based optimization algorithm based deep residual network from retinal fundus images. *Multimedia Tools and Applications*, 1–30.

[22] Balasubramaniam, S., Nelson, S.G., Arishma, M. and Rajan, A.S. (2024). Machine Learning-based Disease and Pest Detection in Agricultural Crops. *EAI Endorsed Transactions on Internet of Things*, 10.

[23] Fister Jr, I., Yang, X. S., Fister, I., Brest, J. and Fister, D. (2013). A brief review of nature-inspired algorithms for optimization. *arXiv preprint* arXiv:1307.4186.

3 Evaluation of Bio-Inspired Algorithm-based Machine Learning and Deep Learning Models

Selvam Durairaj,[1*] Malik Mohamed Umar[2] and Natarajan B.[1]

Natural processes such as neural networks, swarm intelligence, and genetic development have inspired algorithms that exhibit great promise in solving complicated optimization problems in deep learning (DL) and machine learning (ML). A thorough evaluation of bio-inspired algorithm-based ML and DL models in medicine is conducted in this research chapter. This study evaluates and contrasts the performance of multiple bio-inspired algorithms using a range of datasets and goals. Ant colony optimization, particle swarm optimization, genetic algorithms, and artificial neural networks are a few of these. Experimental data are used to assess these bio-inspired models' robustness, scalability, and performance in classification, regression, and optimization tasks. This chapter looks at how bio-inspired algorithms enhance the interpretability and generalizability of ML and DL models. The advantages and disadvantages of these nature-inspired methods are also discussed. The findings show how bio-inspired algorithms can be used to develop intelligent systems of ML and DL in different types of medical healthcare applications.

1. Introduction

1.1 Background

Artificial intelligence (AI) has come a long way in recent years. Deep learning (DL) and machine learning (ML) approaches have transformed many fields worldwide, such as medicine, computation, finance, and agriculture. However, standard training and optimization issues include the ability to be understood, shortage of data, and overfitting. Researchers have developed computer models that are adaptive and self-learning through the use of bio-inspired algorithms, which take inspiration from biological systems and natural processes. Assessing bio-inspired algorithm-based ML and DL models is essential to progressing cutting-edge AI research and technology. By assessing these hybrid models' efficacy, performance,

---

[1] School of Computer Science and Engineering (SCOPE), Vellore Institute of Technology, Chennai Campus, 600127, Tamil Nadu, India.

[2] National Space Science & Technology Center (NSSTC), United Arab Emirates University (UAEU), Al Ain, 15551, Abu Dhabi, UAE.

* Corresponding author: selvam.d@vit.ac.in

Evaluation of Bio-Inspired Algorithm-based Machine Learning and Deep Learning Models | 49

and application, researchers expect to discover new approaches to enhance their interpretability, robustness, and scalability. More intelligent, flexible, and human-like AI systems will be possible due to technology.

Traditional Approaches

SGD (stochastic gradient descent), its variants, and other gradient-based optimization algorithms are widely used in classic ML and DL techniques for both model training and optimization. Even while these techniques are effective in many situations, they frequently need assistance when used on high-dimensional, non-convex optimization-based problems, which results in unsatisfactory solutions and the slowest convergence rates. Additionally, understanding issues plague traditional ML and DL models, making it difficult to understand the underlying mechanics behind their predictions. Additionally, this method uses the diversity and flexibility of biological-based optimization, its limits, and its ability to function in very complex contexts.

Current Trends

The bio-inspired Bio algorithms make the drawbacks of conventional ML and DL algorithms in medical-based applications. It mimics naturally adaptable and self-organization property-based learning, optimizing model training and generalization. The ML and DL-based algorithm models hide some information on the complex optimization problem and change and adjust their environment. This chapter presents the primary approach of the bio-inspired optimization algorithm, which handles various ML and DL-based models.

1.2 Motivation

Bio-inspired algorithms are adaptive and self-learning of natural processes and biological systems with the help of ML and DL, prompting the investigation of AI system growth increasingly robust and efficient. These algorithms cover evolutionary, particle swarm, and genetic optimization, providing unique identity and complex optimization issues based on the convergence speed or processing rate in the ML and DL. The changing circumstances and solutions of new solutions are promising and offer new enhancing bio-inspired optimization algorithms. The new generation of the AL-based model is evolving to medical applications. It will make new high-accuracy systems on the ML and DL model systems.

The hybrid techniques of ML and DL successfully solve issues of ML and DL, such as overfitting and underfitting problems. The data scarcity of the model explores various optimizations and finds hidden high-dimensional data to improve the AI system's accuracy and efficiency.

The hybrid model applies to bank engineering and healthcare, which evaluate ML and DL-based real-world scenarios in miniature and large-scale banking engineering and healthcare industries. The next compares the bio-inspired standard ML and DL architecture and optimization techniques regarding linear and nonlinear and the relative benefits and drawbacks with some constraints. Next, it is highlighted to improve hybrid application requirements involving the process of minimum and maximum objective functions in the optimization techniques.

The alternative goal of bio-inspired ML and DL server AI research and technology is to forward adaptive and intelligent systems with complex problems solved with advanced argumentation of real real-world problem issues in society.

1.3 Objectives

The main objective of ML and DL-based bio-inspired algorithms is to achieve the following three objectives in AI research and technological progress:

I. The hybrid model is explored with a high and enhancing model to make the training, generalization, and optimization in the swam intelligent, neural system, and evolutionary system.

II. If handling complex problems to solve optimization problems, it highlights the high-dimensional data and how to pattern to ML and DL and compare their adapting environment.

III. The hybrid ML and DL model further improves the applications' specific domain. For example, the field of medical domain, particularly cardiac attacks, needs advanced patterning in the different locations of different servers.

Additionally, the bio-inspired optimization algorithm models are used in real-world scenarios to make the interpretability and SCA (sine cosine algorithm) possible. The main goal is for AI research-based intelligent systems to create more flexible and easy ways to handle complex issues and change society in healthcare.

2. Literature Review

2.1 Bio-Inspired Algorithms in Machine Learning

Cloud-fog computing using ML and DL with bio-inspired optimization [1, 2], improving the overall efficiency of cloud and fog computing in the distributing approach. It also effectively handles complex optimization problems because of the valuation of natural activity and swarm behaviour. The computing resources appropriately respond to the system, such as power processing, memory, and network bandwidth, and reduce the optimization throughput and latency. By applying the bio-inspired optimization approach algorithms with ML and DL, the entire machine ensures high reliability, resource utilization, and load balancing, and enhances overall performance. The cloud and fog-based data processing analyzes larger scale data evaluation and analyses by using hybrid cloud architecture.

Cloud environment also improves the intrusion and detection system by using bio-inspired optimization to shield data from online social network threads and security protocols [3, 4]. Combining the ML or DL with a bio-inspired optimization algorithm in the cloud-fog environment makes it possible to create a more efficient and secure distribution solution [5, 6]. Identification of medical cancer diagnosis

[7,8] applies to bio-inspired algorithms that enhance ML application. These algorithms solve the complex problem of biological brain activity and swarm evaluation and improve the efficiency of ML models in detecting cancer using large datasets [9], predicting related features and increasing their reciting accuracy.

Bio-inspired optimization algorithms are used in breast cancer prediction systems, and their image processing and classification tasks are enhanced with the help of GA (genetic algorithm), PSO (particle swarm optimization), and ABC (artificial bee colony algorithm) [10-12]. Feature selection methods of DL detect malignant tumours with high accuracy [13]. Earlier, ML-based broader medical diagnostic of bio-inspired optimization algorithms augmented the sensitivity of models by way of reflecting a biologically based ML system that leads and is accurately detected by using productive diagnostic tools and speeds up the diagnostic system and reduces the incorrect positives and negatives, and enhances patient outcomes. Bio-inspired optimization algorithm-based AI applications are used in feature selection, sentimental analysis, social media spam detection, physiological data analysis, and data mining classification. This type of algorithm-based model improves the optimization fitness functions and behavioural swarm. For example, GA, PSO and genetic programming identify the extensive dataset features and reflect ML models' high accuracy and efficiency.

Bio-inspired algorithms' adaptable and experimental nature effectively differentiate spam from legitimate material, enhancing the efficacy of classifications for social network spam detection. Bio-inspired techniques improve the classification learning process in data mining, leading to more accurate and dependable classification outcomes. Sentiment analysis [14] benefits from bio-inspired algorithms because they enhance the extraction of features and model tweaking, allowing for a more precise interpretation of textual input.

These algorithms make biomedical data analysis more accessible, which helps with accurate disease diagnosis and treatment planning by processing and analyzing complex medical datasets more effectively. Applications for swarm intelligence, which mimic the group behaviour of gregarious animals with algorithms, can enable efficient problem-solving in complex, dynamic environments. When bio-inspired algorithms are integrated, these diverse ML applications yield more precise, effective, and flexible systems, resulting in data processing and decision-making advancements across multiple industries.

ML-based cloud security, network security, spam detection, and task allocation for vulnerability checking are improved in bio-inspired algorithms. This algorithm is the proper solution to complex network security issues because of the naturally inspired swarm intelligent behaviour convergence. In cloud security, using bio-inspired algorithms automatically addresses the vulnerability score of the given population input and provides a more robust architecture [15, 16]. We can predict more responses and accurate unauthorized access in the security system using bio-inspired intrusion detection algorithms with ML or DL models.

In predicting adaptive learning-based spam detection of bio-inspired algorithms, Cloud email and communication platforms are primarily used to distribute malicious content [17]. In the network security view, bio-inspired algorithms improve the security tools gateway and quickly detect the threat response in the network anomalies' traffic control system [18,19]. ML-based security maintains high security, operates in the cloud, and further incorporates the reliability, adaptability, and knowledge-based security solution in bio-inspired optimization-based solutions on a distributed cloud environment.

2.2 Applications of Bio-Inspired Algorithms in Deep Learning

The advance of DL-based medical healthcare mainly uses bio-inspired algorithms for sharing the resources of the healthcare system [20, 21]. Using bio-inspired algorithms in medical healthcare improves the accuracy and efficiency of diagnosis systems. Convolutional neural networks (CNNs) and recurrent neural networks (RNNs) models detect diseases like cancer and cardiovascular issues with high accuracy using bio-inspired GA and PSO optimization [22, 23]. Enhancing the protection of patterns and anomalies of identification on DL in precise detection by using medical images is better than using existing optimization techniques.

The medical healthcare systems of resources regarding equipment, facilities, and medical personnel allocate tasks using bio-inspired optimization techniques [24, 25]. This algorithm is used to distribute resources effectively in the natural processing of ACO (ant colony optimization) and BCO (bee colony optimization). The result of the algorithms' waiting time is less than the exiting of GA and PSO. Bio-inspired optimization algorithms dynamically change the daily administration of staff schedules and equipment based on real-time data and adequately receive the required resources and attention. The intelligent and flexible DL-based bio-inspired optimization combined with the healthcare system and resource allocation enhances its accuracy and treats the system's best outcome.

The cloud and fog-based DL system uses bio-inspired algorithms, making task allocation process, data processing, and resource management in the medical healthcare system easier. The load balancing, resource allocation, and virtual machine placement are optimized in the Bio-inspired algorithms, which improve their performance, latency and computational resource efficiency [26, 27].

In fog computing, the cloud services show how to interconnect to the network edge and manage the distributed node of fog in the edge, tell about bio-inspired optimization techniques, and make flexible and adaptable resources for node allocation tasks in swarm intelligent processing. By enhancing the scheduling of tasks and data caching techniques, evolutionary algorithms, for instance, can lower general response time and bandwidth usage in fog nodes. Applications like Internet of Things (IoT) software and sophisticated city infrastructure that require minimal latency and real-time processing would greatly benefit from this [28].

When DL is combined with bio-inspired cloud or fog-computing algorithms, system efficiency, trustworthiness, and scalability are enhanced. These algorithms, which mimic natural adaptations and self-organizing behaviours seen in the environment, provide innovative solutions to the problematic issues associated with managing large-scale distributed computer environments, consequently contributing to enhanced intelligence and efficient cloud and fog systems [29–30].

2.3 Comparative Studies on Bio-Inspired Algorithms

The effectiveness, efficiency, and applications of bio-inspired algorithms across various domains are investigated through comparative analyses between them and other bio-inspired methodologies and conventional optimization techniques. Bio-inspired algorithms' efficacy, efficiency, and generalizability are assessed through comparative studies with other bio-inspired technologies and traditional optimization techniques. The research provides valuable insights into the pros and cons of various algorithms, which can aid in implementing such algorithms to tackle intricate real-world issues [31]. The various metrics, goals, obstacles, and bio-inspired algorithms are shown in Table 1.

3. Methodology

3.1 ML Models

Computers can collect data by using a collection of techniques called ML. Algorithms such as Support Vector Machines (SVMs), Naïve Bayes, K-Nearest Neighbors (KNNs), K-means, Random Forest, and K-means are widely used because of their versatility and efficiency in a range of situations, as exemplified by Algorithms 1 through 5. Using SVMs separates classes between regression and classification applications in the hyperplane optimization techniques. It facilitates text classification and spam detection.

In nonlinear decision boundaries, KNN is an instance-based learning method that is simple to apply and efficient. The prevalent class of a data point's nearest neighbours determines its category. An unsupervised technique called K-means clustering divides data into k different categories. Two typical applications are picture compression and market segmentation. Lastly, Random Forest is an ensemble learning technique that is excellent at resolving problems with classification and regression. Multiple decision trees are constructed to reduce overfitting and boost accuracy, and the results are aggregated [32].

3.2 DL Models

The DL models make the maximum learning and optimization from biological learning processing on Bio-Inspired methods algorithms. This is an imitation of the self-learning methods in the nature and feature selection. This chapter considers the six models of DL, like ANNs, CNNs, RNNs, and Fuzzy DL and Fuzzy_ ANN, Fuzzy_CNN, and Fuzzy_RNN, as shown in Algorithms 6 to Algorithm

Table 1 Different Bio-inspired algorithms and limitation.

Reference	Algorithm/Method	Metric Types	Objective	Limitations	Future Use
Baburaj, E. (2022) [28]	Genetic Algorithms, Particle Swarm Optimization, Ant Colony Optimization	Accuracy, Computational Efficiency	Neural network-based data mining classification	Computational cost and convergence issues with larger datasets	Hybrid approaches integrating multiple bio-inspired algorithms
Yadav, A. and Vishwakarma, D.K. (2020) [29]	Artificial Bee Colony, Firefly Algorithm	Accuracy, Precision, Recall	Sentiment analysis	Sensitivity to parameter settings	Real-time sentiment analysis applications
Gibson, S., Issac, B., Zhang, L. and Jacob, S.M. (2020) [30]	Genetic Programming, Neural Networks	Detection Rate, False Positives	Spam email detection	High false positive rates in diverse email datasets	Adaptive spam detection systems incorporating real-time learning
Subbiah, S.S. and Chinnappan, J. (2022) [31]	Particle Swarm Optimization, Genetic Algorithms	Prediction Accuracy, Error Rates	Electricity load forecasting	Handling of extreme load variations	Integration with smart grid technologies for better prediction accuracy
Ahsan, M.M., et al. (2020) [32]	Ant Colony Optimization, Artificial Immune Systems	Security Metrics, Response Time	Cloud security enhancement	Scalability issues in large cloud environments	Advanced threat detection systems leveraging hybrid bio-inspired methods
Moizuddin, M. and Jose, M.V. (2022) [33]	Hybrid Deep Learning, Genetic Algorithms	Detection Accuracy, Response Time	Network intrusion detection	High computational requirements	Real-time intrusion detection with reduced computational overhead
de Albuquerque, V.H.C., et al. (2020) [34]	Various Bio-Inspired Algorithms	Diagnostic Accuracy, Sensitivity, Specificity	Biomedical data analysis	Handling of high-dimensional and noisy data	Personalized medicine through enhanced data analysis techniques
Soula, M., et al. (2022) [35]	Firefly Algorithm, Ant Colony Optimization	Resource Utilization, Task Distribution	Task allocation in edge computing	Suboptimal performance under varying network conditions	Dynamic task allocation strategies for heterogeneous edge computing environments

Evaluation of Bio-Inspired Algorithm-based Machine Learning and Deep Learning Models | 55

11. PSO is one technique that emulates the social behaviour of live things by iteratively adjusting candidate solutions based on their performance. GAs mimic natural selection simultaneously by generating populations of possible solutions across several generations. These frameworks are valuable for many applications, including optimization challenges, because DL improves their ability to handle complex, high-dimensional data, and optimize parameters [33].

ANNs, made up of layers of connected nodes or neurons, are the basic models used in DL. On the other hand, RNNs are designed to process sequential input by keeping track of temporal dependencies in a hidden state. This characteristic is critical for various applications, including language modelling and time-series prediction. Fuzzy ANNs, CNNs, and Fuzzy RNNs are created by enhancing these conventional models with fuzzy logic. These models combine fuzzy membership functions and rules to manage imprecision and uncertainty in data and reliable performance is possible in real-world applications with frequently noisy or unclear data. Fuzzy CNNs improve feature extraction in the face of ambiguity, fuzzy ANNs improve generalization from uncertain data, and fuzzy RNNs more skilfully handle imprecise temporal correlations.

Algorithm 1. ML: SVM Model

Steps:

    i) Get the data ready: Standardize or normalize the information.

    ii) Decide the kernel function to use: Select a kernel (RBF, polynomial, or linear).

    iii) Educate the SVM Model

    iv) Adapt the model: For the SVM model to fit, use training data.

    iv) Optimization: To maximize the margin, solve the quadratic optimization problem.

    v) Assess the Model: Use a validation set to adjust hyperparameters (C and gamma).

    vi) Predict: Make predictions on fresh data using the trained model.

Assessing Performance Compute specificity, recall, accuracy, and precision.

Algorithm 2. ML: Naïve Bayes Model

Steps:

    i) Prepare the data: Convert categorical data to numerical format and address missing values.

    ii) Determine Prior Probabilities: Determine each class's prior probability.

    iii) Compute Likelihoods: Determine the probability of each feature for each class.

    iv) Utilize the Bayes Theorem

    v) Integrate the Pasts and Probabilities: Determine each class's posterior probability.

    vi) Forecast: The class with the most considerable posterior probability should be assigned.

    vii) Assessing Performance: Use measures such as specificity, recall, accuracy, and precision.

Algorithm 3. ML: KNN Model

Steps:

   i) Get the data ready: Normalize the data to guarantee that every feature contributes equally.

   ii) Select the Neighbour Count (k): Determine what k is worth.

   iii) Compute Distances: Determine the separation between training and query instances.

   iv) Get the closest neighbours: Determine the closest neighbours using the calculated distances.

   iv) Make Forecasts:

      Classification: Assign the neighbourhood's most prevalent class.

      Regression: Calculate the mean of the k closest neighbours' values.

   v) Analyze Performance: Determine recall, specificity, accuracy, and precision.

   vi) Assessing Performance: Compute specificity, recall, accuracy, and precision.

Algorithm 4. ML: K-means Model

Steps:

Actions:

   i) Set Centroids in Motion: Choose k sites randomly as the starting centroids.

   ii) Assign Clusters: Assign the closest centroid to every data point.

   iii) Revise Centroids: Take the average points in each cluster to recalculate the centroids.

Again:

   iv) Assign each data point to the closest new centroid when reassigning clusters.

   v) Update the centroids by recalculating them.

   vi) Convergence: Continue until there is no discernible change in the centroids.

   vii) Assessing Performance: Use measures such as silhouette score and inertia (within-cluster sum of squares).

Algorithm 5. ML: Random Forest Model

Steps:

   i) Prepare the Data: Convert categorical data to numerical form and address missing values.

   ii) Bootstrap Sampling: Generate several dataset samples using replacement.

   iii) Learn how to use decision trees:

      Grow Trees: Develop an unpruned decision tree for every bootstrap sample.

   iv) Choose a random collection of characteristics to divide at each node using the random feature selection method.

   v) Overall Forecasts:

      Classification: For each tree, utilize a majority vote.

      Regression: Calculate the average of each tree's predictions.

   vi) Analyse Performance: Determine recall, specificity, accuracy, and precision.

Evaluation of Bio-Inspired Algorithm-based Machine Learning and Deep Learning Models | 57

Algorithm 6. DL: ANN Model

Steps:

1) Preparing Data:
    i) Preprocess and load the dataset.
    ii) Make the data more standardized.
    iii) Set training, validation, and testing out of the dataset.

2) Architecture Model:
    i) Set up the sequential model.
    ii) Add ReLU-activated dense layers.
    iii) Put in the last Dense layer using the proper activation function

3) Gathering:
    i) Select an optimizer, such as Adam.
    ii) Choose a loss function (for classification, use sparse_categorical_crossentropy).
    iii) Establish evaluation metrics, such as accuracy.

4) Using the training data, train the model.

5) Use test data to evaluate the model.

Algorithm 7. DL: CNN Model

Steps:

    i) Preparing Data, preprocessing and loading data, then making the data with standardized, validation and test sets.
    ii) The Architecture Model gets the sequential model, Conv2D layers used by ReLU, and layers for MaxPooling2D, and flattened layer to transform the 2D matrix data into a vector.
    iii) ReLU-activated dense layers and set its activation function appropriately.
    iv) Gathering optimizer of Adam, Select a loss function
    v) Use test data to evaluate the model.

Algorithm 8. DL: RNN Model

Steps:

    i) Data Preparation of load and preprocessing data.
    ii) Architecture Model of Assemble the model in sequential order with Insert the layer of embedding, an RNN layer, dense layers activated by ReLU, Dense layer with the appropriate activation function.
    iii) Choose a loss function; for binary classification, binary_crossentropy, utilized and evaluation parameters.
    iv) Accessing training and testing data.
    v) Assess the model using test data.

Algorithm 9. DL: Fuzzy_ANN Model

1) Data Preparation:
    i) Obtain and prepare the dataset.
    ii) Completely standardize the data.
    iii) Create training, validation, and test sets using the dataset.
2) Architecture Model:
    i) Put the model together step-by-step.
    ii) Apply fuzzy activation functions to the fuzzy dense layers.
    iii) After adding the Dense layer, modify the activation function.
3) Gathering:
    i) Select an optimizer, such as Adam, for compilation.
    ii) Choose a loss function: sparse_categorical_cross-entropy is a good choice for classification.
    iii) Specify evaluation parameters, such as accuracy.
4) Use the training data to train the model.
5) Test data should be used to evaluate the model.

Algorithm 10. DL: Fuzzy_CNN Model

Steps:

1) Data Preparation:
    i) Load and preprocess the dataset.
    ii) Standardize the data more thoroughly.
    iii) Use the dataset to create test, validation, and training sets.
2) Architecture Model:
    i) Assemble the model in sequential order.
    ii) Use fuzzy activation functions in layers of Fuzzy Conv2D.
    iii) Extend Fuzzy MaxPooling2D by adding layers.
    iv) Add a flattened layer to convert the 2D matrix data into a vector. Add layers that are thick and have unclear activation functions.
    v) Add the Dense layer at the end and adjust its activation function.
3) Compiling:
    i) Pick an optimizer, like Adam.
    ii) Select a loss function (sparse_categorical_cross-entropy works well for classification).
    iii) Define assessment criteria, such as precision.
4) Directions: Train the model using the training data.
5) Evaluation: Examine the model using test data.

Evaluation of Bio-Inspired Algorithm-based Machine Learning and Deep Learning Models | 59

Algorithm 11. DL: Fuzzy_RNN Model

Steps:

1) Preparing Data:
   i) Preprocess and load the dataset.
   ii) Pad and tokenize sequences.
   iii) Make training, validation, and test sets from the dataset.
2) Architecture Model:
   i) Set up the sequential model.
   ii) Add a layer of fuzzy embedding.
   iii) Add a layer of fuzzy RNN (fuzzy LSTM, GRU, etc.). Include dense layers with hazy activation functions.
   iv) Apply the last Dense layer using the proper activation function (binary classification: use sigmoid, for example).
3) Gathering:
   i) Select an optimizer, such as Adam.
   ii) Choose a loss function (for binary classification, use binary_cross-entropy, for example).
   iii) Establish evaluation metrics, such as accuracy.
4) Instruction: Utilize the training data and train the model.
5) Assessment: Utilize test data to assess the model.

3.3 Bio-Inspired Optimization Algorithm

GA: By generating a population of potential solutions that change over many generations, GAs imitate the process of natural selection. It uses processes including selection, crossover (recombination), and mutation to explore the solution space and raise the population's fitness. To address optimization issues, GAs simulate the process of natural selection. The initial population of potential solutions, referred to as people, is created at random. A fitness function is used to assess each person. Then, to generate a new population, the algorithm uses genetic operators, including crossover, mutation, and selection. The most fit individuals are selected to procreate. Recombination, or crossover, creates offspring by combining elements of two-parent solutions, whereas mutation brings haphazard changes into individuals to preserve genetic diversity. Until the population progresses toward ideal solutions, this iterative process of selection, crossover, and mutation successfully explores and exploits the search space to find the most excellent answer [34].

PSO: It draws inspiration from the social behaviour of fish schools and flocks of birds. In PSO, possible solutions in the search space are represented by a swarm of particles. Each particle modifies its position based on its own best-known position (personal best) and the best-known positions of its neighbours (global best).

ABC: The honey bee's foraging habits served as the model for the Artificial Bee Colony algorithm. It is made up of scouts, observers, and working bees. While observers choose food sources, working bees look for food sources. The honey bee's foraging habits served as the model for the ABC algorithm. It is made up of scouts, observers, and working bees. Worker bees look for food, observers choose food according to its quality, and scouts must investigate new regions more carefully. This cooperation aids in identifying the best course of action.

ACO: Ants' foraging habits serve as the model for ACO. When ants follow a path, they leave behind pheromones, which other ants are more likely to follow based on how strong the trail is. Shorter paths gradually gather more pheromones, which direct the colony toward the best solution.

CSOA: The clever foraging techniques of crows inspire this algorithm. Crows can follow other crows to take food, but they can also hide their food and learn where it is hidden. The step crow optimization algorithm (CSAO) uses this behaviour to explore and exploit the search space effectively.

FA: The Firefly Algorithm (FA) is derived from the way fireflies flash. A firefly's brightness is directly correlated with its appeal, and it diminishes with distance. Fireflies travel in the direction of brighter areas, which aids in the search for space exploration and convergence on the best answer.

MOA: The mating habits and flight patterns of mayflies served as the model for the MOA. The mayfly population in MOA is separated into male and female individuals. While female mayflies move in the search space to select the best possible mate, male mayflies are attracted to female mayflies and modify their positions based on attraction forces. This mimics the processes of discovery and exploitation involved in finding the best answers. To maintain diversity and prevent local optima, the algorithm integrates mechanisms of attraction, repulsion, and mutation, which improves its efficiency in locating global optimal solutions [35].

BA: The Bat Algorithm (BA) is based on bats' echolocation strategies. Bats use echolocation to find prey and to navigate by producing sound pulses and listening for the echoes that return. BA leverages each bat to represent a potential solution and searches the search space using velocity and location updates. The computer adjusts the bats' frequency, loudness, and pulse emission rate to balance discovery and exploitation. Bats' heart rates and noise levels decrease as they find better options; this allows them to focus on a local search for the best options. This dynamic aspect helps BA by avoiding local optima and effectively converging to the global optimum.

GWO: Grey wolves' social structures and hunting techniques inspired the Grey Wolf Optimizer (GWO). The many leadership tiers in GWO are represented by the four groups of wolves: alpha, beta, delta, and omega. Alpha wolves lead the pack in hunting, followed by beta, delta, and omega wolves. As part of an optimization process, wolves encircle their prey and adjust their positions in reaction to alpha, beta, and delta wolves' placements. Because wolves encircle and attack their

Evaluation of Bio-Inspired Algorithm-based Machine Learning and Deep Learning Models | 61

prey during hunting, the algorithm can effectively explore and exploit the search space. GWO effectively approaches optimal solutions by mimicking these natural inclinations.

WOA: The bubble-net hunting technique used by humpback whales served as the model for the Whale Optimization Algorithm (WOA). In this approach, whales are represented as agents searching for the optimal solutions. The algorithm consists of three main stages: finding prey, encircling the animal, and bubble-net feeding. Whales adjust their locations throughout the surrounding prey phase based on the best-known solution. During the bubble-net feeding phase, the whales simulate a spiral movement around the prey by using spiral-shaped travel techniques and shrinking surroundings. Whales improve exploration by randomly looking for better options when they hunt for prey. WOA is a robust optimization technique for solving complex problems by mimicking these clever hunting strategies because it effectively balances exploration and exploitation [36].

3.4 Healthcare Datasets

The Cleveland dataset was selected for study out of the four Heart Disease dataset collection datasets because it had a comparatively lower percentage of missing values than the other two. Out of the 76 features in this dataset, we chose to work with 13 features that had no missing values. There are 303 samples in the Cleveland dataset and 270 in the Statlog dataset. Remarkably, the Cleveland dataset is the only one with six missing values; it was left out of our analysis instead of performing data correction. The constriction of blood vessels is a significant health indicator that is used to classify each sample in the Cleveland and Statlog datasets. If the vessels show less than 50% narrowing, the samples are classified as (i) healthy; if the vessels show more than 50% narrowing, they are labelled as (ii) CAD, which stands for coronary artery disease. The Cleveland dataset's comparatively reduced number of missing values across its 76 variables led to its selection over other datasets in the Heart Disease collection. To ensure robustness and integrity in our research, we limited our work to 13 features from the Cleveland dataset that had no missing data. On the other hand, 303 samples and 55 attributes make up the Z-Alizadeh Sani dataset, which is carefully arranged into many categories like "Demographics", "Symptom and Examination", "ECG", and "Laboratory and Eco". Each sample in this dataset is categorized as either (i) healthy or (ii) unhealthy, a more inclusive categorization that extends beyond the particular vessel-narrowing criteria applied in the Cleveland dataset and enables a more thorough assessment of health issues [37].

4. Result Evaluation and Analysis

4.1 Experimental Setup and Datasets

Importance scores of features were computed using methods on the three datasets of Cleveland, Statlog, and Z-Alizadeh Sani. Ensemble scores of features were computed 216 times, representing each combination of the 16 FS methods; 216 different lists, each showcasing feature scores, were generated. Varying numbers of features (t) are tested for each list, ranging from 1–216. Computational efficiency considerations set M to 25 for the Z-Alizadeh Sani dataset and 22 for the Cleveland and Statlog datasets. For each combination of FS methods, 21 (25 − 16 + 1) and 8 (22 − 16 + 1) combinations of top t features were generated for the Z-Alizadeh Sani and Cleveland/Statlog datasets, respectively. The probabilistic ensemble FS approach is explicitly applied to the Z-Alizadeh Sani dataset. Due to the limited number of features (9–25) in the Cleveland and Statlog datasets, the probabilistic ensemble FS approach needed to be applied. On the Z-Alizadeh Sani dataset, feature sets ranging from 1 to 216 are selected and separately tested in each classification.

4.2 Performance Comparison

In Figure 1, the Z-Alizadeh Sani dataset can be optimized using a variety of bio-inspired algorithms, although the results of ML methods vary noticeably. MOA continuously produces the highest accuracy, outperforming SVM and K-means by 99.85% and 99.34%, respectively. With SVM and Random Forest, the WOA also demonstrates outstanding performance, achieving 98.5% and 98.9% accuracy, respectively. When paired with PSO, Naïve Bayes works exceptionally well, exhibiting resilience and accuracy of 98.2%. By contrast, the accuracy rates produced by the CSOA and ACO are often lower; ACO's performance with the Random Forest model is especially dismal, yielding 79.76%. The best optimization strategies for increasing model accuracy are MOA and WOA, with relatively minor performance benefits from GA and ACO.

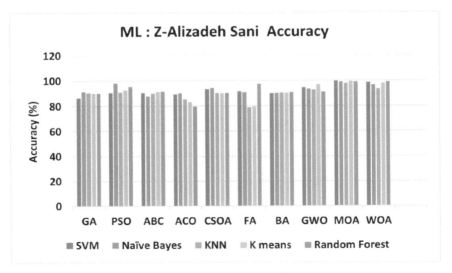

Fig. 1   ML-based Z-Alizadeh Sani Accuracy.

Evaluation of Bio-Inspired Algorithm-based Machine Learning and Deep Learning Models | 63

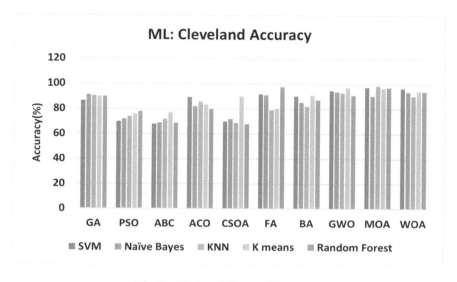

Fig. 2 ML-based Cleveland Accuracy.

In Figure 2, notable variations in accuracy are observed when comparing the performance of different bio-inspired algorithms on the Cleveland dataset. The MOA and WOA consistently yield high accuracies across most models. MOA performs exceptionally well with SVM at 97.2% and achieves the highest accuracy with KNN at 98.4%. WOA also shows strong performance, particularly with SVM and K-means, achieving 96.45% and 96.4%, respectively. In contrast, ACO and PSO typically produce lower accuracies; for example, PSO performs poorly with Random Forest and SVM models, with accuracies of 78% and 70%, respectively. The GA performs moderately, scoring 91.2% for Naïve Bayes and 90.4% for KNN. The CSOA tends to perform poorly, especially with the Random Forest model, showing an accuracy of 68%. Overall, MOA and WOA are the most effective optimization techniques for this dataset, while PSO and ACO demonstrate the slightest improvement in model accuracy.

In Figure 3, accuracy trends are evident in the performance of different bio-inspired algorithms applied to the Statlog dataset. The CSOA exhibits the highest accuracy among various models, offering 99.85% for SVM, 99.06% for Naïve Bayes, and 99.34% for K-means. The FA also performs strongly, particularly with Random Forest at 98.9%. Both CSOA and FA are highly effective in significantly enhancing model accuracy. Conversely, the GA typically produces the lowest accuracies, with Naïve Bayes at 69% and SVM at 68%. ACO and PSO generally perform moderately; ACO performs well with Random Forest, achieving a 97.45% success rate. The MOA and GWO yield good results, particularly with SVM at 94.5%, although they do not reach the peak accuracies CSOA and FA attain. CSOA and FA are the most effective optimization techniques for improving model accuracy on the Statlog dataset, while GA shows the slightest improvement.

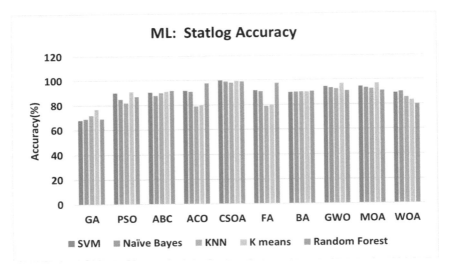

Fig. 3 ML-based Statlog Accuracy.

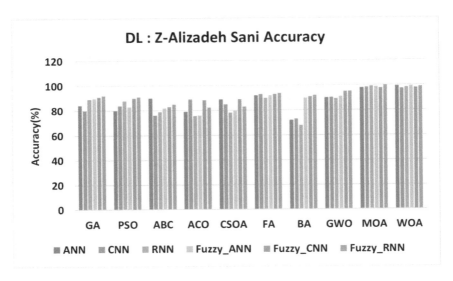

Fig. 4 DL-based Z-Alizadeh Sani Accuracy.

In Figure 4, significant variations in accuracy are observed in the performance of multiple DL models on the Z-Alizadeh Sani dataset, which were improved using distinct bio-inspired techniques. The MOA and WOA consistently yield the highest accuracies across most models. For example, MOA performs remarkably well with ANN at 97.86%, CNN at 98.34%, and RNN at 99.03%. Similarly, WOA excels with ANN at 99.21%, Fuzzy ANN at 99.34%, and Fuzzy RNN at 98.9%. Conversely, the GA and ACO typically produce lower accuracies, with ACO performing poorly, with RNN at 75.45%. PSO and FA exhibit modest performance, with FA achieving 93.78% accuracy with RNN and 93% accuracy with CNN. Overall, MOA and WOA are the best optimization strategies for enhancing the accuracy of DL models on this dataset, while GA and ACO show much lower performance gains.

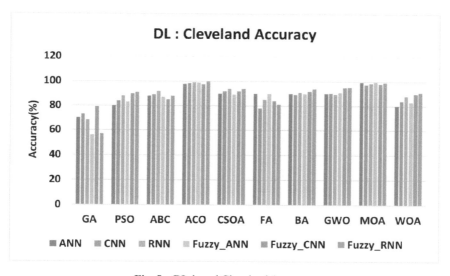

Fig. 5 DL-based Cleveland Accuracy.

In Figure 5, the accuracy of multiple DL models optimized using different bio-inspired techniques on the Cleveland dataset shows significant differences. The MOA consistently achieves the highest accuracies, such as ANN at 99.21%, CNN at 97.34%, and RNN at 98.34%. The WOA also performs well, particularly with CNN at 84% and Fuzzy RNN at 91%. In contrast, PSO and GA typically produce poorer accuracies, with GA performing especially poorly with RNN (68%) and Fuzzy ANN (56%). ACO exhibits superior performance, particularly with RNN (99.03%) and Fuzzy RNN (99.85%). The performance of the CSOA and FA is moderate, with CSOA achieving 94% with RNN and 92% with CNN. In general, MOA and ACO yield significantly better performance gains compared to GA and PSO when it comes to improving the accuracy of DL models on this dataset.

Figure 6 shows the accuracy trends of multiple DL models trained using different bio-inspired techniques on the Statlog dataset. The CSOA stands out with the highest accuracy rates for many models, such as ANN at 98%, CNN at 97%, and Fuzzy ANN at 99%. Strong performance is also demonstrated by the MOA and WOA, particularly with fuzzy RNN at 98% for WOA and fuzzy ANN at 97% for both MOA and WOA. ABC and PSO perform moderately well, with

ABC achieving 95% for both CNN and RNN. The accuracies of the FA and ACO are generally lower, with FA yielding 90% for ANN and 82% for RNN. Regarding accuracy, the GA shows the lowest, with ANN at 80% and CNN at 81%. The best optimization techniques for increasing model accuracy on the Statlog dataset are CSOA, MOA, and WOA, whereas GA and ACO slightly improve performance.

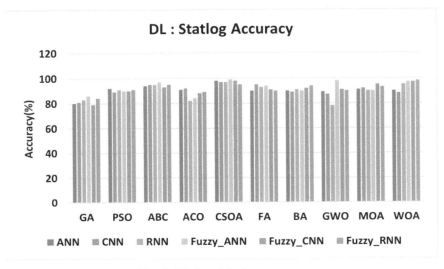

Fig. 6 DL-based Statlog Accuracy.

Conclusion

Their evaluation clarifies the efficacy of bioinspired algorithm-based DL and ML models on many datasets. Regarding increasing the accuracy of DL and ML models, bio-inspired algorithms such as the WOA and MOA consistently beat alternative methods. When optimizing models like SVM, ANN, and fuzzy RNN, these algorithms MOA and WOA perform remarkably well, yielding optimal accuracies on various datasets. On the other hand, conventional methods such as GA and ACO usually result in smaller accuracy gains, suggesting that they need more scope for optimization. While PSO and ABC perform reasonably, their potential is highlighted under specific conditions. The CSOA technique has demonstrated its robustness in increasing model correctness, and it is particularly well-suited for the Statlog dataset. Although GA and ACO yield more moderate benefits, the top optimization techniques MOA, WOA, and CSOA significantly improve model performance. This thorough analysis emphasizes the importance of using suitable bio-inspired algorithms in conjunction with ML and DL to maximize efficacy and precision.

References

[1] Bakro, M., Kumar, R.R., Husain, M., Ashraf, Z., Ali, A., Yaqoob, S.I., Ahmed, M.N. and Parveen, N. (2024). Building a Cloud-IDS by hybrid bio-inspired feature selection algorithms along with random forest model. *IEEE Access, PP*(99), 1–1. IEEE.

[2] Kulhare, R. and Veenadhari, S. (2022). Feature reduction in classification tasks using bio-inspired optimization algorithms. *SAMRIDDHI: A Journal of Physical Sciences, Engineering, and Technology, 14*(04).

[3] Abd Elaziz, M., Ouadfel, S., Abd El-Latif, A.A. and Ali Ibrahim, R. (2022). Feature selection based on modified bio-inspired atomic orbital search using arithmetic optimization and opposite-based learning. *Cognitive Computation, 14*(6), 2274–95. Springer.

[4] Chou, J.-S. and Molla, A. (2022). Recent advances in use of bio-inspired jellyfish search algorithm for solving optimization problems. *Scientific Reports, 12*(1), 19157. London: Nature Publishing Group UK.

[5] Soula, M., Karanika, A., Kolomvatsos, K., Anagnostopoulos, C. and Stamoulis, G. (2022). Intelligent tasks allocation at the edge based on machine learning and bio-inspired algorithms. *Evolving Systems, 13*(2), 221–42. Springer.

[6] Bangui, H. and Buhnova, B. (2022). Lightweight intrusion detection for edge computing networks using deep forest and bio-inspired algorithms. *Computers and Electrical Engineering, 100*, 107901. Elsevier.

[7] Mohamed, T.I.A., Ezugwu, A.E., Fonou-Dombeu, J.V., Ikotun, A.M. and Mohammed, M. (2023). A bio-inspired convolution neural network architecture for automatic breast cancer detection and classification using RNA-seq gene expression data. *Scientific Reports, 13*(1), 14644. London: Nature Publishing Group UK.

[8] Mujawar, S. and Gupta, J. (2022). A statistical perspective for empirical analysis of bio-inspired algorithms for medical disease detection. *In: 2022 International Conference on Emerging Smart Computing and Informatics* (*ESCI*) (pp. 1–7). IEEE.

[9] Priya, R.S.P. and Vadivu, P.S. (2022). Bio-inspired ensemble feature selection (BIEFS) and ensemble multiple deep learning (EMDL) classifier for breast cancer diagnosis. *Journal of Pharmaceutical Negative Results*, 483–99.

[10] Gonçalves, C.B., Souza, J.R. and Fernandes, H. (2022). CNN architecture optimization using bio-inspired algorithms for breast cancer detection in infrared images. *Computers in Biology and Medicine, 142*, 105205. Elsevier.

[11] Praveena, V., Sujithra, L.R., Karthik, S. and Kavitha, M.S. (2023). Bio-inspired ensemble feature selection and deep auto-encoder approach for rapid diagnosis of breast cancer. *Multimedia Systems, 29*(6), 3403–419. Springer.

[12] Mani, R.K.C., Kamalakannan, J., Rangaiah, Y.P. and Anand, S. (2024). A bio-inspired method for breast histopathology image classification using transfer learning. *Journal of Artificial Intelligence and Technology, 4*(2), 89–101.

[13] Ghoniem, R.M. (2020). A novel bio-inspired deep learning approach for liver cancer diagnosis. *Information, 11*(2), 80. MDPI.

[14] Subbiah, S.S. and Chinnappan, J. (2022). A review of bio-inspired computational intelligence algorithms in electricity load forecasting. *In:* O.V. Gnana Swathika, K. Karthikeyan and S.K. Padmanaban (Eds.), *Smart Buildings Digitalization*, 169–92. CRC Press.

[15] Gibson, S., Issac, B., Zhang, L. and Jacob, S.M. (2020). Detecting spam email with machine learning optimized with bio-inspired metaheuristic algorithms. *IEEE Access, 8*, 187914–187932. IEEE.

[16] Ahsan, M.M., Gupta, K.D., Nag, A.K., Poudyal, S., Kouzani, A.Z. and Mahmud, M.P. (2020). Applications and evaluations of bio-inspired approaches in cloud security: A review. *IEEE Access, 8*, 180799–180814. IEEE.

[17] Jundi, Z.Z. (2023). Landscape view of hyperparameter optimization cybersecurity by using bio-inspired algorithm. *In: International Conference on Intelligence Science* (pp. 529–41). Springer.

[18] Narengbam, L. and Dey, S. (2023). WiFi intrusion detection using artificial neurons with bio-inspired optimization algorithm. *Procedia Computer Science, 218*, 1238–46. Elsevier.

[19] Jeyavim Sherin, R.C. and Parkavi, K. (2022). Investigations on bio-inspired algorithm for network intrusion detection: A review. *International Journal of Computer Networks and Applications*, 399–23.

[20] Kala, A. and Vaidyanathan, S.G. (2022). Forecasting monthly rainfall using bio-inspired artificial algae deep learning network. *Fluctuation and Noise Letters, 21*(02), 2250018. World Scientific.

[21] Yadav, A., Yadav, G., Jain, S. and Dwivedi, S.A. (2023). Comparison of ML, deep learning and bio-inspired algorithms in bug triaging. *In: Proceedings of the 2023 Fifteenth International Conference on Contemporary Computing* (pp. 759–65).

[22] Alfarraj, O. (2020). Internet of things with bio-inspired co-evolutionary deep-convolution neural-network approach for detecting road cracks in smart transportation. *Neural Computing and Applications*, 1–16. Springer.

[23] Bouramoul, I.E., Zertal, S., Derdour, M. and Zenbout, I. (2024). Enhancing IoT security through deep learning and evolutionary bio-inspired intrusion detection in IoT systems. *In: 2024 6th International Conference on Pattern Analysis and Intelligent Systems (PAIS)* (pp. 1–8). IEEE.

[24] Moizuddin, M. and Jose, M.V. (2022). A bio-inspired hybrid deep learning model for network intrusion detection. *Knowledge-Based Systems, 238*, 107894. Elsevier.

[25] Baviskar, V., Verma, M. and Chatterjee, P. (2021). Improving classification performance of deep learning models using bio-inspired computing. *In:Proceedings of the 2021 Thirteenth International Conference on Contemporary Computing* (pp. 333–40).

[26] Vijh, S., Saraswat, M. and Kumar, S. (2023). Automatic multilevel image thresholding segmentation using hybrid bio-inspired algorithm and artificial neural network for histopathology images. *Multimedia Tools and Applications, 82*(4), 4979–5010. Springer.

[27] Zhang, G., Ali, Z.H., Aldlemy, M.S., Mussa, M.H., Salih, S.Q., Hameed, M.M., Al-Khafaji, Z.S. and Yaseen, Z.M. (2022). Reinforced concrete deep beam shear strength capacity modelling using an integrative bio-inspired algorithm with an artificial intelligence model. *Engineering with Computers, 38*(Suppl 1), 15–28. Springer.

[28] Baburaj, E. (2022). Comparative analysis of bio-inspired optimization algorithms in neural network-based data mining classification. *International Journal of Swarm Intelligence Research (IJSIR), 13*(1), 1–25. IGI Global.

[29] Yadav, A. and Vishwakarma, D.K. (2020). A comparative study on bio-inspired algorithms for sentiment analysis. *Cluster Computing, 23*(4), 2969-89. Springer.

[30] Gibson, S., Issac, B., Zhang, L. and Jacob, S.M. (2020). Detecting spam email with machine learning optimized with bio-inspired metaheuristic algorithms. *IEEE Access, 8*, 187914–187932. IEEE.

[31] Subbiah, S.S. and Chinnappan, J. (2022). A review of bio-inspired computational intelligence algorithms in electricity load forecasting. *In: O.V. Gnana Swathika, K. Karthikeyan and S.K. Padmanaban (Eds.), Smart Buildings Digitalization*, 169–92. CRC Press.

[32] Ahsan, M.M., Gupta, K.D., Nag, A.K., Poudyal, S., Kouzani, A.Z. and Mahmud, M.P. (2020). Applications and evaluations of bio-inspired approaches in cloud security: A review. *IEEE Access, 8*, 180799–180814. IEEE.

[33] Moizuddin, M. and Jose, M.V. (2022). A bio-inspired hybrid deep learning model for network intrusion detection. *Knowledge-Based Systems, 238*, 107894. Elsevier.

[34] de Albuquerque, V.H.C., Gupta, D., De Falco, I., Sannino, G. and Bouguila, N. (2020). Special issue on Bio-inspired optimization techniques for Biomedical Data Analysis: Methods and applications. *Applied Soft Computing, 95*, 106672. Elsevier.

[35] Balasubramaniam, S., Prasanth, A., Kumar, K.S. and Kavitha, V. (2024). Medical Image Analysis Based on Deep Learning Approach for Early Diagnosis of Diseases. *In:* J.A. Vijay, et al. (Author), *Deep Learning for Smart Healthcare* (pp. 54–75). Auerbach Publications.

[36] Thankaraj Ambujam, S. (2024). Power quality enhancement in the wind energy distribution system using HHO algorithm based UPFC. *Journal of the Chinese Institute of Engineers*, 1–21.

[37] Soula, M., Karanika, A., Kolomvatsos, K., Anagnostopoulos, C. and Stamoulis, G. (2022). Intelligent tasks allocation at the edge based on machine learning and bio-inspired algorithms. *Evolving Systems, 13*(2), 221–42. Springer.

4 | Disease Diagnosis
Traditional vs. Bio-Inspired Algorithm Approaches

Varunsaagar Saravanan,[1] Dawn Sivan[2,3], K. Satheesh Kumar[4] and Rajan Jose[2,3*]

Bio-inspired algorithms (BIAs) are computational methods following natural principles and processabilities. 'Bio-inspired' is a metaphorical expression and refers to the way these algorithms simulate biological functions or claim to target bionic accomplishments, where other conventional algorithms cannot deal with the problem. This chapter compares traditional or conventional approaches with BIAs for disease diagnosis, highlighting their strengths and weaknesses. We discuss the principles and mechanisms of each approach, including their advantages and limitations in terms of accuracy, interpretability, and efficiency. Case studies of successful BIAs applications are presented, and future directions and challenges are discussed. The chapter thus provides a thorough understanding of the role of traditional approaches and BIAs in disease diagnosis.

1. Introduction

Nature, in all its diversities, dynamism, and intricacies, is the ultimate source of inspiration for the resolution of complex issues in Computer Science (CS). During the past years, which have witnessed the great development of this field, research on solving optimization problems by imitating nature has resulted in the birth of Bio-Inspired Algorithms (BIAs). These algorithms have gained much attention because they enable the provision of optimum solutions at much lower computational resources [1, 2]. Bio algorithms belonging to different categories borrow several features from nature in which their structures sum up the characteristic flow of nature. Instructors and researchers often find detailed descriptions of BIAs beneficial because of their high-fidelity of accessibility to solutions. Amongst others, this section compares the performance of Genetic Algorithms (GAs),

---

[1] Lead AI ML, Asianet News Media and Entertainment Pvt. Ltd., Crescent Road, Gandhi Nagar, Bangalore-560070.
[2] Center for Advanced Intelligent Materials and
[3] Faculty of Industrial Sciences and Technology, Universiti Malaysia Pahang Al-Sultan Abdullah, 26300, Kuantan, Pahang, Malaysia.
[4] Kerala University of Digital Sciences, Innovation and Technology, Technocity Campus, Thiruvananthapuram, Kerala-695317, India.
Email: varunsaagar.s@gmail.com; dawnsivan91@gmail.com; satheesh.kumar@duk.ac.in
* Corresponding author: rjose@umpsa.edu.my

Particle Swarm Optimization (PSO), and Simulated Annealing (SA) on well-defined benchmarking problems and real-world medical imaging challenges [3].

The last few years have seen the interest in the so-called nature-inspired algorithms growth due to the dynamic development of machine learning (ML), in particular, convolutional neural networks and deep learning (DL). The further development of the computation capacity and its easy access to individuals and companies has contributed more to this interest. The incorporation of BIAs techniques into the daily use of computers, together with their excellent results, is one of the key reasons that they are on the rise. Traditional methods for diagnosing diseases have seen a paradigm shift with the arrival of artificial intelligence (AI). In the first instance, the initial principles of AI were inspired by natural systems, followed by the establishment of bioscience to highlight problem statements through human anatomy settlement. These transformational learning techniques have now permeated variously in sub-cases such as engineering heights and edge devices. For instance, algorithms such as the Artificial Bee Colony, PSO, Firefly Algorithm, and Differential Evolution, are fundamental elements of the applications, which is proof of biologically inspired methods and their impact on disease diagnosis.

1.1 Overview of Diagnostic Approaches

The process of identifying a disease or condition that accounts for a person's symptoms and indicators is known as medical diagnosis. It entails categorizing a patient's condition into different groups so that medical decisions regarding prognosis and treatment may be made with knowledge. The diagnostic process is a multifaceted, cooperative, patient-centred endeavour that calls for the collection of data and clinical reasoning. This tradition of diagnosing involves the normal processes of interviewing and examining the patient, blood tests, and scans among others. These fundamental ways have some drawbacks regarding to sensitivity, specificity and, especially, the possibility of early diseases' detection. Selecting appropriate diagnostic tests is challenging due to the vast number of available options. Ensuring the quality of medical imaging and laboratory tests is crucial, as these are highly regulated areas in healthcare.

Following are the notable methods applied conventionally for diagnosis:

- **Clinical assessments and history tracking**: Patient history and physical examination is critical in the diagnosis of patients because it allows the physicians to get the first impression. This approach is largely based on the professional experience of the practitioner, and as such, can present fluctuations in the diagnostic process.
- **Laboratory tests**: These include the blood test, urine test, and biochemical tests that determine aberrations that show evidence of disease. As useful as these tests are, they tend to be lengthy to produce and can take significant time and often results are not guaranteed.

- *Imaging techniques*: MRI, CT scan, and ultrasounds are some major recent diagnose techniques which provide non-invasive approaches on internal body scans which include Xrays. But they are often costly, and its precision may be dependent with the resolution of the used apparatus or radiologist's interpretation.
- *Pathology and histology*: Microscopy of tissues is still common in diagnosing many diseases, including forms of cancer, until today. However, this method is time-consuming and requires tissue sampling through one way or the other.

1.2 Role of ML/DL in Disease Diagnosis

ML and DL techniques are reshaping the healthcare industry with many applications. The early diagnosis of diseases is one of these applications which are positively affected. The data analytics today have been made possible, thanks to the high power of the machines and AI, which has led to detecting various diseases, including cancer [4, 5]. Furthermore, they have been useful in studying and finding solutions to diseases with the help of acquiring necessary information, recognizing difficult patterns and answering that can be used for the patient's diagnosis [6]. Thus, ML and DL coupled with telemedicine have the potential for doctors to find and predict diseases with only one patient remotely. The smartness of ML and DL in disease diagnosis includes characteristics such as real-time information collection, high accuracy in recognizing the symptom of a disease from images and genetic data, and detailed prescription of a suitable treatment. It also gives the counsellors insights into the patient's personality and thinking patterns which serve as the basis of their prescriptions for the treatment of mental illnesses. The mechanistic explanation is the way ML and DL are analysing the big data and giving personalized medicine to each patient; this is the "the medicine of the future" concept.

1.2.1 Applications of ML/DL in Disease Diagnosis

- *Early detection and diagnosis*: Diagnostic tests are the basic and most crucial part of doctors' work which is to screen, monitor, and follow up the patient's medical condition; thus, the best treatment plan can be designed. The AI models have indeed shown that they can carry out early detection of illnesses that usually go undiagnosed by traditional diagnostic methods and this has been done with high precision [7, 8]. The other imaging methods like X-rays and MRI are equally good, except that their results tend to be more expensive and time-intensive. However, AI methods could enable early diagnosis, for example, ML and DL is very efficient in inspecting early changes in retinal images [9, 10], which is not possible during standard examination. An enhanced diagnostic technique using telematics, mixed with AI, can eliminate the hurdle of patients travelling to healthcare facilities, places where the risk of viral transmission is higher, for consultations.

Disease Diagnosis | 73

- ***Imaging and radiology*:** Medical imaging is the leading edge where the ML and DL technologies have produced massive progress, capable of the autonomous analysis of medical images such as Xrays, MRIs, and CT scans, which allows a rapid discovery of anomalies that could signal diseases like cancer, TB, and neurological disorders to a doctor. However, though AI has excelled in being expert-like, it has not yet surpassed human capability for innovation and ethical decision-making.
- ***Genomics and precision medicine*:** The study of genetics has been very beneficial to reinforcement learning (RL) and DL, especially as the therapy of precision medicine. These algorithms, using whole genetic data, could recognize mutations and genetic markers which show a connection of the disease with different genes. This action makes it very easy for personalized treatment plans to be introduced to the genetic uniqueness of an individual, thereby increasing the effectiveness of the treatment.
- ***Electronic Health Records* (*EHRs*):** The EHR data helps the AI models. These AI tools could process and find patterns and correlations that may present the development or increase in illness from the EHR database. Semantic technology, which is a class of natural language processing (NLP), plays a crucial role in reading those raw text, so that we can build predictive models to the occurrence of diseases such as heart disease and diabetes.

2. Traditional Approaches in Disease Diagnosis

Traditional methods such as statistical methods and rule-based systems are the usual ways of diagnosing a disease.

2.1 Statistical Methods

Even though there are methodologies for the elaboration in traditional diagnostic techniques, maths and statistical theories are to be employed to analyse the medical data. The main principles that are represented in this phase are the following:

- ***Descriptive statistics:*** Summarized in detail, they give a true picture of the time it takes for every patient to get affected with the disease and the distribution of the patients from different races, the ages of the patients, and other information.
- ***Inferential statistics:*** This is the core statistical method used to generalize from the sample data to the larger study population. Techniques such as hypothesis testing, and regression analysis are common.
- ***Bayesian inference:*** It uses Bayes theorem to update the probability of a hypothesis and new evidence, aid in refining diagnostic probabilities.

2.2 Rule-based Methods

In rule-based or expert systems, the original set of rules in making diagnostic decisions come from the clinical guidelines and expert knowledge. The important constituent parts of such methods are:

74 | Bio-inspired Algorithms in Machine Learning and Deep Learning for Disease Detection

- **Knowledge base:** An organized area where here all the rules and facts related to diseases and their symptoms are stored.
- **Inference engine:** The part of the computer system that scans the rules with logical processing by which patient data is related to the knowledge base and consequently gives the diagnoses.
- **User interface:** The patient can enter data into it and the system can offer the diagnostic recommendations on the screen.

2.3 Contrasting Traditional and BIA Methods

2.3.1 Foundation

- **Traditional approaches:** The approach of a medical expert, who is a source of data with similar studies and diagnosed cases that have been carried out during their career has been the steady technology used in medical diagnostics. From the outset, these practices have been issued as analytical and clear protocol by experienced healthcare professionals.
- **BIAs:** BIAs mimic the processes of natural sciences, i.e., evolution, swarm behaviour, and neural networks. They borrow from living species and the way they work their specific infrastructure to figure out difficult problems. In addition to this, new methods of the traditional method implementation are also possible.

2.3.2 Methodology

- **Traditional approaches:** Mostly, these methods are designed to meet statistical and logical requirements, namely, the basics of statistics, and the prevalence of patterns in testing procedures. Forms of these have consequences causing exponential growth.
- **BIAs:** However, in the case of BIAs, they are much more interested in the real-time adaptive multistep optimization and iterative learning. The results of this are the models get updated more frequently as new data come in so that the outputs that we get are in line with current real-world data. The method involves letting the tools flexibility and their ability to take on more complicated tasks.

2.3.3 Data Handling

- **Traditional approaches:** These methods frequently rely on primary data, i.e., numbers from tests and physicals, to draw conclusions. In most cases, the data are accurately catalogued and heir to stricter formats, resulting in easier data analysis employing traditional statistical methods.
- **BIAs:** BIAs are proficiently handling a high-dimensional data including images, genetic information, and movies. Their versatility in the treatment

and learning of various specific data types allows far more intricate and more nuanced diagnostic capabilities.

2.3.4 Decision-Making

- **Traditional approaches**: With the implementation of traditional methods, the interpretation of input into the diagnostic is fixed, and there is a clear path from the input to diagnosis. The result is generally an easy perfect solution that follows data at the start and defines the rules.
- **BIAs**: BIAs can provide the users with several possible results, adding the advantage of uncertainty and confidence in the diagnosis. This feature of probability is a specification of the complexity of biological processes, and it can also absorb the natural variance of medical records.

2.3.5 Adaptability

- **Traditional approaches**: These techniques are, in general, less adaptable to the newly arrived data or the change of the pattern of the disease in the organism. Once settled, the protocols and guidelines are very hard or impracticable to update, which upsets the treatment of emergent medical know-how.
- **BIAs**: Alterations in adaption, BIAs can be modelled with new information and changing environments. For this reason, they can alter the diagnosis they give, as they adjust the criteria they need for the correct diagnosis using new data revealed.

2.3.6 Complexity

- **Traditional approaches**: When clearly well-defined conditions are in question, traditional modes can be the easiest. On the other hand, they may respond more slowly or be less accurate if they are dealing with complex or very rare diseases. Their characteristic of being linear and rule-based is their negative side and, due to this, they are not very efficient in diagnosing diseases that are less connected to the already established category.
- **BIAs**: These types of AI models can come to terms with high complexity, they can find very fine things, such as revealing and establishment of subtle patterns and relationships. Their dry runs over learning cycles allow them to skilfully handle the most intricate tasks of diagnosis.

2.3.7 Accuracy and Sensitivity

- **Traditional approaches**: These ideas can pick out, diminish, and follow different criteria depending on human error and diversity. The use of predefined rules and protocols as their main issue can make such technologies sensitive to only a few things which can make them exceptionally vulnerable, especially those that are complicated.

- ***BIAs***: BIAs, by processing a lot of large datasets and identifying detailed patterns, can not only find minute details that are not detected by other methods but also give good quality results in case the disease/infection is difficult to diagnose. For example, convolutional neural networks (CNNs) have been found to be operating at a much superior level in patients' analysis using medical images than traditional image processing systems.

2.3.8 Speed and Efficiency

- ***Traditional approaches***: Evaluation of a patient's condition using traditional methods that are longer, e.g., lab tests that take several days for cultures or histopathology, can be considered time-consuming by today's standards. Error-free the whole time is not likely if people are the only ones that do the meaningful activities, like data analysis and explaining what the results found by the diagnostic tools were.
- ***BIAs***: BIAs can process and analyse data immediately, hence quicker to give the results. Their facility to shift the data processing assignments into automated mode has a very positive impact in the sense that it leads to an increase of the productivity and hereby, decreasing the time of diagnosis.

2.3.9 Scalability and Adaptability

- ***Traditional approaches***: Scalability could be a problem when sections are missing, for example, if one does not have the necessary equipment and staff. Lack of the necessary resources such as those needed in this case can be the major roadblocks to the general application of such methods.
- ***BIAs***: BIAs are the most adaptable beasts in the zoo of technology, which are optionally on cloud-based propagation platforms deployed in many health institutions giving an opportunity to everyone to enjoy all the benefits of one incredible technology. Their ability to quickly and accurately sift through massive amounts of data through new technology has made possible their being used on a larger scale.

2.3.10 Cost

- ***Traditional approaches***: The methods are expensive due to the expenses of equipment, reagents, and labour. It is necessary to take care of the diagnostic protocol's upgrades and replacement of parts.
- ***BIAs***: The initial investment in development and training followed by automation and decreased manual labour costs in the future lead to the eventual economy of funds. Therefore, this makes their impact on healthcare very beneficial in the long run.

2.3.11. Application Range

- **Traditional approaches:** These methods are the most fitting for the different conditions and have the proof validated from the clinical research use.
- **BIAs:** BIAs could be composed by using multiple sources of data, such as genomic and proteomic information, to build the most relevant treatment to the rare and complex diseases. Being multifaceted allows them to build the diagnosing instruments with a specialization of medical ailments.

3. Bio-Inspired Algorithms (BIAs) in Disease Diagnosis

BIAs is a sort of new method of innovation, which takes ideas from nature, and really adds to the generation of new solutions to complex issues. The use of bio-inspired algorithms brings efficiency, sensitivity, and flexibility to a new level.

3.1 Different Types of BIAs

This section studies the different BIAs and illustrates their functions, comparison, and advantages and disadvantages.

3.1.1 Evolutionary Algorithms

Evolutionary Computation mechanisms mimic natural molecular biology and are the primary optimization problem solving approach in a stochastic fashion [11]. The population of these solutions evolves along the generations. Each one of the individuals, or the solutions, emerge from selection, crossover as well as having a point mutation that renders their offspring. Then, it's all about the current fitness of each participant, which in turn, affects the forthcoming generation.

For instance, one can use GAs to select features and set the parameters of a ML model to reach a high level of accuracy in disease diagnosis. The GAs use methods like selection, crossover, and mutation to come up with optimization solutions, which evolved. Regarding the diagnosis of diseases, GAs could optimize the feature selection and parameters to use in a machine learning model.

Genetic Programming (GP) formalizes the paradigm of GAs by taking out an evolutionary part. Specifically, GP makes use of the mutation process. It is critical to design the GP about medical images to recognize the patterns of a chosen area in a patient or to make the GP functional in the development of diagnostic rules.

3.1.2 Swarm Intelligence

Swarm Intelligence (SI) is a method based on the cooperative behaviour of social organisms such as birds, fish, and insects [12]. A few to list are:

- **Ant Colony Optimization (ACO):** Examples of ACO are where it imitates the foraging actions by ants, where they lay down pheromones on favourable paths. It is a machine learning technique that can be applied to medical diagnostics for feature selection and clustering which improves the identification of features in documents with high dimensionality [13].

- **Particle Swarm Optimization (PSO):** The PSO model is based on the patterns that birds usually follow, i.e., flocking, and the behaviour patterns of fish as well. The particles that represent a greater number of potential solutions begin to change their location by using both their personal and collective experiences [13]. Through the use of PSO, neural network architectures and parameters are optimized and therefore, more precise diagnosis is obtained.
- **Firefly Algorithm (FA) and Artificial Bee Colony (ABC):** The simulation methodologies of the fireflies and bees are proved as optimization processes for various problems [14]. Furthermore, their benefits have been on the table a lot of times, starting on the fields like medical diagnosis. They are especially effective in finding optimal solutions.
- **Fish Swarm Algorithm (FSA):** Inspired by the movement of fish, this algorithm is specially designed for the mentioned purposes and has proved effectiveness in the mentioned features. Often it is used as a powerful instrument to optimize the diagnostic scenario by doing the search in the parameter space more efficient way. It can be discordant to the other method that does the optimization of this, and it can be the one that does it better.

3.1.3 Artificial Neural Networks (ANN) and Deep Learning (DL)

ANNs and DL models are ways that are influenced by the structure and working of the human brain. Networks include thousands of interconnected neurons that perform the information processing procedure.

- **Artificial Neural Networks (ANNs):** The main characteristic of ANNs is that they can be used in the various prediction tasks. The positive aspect is that it can describe details that traditional methods cannot find. Hence, the nonlinear and intricate nature of the given relationships can be determined.
- **Deep Learning (DL):** DL is a subfield of ANNs, meaning that the models that are nowadays being explored are deep networks having several levels that have been trained for data recognition at different levels of abstraction. Two of the DL techniques, the CNNs and Long Short-Term Memory (LSTM) networks, prefer to the new deep learning models. CNNs are best with image processing as they are highly functional meanwhile LSTMs demonstrate preferable results when being tasked with the forecasting of sequences such as patient history or time-series data obtained from wearable devices.

3.2 BIA Mechanisms in Diagnosis

BIAs are based on the approach of duplicating natural processes and outcomes to solve various complex optimization problems. The main mechanisms involve:

- **Evolution and selection:** This is utilized in evolutionary algorithms where solutions are shaped over generations through mutation and crossover with the best individual being passed on to next generation.

Disease Diagnosis | 79

- *Insect gang working*: Engaged in SI algorithms, where the simple agents collaborate and together concentrate on fast convergence in the optimal solutions.
- *Neural adaptation*: In ANNs and DL, neurons change their weights depending on input data and feedback, which leads the network to pick up complicated patterns.

3.3   BIA Applications in Diagnosis

Bio-inspired algorithms have been put into practice in various medical diagnosis tasks with grand achievements due to these:

- *Attraction of features*: It is part of the characteristics of ACO and the other SI algorithms that efficiently explore dimensions of medical data, thus, they effectively help in the identification of the most important attributes of the data for classification of diseases.
- *Image processing*: It is the area where the analysis of medical images, for example, X-rays, and MRIs are potential targets for the CNNs that are optimized by BIAs. This makes it possible to make the detection and classification of the problems such as tumours and lesions.
- *Predictive modelling*: These create models by using patient data to predict the outcomes of a certain disease. ANNs and DL models use EHRs, wearable device data, etc., and other patient information to perspicaciously forecast disease progression and are helpful in identifying treatment options accordingly.
- *Genomic analysis*: AI has been used as a method to identify important genetic factors for diseases for the identification of new drugs and drug targets at the gene level, thus improving personalized medicine by treating diseases based on genetic information of individual patients.

3.4   Comparative Advantages and Limitations of BIAs

3.4.1   Advantages

- *High accuracy*: BIAs together with DL models can reach the desired accuracy by learning patterns and connections in the data.
- *Adaptability*: BIAs have the capability to adapt to new data types such as continuous change in pathology patterns through dynamic learning thus they continue to improve and develop their diagnostic capabilities.
- *Handling complex data*: BIAs displayed their utmost qualities in processing and analysing very high-dimensional, heterogeneous data including images, genomic sequences, and physiological signals.
- *Automation and efficiency*: BIAs are intelligent and automate diagnostic systems by which doctors can save time and hence reduce possible human errors during diagnostics.

- *Optimization efficiency*: AI-built systems can allocate the most efficient ways to complete the task in spacious search spaces what is critical for the development of effective disease diagnosis.
- *Parallelization*: The BIAs are devised having parallel computational capability which provides the speed for large dataset analysis and reduces time consumption.

3.4.2 Limitations

- *Interpretability*: Most BIAs, especially DL models, are opaque, and they work like "black boxes", meaning that one cannot comprehend their decision-making procedures. Through the lack of this, one may have trouble gaining the respect and trust of the patient community.
- *Computational demands*: Training and deploying BIAs, particularly deep learnings, depends mainly on the type of computer resources available, which are often expensive, and this can therefore constrain the broad involvement of such systems, especially if we take resource-limited settings into consideration.
- *Data dependence*: BIAs are among the most compromise-free ones for they demand the most accurate data possible to be able to effectively work. Raw data annotation (preparation but not analysis stage) can be of no less burden than data collection.
- *Overfitting*: BIAs may sometimes be subject to the overfitting problem to the training data, which would result in poor generalization of a test data. For this reason, techniques such as regularization and cross-validation are the must-haves to mitigate this risk.
- *Parameter sensitivity*: The performance of BIAs can change due to the choice of certain parameters within them. That is why the correct adjusting and quality determination of these parameters should take place.
- *Scalability issues*: BIAs work well on a few select issues, but they might have difficulties with a high number of data or complicated diagnostic tasks.

4. Comparative Analysis

The diagnosis of diseases is the area of science that is always changing due to the development of new techniques and methods. So, traditional / conventional diagnostic methods and bio-inspired algorithms (BIAs) will collaborate to bring new viewpoints forward for their respective advantages and disadvantages. This section introduces a full-blown comparative study that shows the outcome performance, readability, and efficiency tests within certain scores, bottom lines, iterative steps, the ensemble learning technique, as well as the way of hybridization.

4.1 Performance, Interpretability and Efficiency Benchmarks

4.1.1 Performance

The performance of success criteria in disease monitoring encompasses parameters such as sensitivity, specificity, precision, and the area under the curve (AUC).

Traditional approaches rely on the vetting of doctors and protocols that have been through a lot of trials and errors to make them accountable. Nevertheless, these protocols may fail to mesh well with data that is too high in dimensions and complexity. On the other hand, BIAs often outperform the human inaccuracy in their power to find subtler patterns of the datasets.

4.1.2 Interpretability

Interpretability is an important factor that provides diagnostic tools with the opportunity to be used in clinical settings. Traditional methods involve interpretable factors, which typically are provided with simple, rule-based decisions or statistical correlations that are easily comprehensible and can be verified by physicians. However, BIAs, especially DL models, are considered as "black boxes" even though they offer any interpretability. However, the recent developments in interpretability methods, for example, the Automated Interpretability Agent (AIA), produce function descriptions and infer function structures, which thereby, make AI systems more transparent. Methods like feature importance scores and visualization of activation maps in CNNs are being altered to make them more interpretative in the future [15].

4.1.3 Efficiency

Efficiency deals with the pace of data processing and the number of computational resources that are utilized. Traditional techniques are much more hardware efficient and can work more quickly than the speed of execution, they are hence best for real-time applications and the cases where they have limited computing resources. However, these protocols are far from perfect and may pose greater time demands because they can be lengthy and require more tests and consultations. On the contrary, the procedure of training BIAs, in particular DL models, can be computationally heavy and time-consuming, as it entails the use of sizeable hardware resources, for example, GPUs (graphics processing units) or TPUs (tensor processing units). Nevertheless, when they are completely trained, these models can deal with large datasets rapidly and give instantaneous diagnostic results. Feature selection methods in BIAs remove redundant features which in turn gives computational complexity lessening and finally they create efficiency [15].

4.2 Potential Examples for Hybrid Approaches

Hybrid approaches that integrate BIAs with traditional diagnosis can utilize both the strengths in novel ways. Following are the examples:

- *Early fusion strategies*: These strategies are based on combining several data types to improve diagnostic accuracy using EHRs and multi-omics data.
- *Feature selection*: The BIAs used here will identify the key features which can be included in the traditional diagnostic methods to make them more

interpretable and efficient. They are built in harmony with the systems of nature regarding the sensor logic thus not altogether uncommunicative from a human perspective.

- *Automated interpretability:* Some AI developers have begun efforts to create AI diagnostic tools. Thus, the quest of AI-based systems to be transparent and trustworthy is engaged and the above interpretability methods are chosen.

5. Case Studies of BIAs in Diagnosis

BIAs have proven to be extremely successful in various sectors of medicine, cardiology, oncology, and neurology [16, 17, 18]. This section details the case studies involving BIAs in these applications and methodologies applied, comparing the results of traditional solutions with those of BIAs, and future research development based on these case studies.

5.1 BIA Successes in Cardiology, Oncology, and Neurology

5.1.1 Cardiology

- *Arrhythmia classification*: ANN models were trained to identify different cardiac arrhythmias from the ECG signals with high accuracy. The models can decode even the most intricate structures of the heart's electric current, thus, by these means, they outstrip the traditional rule-based systems.
- *Heart failure prediction*: GAs have been utilized to help find different combinations of patient-specific variables to assess which one gives the best results in predicting cardiovascular diseases. These earlier detections result in immediate treatments and better patient outcomes.
- *Coronary Artery Disease (CAD) detection*: The combination of GAs and ANNs exerted the detection of CAD. The GA was useful in the process of choosing the characters that are of most importance in a patient's data, then those data were used in the chosen ANN for classification.

5.1.2 Oncology

- *Cancer diagnosis*: Medical images can be effectively analysed with ML techniques to detect an illness before showing first symptoms. Sometimes these tools can disclose what is hidden from the human eye.
- *Personalized treatment planning*: The radiation therapy could be optimized by including ACO. This new method reduces normal tissue irradiation and enhances the dose received to tumours which also makes treatment safer and more effective.
- *General cancer prediction and diagnosis*: BIAs technology could select the best features in quite complex data sets. Occasionally, dynamic data redesigned with PSO resulted in a better performance of cancer prediction models.

5.1.3 Neurology

- **Epileptic seizure forecasting**: Neural networks have been applied to analyse EEG data, make predictions, and at the same time identify the onset of epileptic seizures. This function serves as a tool in finding timely interventions to the patient's safety, which would have a significantly positive impact on his prognosis.
- **Alzheimer's disease detection**: ML algorithms like LSTM have been employed using patterns identified in neuroimaging information (MRI, PET scans) for the detection of Alzheimer's in its early stage. Hence these models offer medication before an event occurs and this stops the event.

5.2 Research Directions from Case Study Insights

- **Enhancing Interpretability**: Investigate methods that could improve the interpretability of BIA models, making it easy to use for physicians and to allow its widespread use in clinical practice, thus boosting the trust and adoption of BIA at advanced levels in medicine.
- **Integration with EHR systems**: Surpass barriers that slow down the development of healthcare records by learning how to seamlessly use BIA technology for improving patient outcomes, which are achieved with predictive analytics. In establishing standards of EHRs, consider the use of the data interfaces and the necessary networks for successful data transfer among other systems to ensure that an EHR system reaches its optimum level.
- **Personalized medicine**: Technology when combined with new generation BIAs will make it possible for us to use AI in a way that slows down the growth of cancer or, in some cases, totally medicates it in very rare occurrences, tailoring the therapy using their genetic information and testing. Regression of cells can be modified with the use of GAs which optimizes the effect of treatment and DL can be used to predict how effective a person would be to the treatment's effects.
- **Multimodal data integration**: The data aggregation of proteomic, genomic, imaging, and clinical data is an onus to provide multifaceted diagnosis. The purpose of the hybrid interpretable models is to correct and consolidate multimodal information, thus obtaining more accurate diagnostic and patient outcomes in the clinical graphical presentation. BIA models should be equipped with the functionality of real-time diagnostic aiding in the clinical areas.
- **Automated data preprocessing techniques**: The part which signifies that the process of bio-inspired algorithms is reliable and efficient is that data is pre-processed well. The steps involve advanced data cleaning, normalization, and transformation methods.
- **Explainable AI**: Find new ways to ensure that BIA models are clearer and understandable and so that the logic behind their decisions is transparent to clinicians. This, in turn, is done through a seamless integration of explainable

AI techniques to bring better transparency in the predictions made by the models.

- *Real-world validation*: Besides the experimental approach, we should also conduct larger-scale studies to involve different clinical settings and a variety of patients. The performance of the model under real-world conditions is a key point of the combination of these models with clinical protocols.
- *Ethical considerations*: The question of BIA use in healthcare should be considered from an ethical point of view, liking fairness, transparency, and blame on an algorithmic decision-making process. In the end, we will have to put ethical principles in place to protect patient rights and remain the honest use of AI tools.
- *Continuous learning*: Formulate BIAs that can adapt to the developing data and become more and more efficient so that they are kept in the clock with the dynamic global developments in the specific medical practices. This requires the development of systems that can feed new knowledge to their own and recalculate their prediction models accordingly.

6. Recent Advances in BIAs

With the help of recent advancements in BIAs, the field of disease diagnosis has gone to new extents. Transfer learning, few-shot learning, and large language models (LLMs) are the cutting-edge technologies responsible for the huge jump in the accuracy and efficiency of diagnostic models. The broad significant role played by these techniques is showing in their setting, applications, and other possibilities that are outreach and treatment applications of the future.

6.1 Transfer Learning

Transfer learning has become a very important method in AI, among others, thanks to the sky-high direction deep learning has gone, as well as the creation of immense datasets that are now available. This process is accomplished through the refining of a pretrained model on a fresh, yet identical task, thus the system can be used at its best even if the dataset is, in addition, a different target from the prior pretrain dataset. Such methodology is now commonly applied in different deep learning projects; these include purposes like computer vision and especially in the natural language processing (NLP) aspect. The use of transfer learning in minimizing long-time model training, increasing performance, and reducing the amount of data required is now evident in the field of technology, for example, the health sector, games designing, and language translation [19].

6.2 Few-shot Learning

Few-shot learning is a method which seeks to train models to generalize after seeing as few examples as possible; there are usually between 5 and 20 photos for each category. In cases where data is limited, this procedure is particularly suitable, as it allows models to be instructed and to make decisions even with little data. Few-shot learning has become a novel technology and as such is particularly important in medical imaging for tasks such as classification and segmentation, which have been very effectively addressed as they say by data limitation problems [20].

6.3 Large Language Models (LLMs) in BIAs

Despite all the benefits of the LLMs that exist, they can also be used, by fully incorporating them into BIAs, to process and produce text that is very similar to human beings. These models that are optimized and transferred through different methods such as the utilization of the data in the identification of the patient as suffering from diseases or the solution of some steps; the diagnosis phase as the focal one. In sum, by combining LLMs with transfer learning and few-shot learning, the time of the entire complex medical process from non-fully labelled examples to the attainment of an accurate result may be greatly reduced [21-22].

Conclusions

The BIAs inclusion in the disease diagnosis represents a magnifying glass over the traditional approaches. This part of the chapter focuses on the basic findings by considering the possibilities of the use of ML and DL in the new areas and the discussion of the challenges brought by big data, interpretability, ethics, and legal issues, along with the strategies for continuous improvement.

BIAs are a breath of fresh air in the much-needed refining of the accuracy and speed of the diagnostic process of diseases. Nature-inspired these algorithms have been deployed through cutting-edge ML and DL processes that are designed to tackle even the most challenging medical problems. BIAs, when used with DL models, have shown unbeatable performance in the detection of diseases such as cardiac conditions and multiple sclerosis lesions, which are services that other businesses cannot provide. The role of BIAs is evident in their diagnostic accuracy strengthening role, which is done through the tight coupling of the AI model to a particular medical imaging system, and in the end, the model can find tailoring it to a specific patient, which consequently drives the gaining of more accurate and consistent results by patients.

Transfer learning and few-shot learning techniques have made it possible for model performance to improve with less data, and so have become useful in medical imaging and other diagnostic tasks. Furthermore, LLMs have been effectively used to decode complicated information from which medical professionals can make diagnoses as well as make decision support systems more efficient.

The integration of ML and DL in the diagnosis of diseases enables the practice of early detection of diseases and use of personalized medicine through accelerated data processing and visual decision support delivery, thereby enhancing patient outcomes and prognosis in the process. The potential of these breakthroughs is high; thus, one can expect the future to easily catch up with the situation when somebody gets an illness and the treatment becomes faster, more efficient, and more personalized than before, which changes the atmosphere for the patient from heightened anxiety to a peaceful state of knowing that the ailment will be solved in the best and easiest ways available today. The point that is involved in this fusion is to increase the accuracy of diagnosis, decrease medical costs, and ultimately extend patient's lives.

References

[1] Kar, A.K. (Oct. 2016) Bio inspired computing: A review of algorithms and scope of applications. *Expert Syst. Appl.*, *59*, 20–32. doi: 10.1016/j.eswa.2016.04.018.

[2] Darwish, A. (Oct. 2018). Bio-inspired computing: Algorithms review, deep analysis, and the scope of applications. *Future Computing and Informatics Journal*, *3*(2), 231–46. doi: 10.1016/j.fcij.2018.06.001.

[3] Al-Tawil, M., Mahafzah, B.A., Al Tawil, A. and Aljarah, I. (Mar. 2023). Bio-Inspired Machine Learning Approach to Type 2 Diabetes Detection. *Symmetry (Basel)*, *15*(3), 764. doi: 10.3390/sym15030764.

[4] Hunter, B., Hindocha, S. and Lee, R.W. (Mar. 2022). The Role of Artificial Intelligence in Early Cancer Diagnosis. *Cancers (Basel)*, *14*(6), 1524. doi: 10.3390/cancers14061524.

[5] Khan, O.T. and Rajeswari, D. (Jan. 2022). Brain Tumour Detection using Machine Learning and Deep Learning Approaches. *In: 2022 International Conference on Advances in Computing, Communication, and Applied Informatics (ACCAI)*, IEEE, (pp. 1–7). doi: 10.1109/ACCAI53970.2022.9752502.

[6] Ahsan, M.M., Luna, S.A. and Siddique, Z. (Mar. 2022). Machine-Learning-Based Disease Diagnosis: A Comprehensive Review. *Healthcare*, *10*, (3), 541. doi: 10.3390/healthcare10030541.

[7] Sai Krishna, K., Kangkan Jyoti Sarma, Kalyan Devappa Bamane, Jhakeshwar Prasad, Mohit Tiwari, & Karthikeyan, T. (Nov. 2023). Alzheimer Disease Detection using AI with Deep Learning based Features with Development and Validation based on Data Science. *Journal of Advanced Zoology*, *44*(S4), 91–99. doi: 10.17762/jaz.v44iS4.2174.

[8] Romalt, A.A. and Kumar, M.S. (Apr. 2022). Data Mining Approach for Diagnosing Heart Diseases through Deep Neural Network. *Periodico*, *91*(4). doi: 10.37896/pd91.4/91423.

[9] Schmidt-Erfurth, U., et al., (Jan. 2022). AI-based monitoring of retinal fluid in disease activity and under therapy. *Prog. Retin. Eye Res.*, *86*, 100972. doi: 10.1016/j.preteyeres.2021.100972.

[10] Ibrahim, M.R., Fathalla, K.M. and Youssef, S.M. (Jul. 2022). HyCAD-OCT: A Hybrid Computer-Aided Diagnosis of Retinopathy by Optical Coherence Tomography Integrating Machine Learning and Feature Maps Localization. *Applied Sciences*, *10*(14), 4716. doi: 10.3390/app10144716.

[11] Telikani, A., Tahmassebi, A., Banzhaf, W. and Gandomi, A.H. (Nov. 2022). Evolutionary Machine Learning: A Survey. *ACM Comput. Surv.*, *54*(8), 1–35. doi: 10.1145/3467477.

[12] Shagor, R.K., Faisal, F., Nishat, M.M., Mim, S.A. and H. Akter, H. (Oct. 2023). Implementation of Bio-inspired Algorithms in Designing Optimized PID controller for Cuk Converter for Enhanced Performance: A Software based Approach. *EAI Endorsed Transactions on AI and Robotics*, *2*. doi: 10.4108/airo.4038.

[13] Devika, G. and Gowda Karegowda, A. (2023). Bio-inspired Optimization: Algorithm, Analysis and Scope of Application. doi: 10.5772/intechopen.106014.

Disease Diagnosis | 87

[14] Jakšić, Z., Devi, S., Jakšić, O. and Guha, K. (Jun. 2023). A Comprehensive Review of Bio-Inspired Optimization Algorithms Including Applications in Microelectronics and Nanophotonics. *Biomimetics*, 8(3), 278. doi: 10.3390/biomimetics8030278.

[15] Schwettmann, S., et al., (Sep. 2023). FIND: A Function Description Benchmark for Evaluating Interpretability Methods. arXiv:2309.03886v3.

[16] Sharma, M., Bansal, A., Gupta, S., Asija, C., and Deswal, S. (Feb. 2020). Bio-Inspired Algorithms for Diagnosis of Heart Disease. *In: International Conference on Innovative Computing and Communication, 2019* (pp. 531–42). doi: 10.1007/978-981-15-1286-5_45.

[17] S.S.J. and P.K.S.C. (Dec. 2019). Image Enhancement using Bio-inspired Algorithms on mammogram for cancer detection. *In: 2015 International Conference on Emerging Research in Electronics, Computer Science and Technology (ICERECT)*, (pp. 11–16). IEEE. doi: 10.1109/ERECT.2015.7498979.

[18] Alanis, A.Y., Arana-Daniel, N. and López-Franco, C. (2018). Bio-inspired Algorithms. *In: Bio-inspired Algorithms for Engineering*. Elsevier. pp. 1–14. doi: 10.1016/B978-0-12-813788-8.00001-9.

[19] Raghu, M., Zhang, C., Kleinberg, J. and Bengio, S. (Feb. 2019). Transfusion: Understanding Transfer Learning for Medical Imaging. arXiv.1902.07208v3.

[20] Gollagi, S.G. and Balasubramaniam, S. (2023). Hybrid model with optimization tactics for software defect prediction. *International Journal of Modeling, Simulation, and Scientific Computing*, 14(02), 2350031.

[21] Balasubramaniam, S. and Gollagi, S.G. (2022). Software defect prediction via optimal trained convolutional neural network. *Advances in Engineering Software*, 169, 103138.

[22] Snell, J., Swersky, K. and Zemel, R.S. (Mar. 2017). Prototypical Networks for Few-shot Learning. arXiv.1703.05175v2.

5 | Algorithmic Heartbeat with Bio-Inspired Algorithms in Cardiac Health Monitoring

Ashwini A.,[1*] Kavitha V.,[2] Balasubramaniam S.[3] and Seifedine Kadry[4]

Cardiovascular diseases hold the first position as the leading cause of death globally, therefore, the need for early diagnosis as well as prompt intervention and management to avoid or minimize the effect the diseases could have on human health is inevitable. This chapter holds applications, benefits, and challenges of cardiac health monitoring using bio-inspired algorithms. The first part of the chapter is based on an approach whereby a bio-inspired algorithm is explained in a detailed manner. The intelligence that just imitates biological life as including genetic evolution, swarm intelligence and neural networks in cardiac data is made concentrated and has superior accuracy in anomaly detection. The chapter is followed by stripping down into the key functional fields of these bio-inspired algorithms for cardiac health monitoring, and robust classification. Perspectives of human-like algorithm use in real-life clinical cases are also addressed, as related to data privacy, comprehensibility and regulation. This section will be descriptive about the deep dive into Algorithmic Heartbeat in which biologically inspired algorithms are used to monitoring patients' heart health. It lets people realize the place from which this developing field of bio-inspired algorithms can thrive in cardiac health monitoring which provides the platform for innovation.

1. Introduction to Bio-Inspired Algorithms

Bio-inspired algorithms are computational methods from which natural processes and biologic systems are taken as inspiration to solve problems, which can be very difficult. These algorithms are imitating the very same properties of a natural platform like efficiency, adaptability, and robustness by using techniques such as evolution, swarming behaviour, and neural networks. Through mingling these biologic patterns, bio-inspired algorithms have a strong potential to efficiently resolve a lot of optimization, data analysis, and recognition tasks [1]. They

---

[1] Department of Electronics and Communication Engineering, Vel Tech Rangarajan Dr. Sagunthala R&D Institute of Science and Technology, Avadi, Chennai, Tamilnadu, India.
[2] University College of Engineering, Kancheepuram, Tamilnadu, India.
[3] School of Computer Science and Engineering, Kerala University of Digital Sciences, Innovation and Technology (Formerly IIITM-K), Digital University Kerala, Thiruvananthapuram, Kerala, India.
[4] Department of Applied Data Science, Noroff University College, Norway.
* Corresponding author: a.aswiniur@gmail.com

have a wide range of fields of application—engineering, computer science, and healthcare—which all benefit from the technologies and the problem-solving skills gained by their application.

The most widely recognized bio-inspired algorithm is the genetic algorithm (GA) that is an emulation of the functioning of biological evolution based on the fact of natural selection. The building blocks of GAs are the following mechanisms as selection, crossover, and mutation that create many generations of solutions to optimization problems. However, in recent time, it is trending for utilitarian purpose of bionic algorithms to improve cardiac healthcare and diagnosis. This manner is not only valuable for stumbling upon optimal or suboptimal options in large-scale or complex problem spaces, but also effective and precise. Other than this, the swarm intelligence idea is another of those that are derived from social insects such as the ants and the bees. For instance, the ACO (ant colony optimization) and the PSO (particle swarm optimization) strategies, which are the algorithms derived from the behaviours of insects and their swarms, mimic such distributed characteristics for problems such as routing, scheduling, and resource allocation. Figure 1 shows the cardiac disease prediction system using the bio-inspired algorithms.

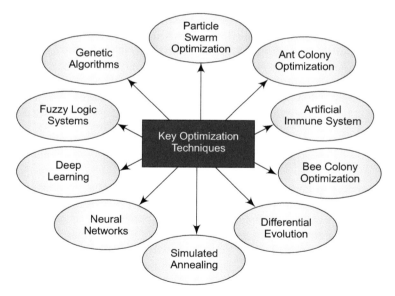

Fig. 1 Flow diagram of cardiac disease prediction using the bio-inspired algorithm.

Neural networks, in the wide range of that—artificial neural networks (ANNs) and its advanced version, deep learning is included and they serve as the machine algorithm that mimics the structure and functions of a human brain. These networks are made up of interconnected submissions (neurons) which use and transfer information, allowing machines to learn from data, identify uniqueness', and make decisions [2]. The base on which these algorithms are built and the substitution of the natural processes with algorithmics are indicated as the bases for biologic systems. We would put into words where these algorithms take their root and why they use GAs that reproduce nature's choice and neural networks that resemble the human brain. Deep learning, with its neural networks composed of multiple layers, has brought to the universe completely new system; it is areas like image and speech recognition, natural language processing, and autonomous systems that have been revolutionized. The neural network has been able to retrieve solutions from the brain's ability to learn-and-adapt [3]. Therefore, using the neural network is one of the most indispensable cornerstones in modern artificial intelligence and machine learning. These algorithms signify an evolutionary breakthrough of biological and computational sciences, achieving the goal of finding a practical solution.

2. Biological Analogies in the Design of Heartbeat Algorithms

The concept of the biological analogies in the development of the heartbeat algorithms is based on the usage of the same concepts and processes that have been long known of in the biological systems to inspire and inform the design of computational methods that will serve the same purposes of analysing and diagnosing heart conditions. Analogies are derived from different natural processes, such as evolution, cellulose behaviour, mind imitation, immune reaction, and human reasoning, in order to build algorithms that copy features from these kinds of biological processes which are effective and adaptive, and which are also able to solve problems.

2.1 Genetic Algorithms: Mimicking Natural Selection

GAs translate into imitating the process of natural selection, a fundamental tool with which evolution takes place. Considering that heartbeat algorithms for monitoring the cardiac health can be utilized to optimize the choice of features through niches from vast datasets like ECG signals, medical imaging, and patient records, GAs are suitable for this purpose. Firstly, the GA starts by employing a pool of potential solutions, each one being represented by a chromosome. These solutions are quite successful thanks to their selectivity criterion, that is, how well they function in recognizing conditions of a heart [4]. Crossover and mutation procedures use exchange and slight modification of existing solutions to generate new ones, imitating the natural way of reproduction and variation. Auditing of age-related populations, leads to a gradual turnover of suboptimal or close-to-optimal populations where the identification of the key biomarkers and diagnostic patterns is highly accurate and efficient.

2.2 Swarm Intelligence: Emulating Collective Behaviour

Swarm Intelligence techniques are rooted in the collective behaviours of species like ants, bees, and birds, whereby there is always information exchange. ACO and Particle Swarm Optimization (PSO) happen to be the most frequently-utilized main examples. In cardiac health monitoring, ACO can be used to manage the skyline of big data salinity, which is a practice of extracting shortest diagnosis paths in the complex medical networks. In ACO, ants draining pheromones on the paths which they frequent; moreover, pheromones grow stronger as the quality of the path increases. Over time, shorter paths and the ones with more effectiveness supply their pheromone trail and this way attract the next ants to the most beneficial way of walking. In the same way, PSO reproduces the natural social behaviour of birds when it is a flocking and fish when it is schooling. Every particle (reminds the particles which potential methods can be used) moves, using its own past experience and the experience acquired from neighbouring particles. The close and collaborative nature of this methodology contributes greatly to the recommended reiteration and amendments of disease diagnosis models [5]. At the same time, the precise navigation through high-dimensions with the aid of this approach improves the accuracy with which heart disease is predicted.

2.3 Neural Networks: Replicating Brain Function

Neural networks, ANNs, and deep learning models are based on the way either whole or separate parts of brain work. The main structures of these networks are based on inputs that each neuron (a node) individually processes and then passes the result over to subsequent layers. In cardiac health monitoring systems, neural networks can be trained to identify irregularities in ECG signal patterns, images, or other indicators of health. The use of convolution neural networks (CNNs), which are types of deep learning models, is effective for processing data from images such as an echocardiogram or MRI scans. CNNs consider convolutional layers as a method of automatically learning the spatial structure of objects where the level of detail is important in the process of anomaly detection, e.g., arrhythmias or the extra-pericardic structures are analysed [6]. Recurrent neural networks (RNNs) and the likes (e.g., LSTM [long short-term memory] networks) are the prevalent choice as models for time-series data, given that they can accommodate a type of dependency inherent in time-series data, and that they can hence predict future ECG readings or cardiac activities relying on the previous ones.

2.4 Immune System Algorithms: Mimicking Biological Defence Mechanisms

The algorithms of artificial intelligent systems are based on the recognition and reaction capability of the human immune system as it always operates to detect and eliminate the pathogens. In cardiac health monitoring, these algorithms can be applied to differentiate both normal and abnormal patterns of heart-related data and, in addition, response to the abnormal ones. One scenario is when negative selection algorithms will have the ability to identify changes in normal functions of the heart—they will create detectors that recognize non-self (abnormal) data and will show tolerance to self (normal) data. This is exactly similar to the immune system which guides it to distinguish between harmful invaders and the body's cells making it more helpful in the early recognition of distortions in heartbeats or other cardiac indicators.

2.5 Evolutionary Strategies: Drawing from Natural Evolution

As a specification of evolutionary algorithms, progressive strategies study adaptation and solutions optimization using natural generative processes. Their effect in the case of the application of machine learning to cardiovascular health monitoring will be to improve the efficiency of the models based on parameters and architecture [7]. However, it is done through the simulation of natural selection, where well-adapted individuals selected for reproduction lead to iterative success the predictive efficiency of diagnostic algorithms. Adopting such a fine-tuning approach will be worthwhile when dealing with complex algorithms like neural networks, which helps to obtain the highest possible accuracy and the conditions to predict cardiac abnormalities.

2.6 Fuzzy Logic: Inspired by Human Reasoning

The evolution of fuzzy logic systems emulates the cognition methodology which is based on imprecision and ignorance of the human brain. In cardiac health monitoring, fuzzy logic is used for interpreting unclear data such as a wide range of symptoms or grey short test results area. Fuzzy logic controllers can take in more than one input, e.g., blood pressure, cholesterol level, and ECG readings to determine the overall degree hard matters javascript of risk for heart disease. The iterative reasoning system enables an approach that is not just simply tagging for binary logic but providing individualized and dynamic diagnostic outcomes [8].

By extending the ways in which these biological strategies are implemented, they provide a wide-range of potentials for developing highly starling and precise heartbeat algorithms that can be deployed to improve the accuracy, efficiency, and reliability of heart monitoring systems. Through employing the fundamentals of natural selection, group behaviour, cognition, immune defence, variations, and human mindfulness, these nature-inspired algorithms present creative resolutions of some of the most difficult issues in cardiac diagnosis [9].

3. Different Optimization Techniques

In the case of cardiac health monitoring, as well as diagnostics, several nature-inspired optimization methods can be used during the system design phase to improve performance and the accuracy of algorithms [10]. The filtering processes of cancer diagnosis which include feature selection, parameter optimization, and the efficiency of the model are enhanced by these techniques. Figure 2 shows some of the key optimization techniques used in Algorithmic Heartbeat with Bio-Inspired Algorithms.

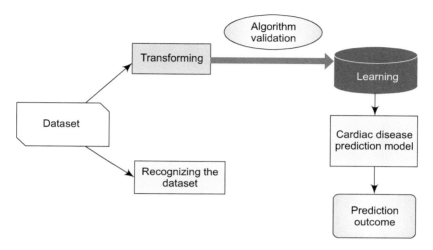

Fig. 2 Key optimization techniques.

3.1 Genetic Algorithms (GAs)

GA is the way of improvement by the rule of nature selection and genetic mutation. At the outset, they work with the set of population whose each individual contains the specific chromosomes symbolizing diverse combinations of features or model variables [11]. The fitness of each solution is determined by how accurately it diagnoses various heart conditions, whereby true positives, false positives, and false negatives, among others, are employed to assess the effectiveness of the solutions. Through the period of repetition, such population undergoes evolution by step to step up the efficiency of the process of diagnosis to become better and better. Through this process, GAs are made to be effective searchers in the relatively large and complex candidate solutions spaces, discovering optimal or near-optimal solutions and parameter values for pliable models for cardiac health monitoring. Through the process of intergenerational transfer of information and machine-learning, the evolution happens, which makes a GA more able to capture this information and predict anomalies and diseases in a more reliable and less-error fashion. In cardiac health monitoring, GAs can be used for:

- *Feature Selection*: Discovering an appropriate set of features from volume datasets such as ECG signals, CT images, and patient data to have a diagnostic precision [12].
- *Parameter Optimization*: To accurately tune the machine learning model's hyperparameters in order to obtain the best performance.

3.2 Particle Swarm Optimization (PSO)

PSO is proven on a premise, the social behaviour of the birds flocking or the fish schooling. The process unites any problem by means of iterative techniques that enhance the candidate solution in regards to the certain of quality characteristics. PSO, a bio-inspired algorithm that mimics the collective behaviour of a swarm like animal groups such as bird flocking or fish schooling, is an approach that is being looked into and used to optimize complex problems like cardiac monitoring [13]. It is very useful in the case of patient's cardiac health monitoring for the improvement the parameters of diagnostic models and the accuracy of prediction models in cardiovascular diseases.

Every single particle in the swarm takes on a solution, e.g., be a good choice of one or few parameters or attribute subsets. Implying they add together, are pushed through the solution space being positioned in line with their own experiences and those of neighboured particles. The movement of particles is guided by two main components: not only cognitive and social, but also physical and emotional [14–17]. During the cognitive stage, each particle is forced to move towards their best known position (social best) while during the social phase, the swarm is mandated to move towards the best-known position of the swarm (communal optimum). Via such mechanism, particles seek and use the solution space, one after another till they finally reach the optimum or near-to-optimum solutions. In cardiac health monitoring, PSO can be used for:

- *Parameter Tuning*: The settings of neural networks and other models of machine learning are optimized.
- *Clustering*: Clustering together the similar cardiac data is to see clear pattern or anomaly detection better.

3.3 Ant Colony Optimization (ACO)

ACO is based on the ant cannibalizing strategy. With ACO bio-inspired algorithms solving optimization problems related to heart disease diagnosis and monitoring that optimize the scavenging behaviour of ants is the basis [18]. The ACO gives particular emphasis to problems where the ideal route is the overflow of complex and multi-dimensional spaces. Within the arena of cardiac health surveillance, the ACO can then be explored to foster data analysis, feature selection, and diagnostic accuracy. ACO is remotely led on the principle of ants foraging and laying down pheromones to mark their ways. The pheromone trails that these ants leave are in fact leading other ants towards the shortest and most efficient paths that will bring them to the sugar source. Pertaining to the computational settings, ACO algorithms simulate this process in the way that artificial ants are moved from one possible solution to another and virtual pheromones deposited that indicate the degree of quality of the solution [19]. It is used to find optimal paths through graphs and can be applied in cardiac health monitoring for:

- ***Path Optimization***: Establishing the quickest and most productive journey through labyrinthine medical entities.
- ***Data Classification***: Adding additional features and removing irrelevant ones in order to optimize the classification accuracy for heart disease data.

3.4 Artificial Immune Systems (AIS)

AIS are imitating the process of human immune system and they are used for anomaly detection. Besides, they can recognize the patterns. This is however very efficient in identification of patterns, anomaly detection, and robust decision-making. In the respect of cardiovascular health monitoring, AIS can be applied to catching anomaly trends of heart files, avoiding the later disease and guaranteeing medical help on time [20].

AIS algorithms imitate such human defensive systems that protect the body by identifying and counteracting the pathogens with adaptive approaches and quick responses. Lymphocyte activation occurs by the principles of negative selection, clonal selection, and immune networks [21]. These atoms together empower the system to identify and recall patterns, classify data as self or non-self, and make improvements when presented with fresh threats. In cardiac health monitoring, AIS can be applied for:

- ***Anomaly Detection:*** The recognition of abnormal patterns in ECG queues and other cardiac data which can suggest heart disease entrance.
- ***Fault Tolerance:*** Affirming the reliability of systems by detecting and using the process of data.

3.5 Bee Colony Optimization (BCO)

The BCO system is a data-driven design approach that mimics the foraging behaviour of honeybees. The procedure takes after the way they communicate and search for nectar with each other [22]. They could logically recognize the best route of foraging in that way. The process of cardiac health monitoring leverages the application of BCO for optimal feature selection, data clustering, and the parameters' tuning of diagnostic models in the featured case. BCO algorithms mimic the flight patterns of the honeybees in their quest for pollen and nectar. This simulation involves artificial bees that explore the search space, and the information they share on the solution quality is particularly their task. The algorithm typically involves two types of bees: carrying, and bees taking care of. Working bees go out to explore the options and they return to the hive to lead fellow bees to sources of food using their intuition and dancing. Beaded-up bees follow these consecutive dances, and they have higher chances of clicking on bees whose answers are correct [23]. Along with that function, scout bees forage new areas of the search space, avoiding trap in local optima which limits the algorithm's startup. It can be used in cardiac health monitoring for:

96 | Bio-inspired Algorithms in Machine Learning and Deep Learning for Disease Detection

- *Data Mining*: Accomplishing good classification results due to dataset size and feature extraction.
- *Resource Allocation*: Improving the antiquated medical equipment and avoiding such situations.

3.6 Differential Evolution (DE)

DE is the class of algorithms conquering the space of continuous optimization problems and known for its level of accuracy, adaptability, and applicability to the nonlinear, non-differentiable, rather multimodal objective functions [24–27]. DE explores the candidate solutions via a population of which every individual is represented as a vector from a feature space. The algorithm optimizes the found solutions in the iterative way via application of mutation, crossover, and selection breaks.

- *Mutation*: Each candidate solution undergoes mutation, where DE creates a carrier vector carrying the weighted difference between two different vectors of the population, chosen at random. This way, the population exhibits the population effect.
- *Crossover*: The algorithm then adds the mutant vector to the original candidate solution in order to get a trial vector. Make sure you thoroughly explain the various impacts of global trade on different countries [28]. At this level, multi-locality becomes the natural force as multifary inheritance makes an offspring possess the qualities from multiple parents, hence keeping the diversity intact.
- *Selection*: Therefore, the algorithm analyzes the result of the change in the solution vector and then compares it to the initial candidate solution [29]. The trial vector advances to the next generation if it provides a more suitable solution (selection is executed according to the given criteria, e.g., the lowest error in predictions) replaces the original solution in the population.

3.7 Simulated Annealing (SA)

SA (Shariah-aligned) follows the concept of annealing in metrology. It is finding a best scalar value via which the assumed function can be appropriately approximated, that is, the issue of finding a global optimum solution can be partly overcome. It is utilized to figure out brilliant approximations to the global optimum point of a function within an enormous search space. SA is particularly helpful in the cases in which the precise optimal solution or Euro-critical/Euro-scale scenarios are mathematically impossible or computationally not profitable.

The SA acting through many expeditions of exploration within the search space, this allows the algorithm to introduce both uphill movement (improving objective function value) and downhill movement (deteriorating objective function value) based on a probability distribution. In every loop, the algorithm randomly selects a neighbouring solution, evaluates its objective function value, and then possibly embeds it into the overall solution [30]. If this new solution is the best from the current solution, that solution becomes the new current solution. If the newly suggested solution is not optimal, and this happens with a certain probability which is determined by the cooling schedule and reduces the probability of acceptance of worse solutions with progression, SA may just accept it [31]. This make the SA to move outside local optima and continue looking at the search space until a global optimum is attained. In cardiac health monitoring, SA can be applied for:

- *Model Optimization*: Parameter fine-tuning of the diagnostic algorithms to achieve the over fitting and generalization or/and the follow the rule of biases reduction to achieve the point.
- *Feature Selection*: Determining what are the most significant features that can bring the heart disease diagnosis to be accurate.

3.8 Neural Networks and Deep Learning

Deep learning models are closely related to—themselves—the construction and the functioning of our brain. Due to the ability to process large amounts of data swiftly, neural networks and deep learning are biology-based algorithms specially developed to assist specialists in timely cardiac diseases detection, diagnosis, and prediction [32]. The algorithms find these data easy to process, especially those that are complex and can be represented in a high-dimensional form like electrocardiogram (ECG) signals, medical images, patient records, etc. Through incorporating neural network architectures that are built on the deep learning algorithms, bio-inspired systems can spot significant patterns and relationships within the cardiac data, increasing the accuracy and timeliness of diagnoses. Optimization techniques in this context include:

- *Back-propagation*: Solving the training of neural networks is by optimizing weights with the aim of minimizing the error in predictions.
- *Regularization Techniques*: Choosing overfitting methods like dropout, weight decay, and batch normalization is of great importance for preventing overfitting.

3.9 Fuzzy Logic Systems

Fuzzy logic originates in the human mind. It is a derivative of the way of human logic of reasoning and decision-making processes. FSL are mostly helpful under the condition when there are no reliable and exact data or the possibilities to interpret it in more than one way. In the particularity of cardiac health monitoring, FLS can aid in the diagnosis of risks, support treatment and establish medical priority based on the fuzzy rules grasped from the doctor's knowledge [33]. FLS operate by using fuzzy programming theory achieving communicating the human linguistic variables and fuzzy rule to emulate human decision-making process. Such systems use linguistic labels (for example, 'very low', 'low', 'middle', 'high', and 'very high') in which variables take these abstract terms, hence reasoning in them is flexible, simple, and intuitive.

FLS consist of three main components: examination, sifting, classification, and clarification. During fuzzification, crispy data that returns its integer inputs is converted into fuzzy sets by way of membership functions [34]. Thus, the rules of the system are passed forward to the fuzzy sets with the final result of being the output. Lastly, the defuzzification stage crudely turns the fuzzy outputs into a crisp result which is interpreted and acted upon. In cardiac health monitoring, fuzzy logic systems can be used for:

- **Risk Assessment**: Integrating the multiple factors or indicators which are somewhat inaccurate to assess the total risk of heart disease.
- **Decision Support**: Hardware capacities must have the ability to handle nuanced diagnostic proposals based on fuzzy rules originated from medical professionals.

Using this biomimetic innovation, the cardiac health monitoring systems for patients can become more precise, efficient, and stable in detection and prevention of heart diseases. This approach includes techniques that take advantage of the natural tendency of processes to solve the issues that are involved in the analysis of medical data that are both complex and challenging.

4. Neural Networks with Bio-inspired Computing

Bio-inspired Computing with ANN nets in cardiac health monitoring combine the strength of ANNs with the rules from natural systems, so as to improve the detection, diagnosis, and individualized treatment of the heart diseases. It is exactly evident that ANNs models, in conjunction with the human brain, which are initiated and used to learn complex patterns and connections from more large volumes of data. By employing GAs, swarm intelligence, or evolutionary strategies, which are bio-inspired computing techniques, these neural networks could still aim for the performance improvement and adaptation in cardiac health monitoring applications.

Another significant advantage of interfacing bio-inspired computing with neural networks for cardiac health monitoring is the capability to deal with the usually strong complexities and unpredictable nature of the data. For instance, GAs can enhance the network architecture of the neural networks in the manner that helps the structure and the other parameters to work effectively in dealing with different data of cardiac types which includes electrocardiograms (ECGs), medical pictures, and patient's data. Furthermore, swarm intelligence algorithms would play an essential role in detecting similarities between heterogeneous data sources. In this way, neural networks will be able to get more sophisticated insights by using multimodal data sources and promoting diagnostic precision.

On the other hand, bionic computing analogous to neural networks can strengthen the reliability of models using the neural network approach in cardiovascular monitoring. Having these strategies, the computation power can be spared to tackle the task of marker selection when several biomarkers or physiological parameters of the heart diseases are available. Addition of genetic information yields much better results and assistance in the classification of neuronal networks models. Besides that, this allows medical specialists to have a deep understanding of the mechanisms of cardiac problems which helps them in applying the personalized treatment programmes.

Therefore, the sophisticated interaction with bio-impellent computing and neural networks brings adaptable and autonomous cardiac monitoring systems with the ability of continuous learning and self-improvement. Through the use of mimicking biological systems such as self-organization and self-change, these hybrid methods have an ability to adjust themselves to a dynamic environment of clinical setups, to a change in a patient's condition, and to a new diagnostic requirement over a period of time [35]. This proverbial nature of capability means that the cardiac health monitoring systems stay state-of-the-art through increased innovation and medical knowledge, generating optimal patient results, and unmatched care thus providing.

5. Swarm Intelligence for Heart Health Monitoring

Swarm Intelligence with Bio-inspired Computing which proposes the use of collective behaviours of decentralized systems to monitor cardiac system of human body, mimicking the behaviours of social insect colonies from the nature, to create the more efficient process of monitoring is a new approach. The fusion of swarm intelligence with bio-inspired computing leads to such newly devised method, which leads more warranted and productive heart health diagnostics, triggering earlier detection of cardiac conditions.

The algorithmic framework referred to as swarm intelligence includes two well-known algorithms namely, ACO and PSO which are also known as the behavioral algorithms that involve the behavior of the ants, bees, etc., amongst various social entities to solve optimization problems. Through displaying cooperative network activities and decentralized decision-making patterns similar to the natural systems, the swarm intelligence algorithms are capable of resolving sophisticated set of data, identifying cardiac biomarkers and optimizing diagnostic models used in the heart disease monitoring. When married with natural programming approaches like GAs and evolutionary approaches, the process becomes even more adaptive and optimal [36].

GAs use peer intelligence for evolutionary operations on the parameters and structures of swarm intelligence algorithms, which allows them to dynamically change their behaviour as the monitoring environment evolves. Regarding the evolution tactics, the technique can also optimize the feature selection process, discovering more effective data subsets which can precisely diagnose heart problems. The conjunction of swam intelligence and bio-inspired computing allows to design intelligent cardiac monitoring systems that do not only detect trends, but also can efficiently deal with new information. These systems have the capacity to manipulate and process the huge amounts of cardiac data from various sources, like ECGs, radiographs, and patients' histories, with great precision thus they can provide timely and accurate diagnosis [37].

Furthermore, utilizing the logic of self-control decision-making and collective intelligence, swarm intelligence having a bio-inspired computing promotes the mutual cooperation between healthcare specialists, researchers and engineers to carry on the massive health monitoring projects related to cardiac health. Swarm Intelligence Guided by Bio-computing Heart Health Monitoring is a nascent an approach that can be a game-changer for cardiac diagnostics due to its scalability, adaptability, and efficiency in overcoming the challenges of cardiovascular disease detection and management. The cardiac health monitoring can be improved by employing an intelligence system of nature and is mixed with advanced computational approaches, and thus make it a revolutionary approach to be more targeted towards the patients and the healthcare delivery systems.

6. Genetic Algorithm in Feature Selection

GA for Heart Health Monitoring with Feature Selection based on Biology Computing as a Computational Technique for the Optimization of Relevant Features within Complex Heart Data, can include any type of Electrocardiogram (ECG), Medical Images, and Patient Data. GAs constitute one of the searching algorithms drawing on the ground-based mechanisms such as natural selection and evolution of genes to identify subsets of features that can successfully diagnose and predict the types of cardiac conditions by the patterns utilized. Regarding feature selection for heart health monitoring, GAs consist of generating chromosomes as feature subsets which outline the population.

Chromosome for each, representing the possible solution, a set of features, from the original dataset, will be the constituent. These subsets are employed to model the typical cardiac diseases by using measurements including sensitivity, specificity, and predictive accuracy. The population of feature subsets is continuously improved over multiple generations through the processes of selection, crossover, and mutation with the aim of providing the best. In the process of selection, generally, fitter feature subsets that are responsible for proficient classifications would be more likely to be chosen as parents for further reproduction. Crossover operations are the process where the selection of bits are performed between groups of parents to develop new offspring with a unique combination of bit-elements. Mutation includes operations like swapping, inserting, and deleting the features and thus the algorithm is able to search new regions of the solution space and it is less prone to the unwanted local optimum solutions.

The bio-inspired nature of GAs possesses them the capability to pin-pointedly deal with the intricacies and ambiguities with cardiac data by incorporating noise, variability, and high dimensionality. Through copying the natural selection process, genetic algorithms solve the search for feature subsets which is, at the same time, the most discriminative information for diagnosing various forms of cardiac diseases. Coming up next, through exploiting bio-inspired computing techniques such as parallelization and neural-engineering in addition to other optimization methods genetic algorithms can improve their overall performance on the process of feature selection in heart health monitoring.

To summarize, it is Genetic Algorithm in Feature Selection with Bio-inspired Computing that we propose for the monitoring of the health of the heart, which is the robust and efficient method to the identification of informative features from the cardiac datasets. Through incorporation of elements of natural evolution along with state of the art computational techniques, this method makes possible the design of tested and accurate diagnostic models for heart diseases screening and treatment, with the final goal of better health outcomes and more efficient medical services delivery.

7. Bio-inspired Data Fusion

Bio-inspired Data Fusion for Heart Health Monitoring integrates principles from biological systems with advanced data fusion techniques to enhance the accuracy and reliability of cardiac diagnostics. Drawing inspiration from the collective behaviours observed in natural ecosystems, bio-inspired data fusion approaches aim to intelligently integrate heterogeneous cardiac data sources, such as ECGs, medical images, genetic profiles, and patient records, to provide comprehensive insights into heart health.

The main feature of bio-mimicry is that it is capable of imitating the cooperation that is happening and the decentralized decision-making that ants and bees are known for. Just like ants, which employ a network of pheromone trails to solve complex tasks in groups, bio-inspired data infusion approaches capitalize on parallel computing models to cooperatively process and fuse data on cardiac originals from various sources. This distributed design adds up to reliable data exchange and aggregation of cardiac monitoring system components leading to a robust and accurate diagnosis.

Not only this, but optimizing the fusion process by incorporating natural principles of selection and evolution into bio-inspired data fusion techniques is one of the bio-inspired data fusion techniques. GAs, for instance, may go ahead and dynamically make the fusion rules' as well as their weights anew in response to the system's performance. The fusion algorithms that mimic the setting of natural evolution iteratively optimize the fusion strategy to deliver the highest likelihood of producing a validated and comprehensive decision-making system based on the combined cardiac data. Table 1 shows the performance analysis of bio-inspired algorithms for cardiac health monitoring.

Table 1 Performance analysis of bio-inspired algorithms for cardiac health monitoring.

Methods	Disease	Accuracy
Naïve Bayes	Heart Disease	86.91%
Bagging	Heart Disease	85.94%
SVM	Heart Disease	87.46%
Genetic Algorithm	Heart Disease	90.53%
Genetic Algorithm +SVM	Heart Disease	91.52%
MLP	Heart Disease	86.17%

One more area of bio-inspired data fusion towards precise heart health monitoring is its capability of dealing with uncertainties and confusion that come with medical data. Learning from the characteristics of living systems that are flexible and adaptable, they derive the fuzzy logic and the probabilistic reasoning to get them close to imprecise and uncertain situations. These bio-inspired approaches, having built the concerns of uncertainty in clinical cardiac data act as nuanced and rational diagnostic assessments, by contributing to the reliability of clinical decision-making in cardiac monitoring. This holistic and interdisciplinary Bio-inspired Data Fusion approach for cardiovascular care expresses a sentiment that can be explored through principles of life sciences, computational intelligence and data science to improve diagnostics. By employing heterogeneous data sources where collective behaviours are mimicked and uncertainties are addressed, bio-inspired fusion techniques offer a potential for enhancing the accuracy, reliability, and efficacy of cardiac patients' monitoring, ultimately leading to better patient outcomes and more personalized treatment.

8.   Ethical Consideration and Challenges

The following denotes the ethical considerations and challenges when deploying the bio-inspired algorithms in cardiac monitoring.

Bias and Fairness

Such biologically-inspired computing algorithms may be programmed by the present data biases inadvertently, thus resulting in the chance for the algorithms to have unfair or discriminatory results specifically for marginalized people. Ethical considerations contain understanding and weakening biases in data, maintaining diversity and inclusivity in dataset collection process, and routinely auditing algorithms to make sure the correctness of efficiency in decision-making processes.

Transparency and Interpretability

Sometimes the degree of concealment of bio-inspired computing algorithms such as deep learning models becomes a challenge when making determinations on how the decisions are arrived at. Transparency and interpretability of these algorithms are very important in case of the clinicians and patients to rely on the reliability of diagnostic suggestions. The emphasis should be on the technique that will display the prediction outcomes of the model and furnish understanding on the reasons for certain decision.

Accountability and Liability

However, as preferential assigned algorithms become more vital in clinical decision making, the responsibility and liability in cases of errors or adverse results need to be clarified. Implementing details for accountability, such as the roles and responsibilities of developers, healthcare providers, and regulators, will help to decrease risks and provide oversight across the entire product deployment cycle.

Equitable Access and Affordability

Provision of bio-inspired computing technologies for remote heart health monitoring should be used equitably to avoid compound exacerbation in the gaps of healthcare access and outcomes. Ensuring cost solutions, infrastructure as well as resources supply adequacy is a powerful weapon to democratize access to advanced disease diagnosis and make sure that no one with low social status is left behind.

Informed Consent and Autonomy

Respecting patient autonomy and information authenticity for the co-operation of free and independent agents at work, which is the basis of ethical principles in healthcare. The need for patients to make informed choices about their participation in information for diagnostic purposes cannot be overemphasized. In this case, security, benefits, and implications of sharing of their health data should be understood.

Regulatory Compliance and Standards

Integration of regulatory standards as well as the design, mode and interactions of bio-inspired computing technologies should be the goal with the aim of accomplishing safe and reliable treatment. Making alliance with regulatory bodies and professional organizations, which calls for the set-up of ethics standards and best-practice rules, is important.

Through the discussion of these ethical problems and issues inherent in bio-inspired computing for heart health monitoring, all stakeholders have a role to play to ensure responsible and ethical operation of these technologies and therefore they can result to trusted, equitable, and accountable in the use of these cutting-edge technologies for improving patient outcomes and advancing healthcare delivery.

Conclusion

Finally, the bio-inspired computing joins into the health monitoring of the heart is on its way to be a powerful innovation in healthcare sector where it could provide revolutionary detect, diagnose, and manage cardiovascular diseases. Natural systems and biological processes serve as a reference point for new concepts of bio-inspired computing methods which lead to novel approaches for process analysis of complicated cardio data, improve diagnostic techniques and provide better patient outcome. Bio-mimic computing algorithms, inclusive GAs, swarm intelligence, and neural networks, for instance, which possess the power to process heterogeneous data sources, biomarkers identification, as well as diagnostic models optimization, are tools for smart minds to solve the above-mentioned task. These algorithms act on the principles of evolution, collective learning, and neural processing while being adaptive to successfully navigate the large solution spaces for finding the patterns, they bring accuracy to cardiac health monitoring.

Moreover, ethical implications as well as challenges in the use of bio-inspired computing computer for heart health monitoring emphasize the responsibility, transparent, and patient care-centred innovation. Protecting privacy, avoiding bias, practicing transparency, and fostering an equitable system are vital to check that these technologies adhere to the ethical principles, respect patient self-determination, and promote equal access to high-quality healthcare. In brief, bio-inspired computing is the promising field that can create the paradigm shift to heart health monitoring, which will certainly make the diagnostic devices more personalized, accurate, and efficient. Through the interdisciplinary coordination, compliance to regulations and establishment of ethical governance, the stakeholders could leverage bio-inspired computing to the highest possible potential while preserving data privacy, maintaining fairness and building the trust of the people. To sustain further development in bio-motivated computing, there must be prior research, development, and implementation. In due course, bio-inspired computing will create a better diagnostic system for the cardiac health worldwide and will finally pave the way for a healthier future.

References

[1] Omer, R.M.D., Al-Salihi, N.K., Rashid, T.A., Aladdin, A.M., Mohammadi, M. and Majidpour, J. (Jun. 2024). Discovering the Power of Artificial Cardiac Conduction System (ACCS): Harmony in Bio-inspired Metaheuristic. *arXiv preprint arXiv:2404.02907*.

[2] Digumarthi, J., Gayathri, V.M. and Pitchai, R. (2023). Recognition of Cardiac Arrhythmia using ECG signals and Bio-inspired AWPSO Algorithms. *Iraqi Journal of Electrical and Electronic Engineering*, 20(1).

[3] Ding, W., Abdel-Basset, M., Eldrandaly, K.A., Abdel-Fatah, L. and De Albuquerque, V. H.C. (2020). Smart supervision of cardiomyopathy based on fuzzy Harris Hawks optimizer and wearable sensing data optimization: A new model. *IEEE Transactions on Cybernetics*, 51(10), 4944–58.

[4] Baviskar, V., Verma, M. and Chatterjee, P. (Aug. 2021). Improving Classification Performance of Deep Learning Models using Bio-Inspired Computing. *In: Proceedings of the 2021 Thirteenth International Conference on Contemporary Computing* (pp. 333–40).

[5] Rundo, F., Ortis, A., Battiato, S. and Conoci, S. (2018). Advanced bio-inspired system for noninvasive cuff-less blood pressure estimation from physiological signal analysis. *Computation*, 6(3), 46.

[6] Munagala, N.K., Langoju, L.R.R., Rani, A.D. and Reddy, D.R.K. (2022). A smart IoT-enabled heart disease monitoring system using metaheuristic-based Fuzzy-LSTM model. *Biocybernetics and Biomedical Engineering*, 42(4), 1183–1204.

[7] Balasubramanian, S., Naruk, M.S. and Tewari, G. (2023). Electrocardiogram Signal Denoising using Optimized Adaptive Hybrid Filter with Empirical Wavelet Transform. *Journal of Shanghai Jiaotong University (Science)*, 1–15.

[8] Khan, M.A. and Algarni, F. (2020). A healthcare monitoring system for the diagnosis of heart disease in the IoMT cloud environment using MSSO-ANFIS. *IEEE Access*, 8, 122259–122269.

[9] de Lannoy, G., François, D., Delbeke, J. and Verleysen, M. (Jan.2010). Feature relevance assessment in automatic inter-patient heart beat classification. *In: International Conference on Bio-inspired Systems and Signal Processing*, 2, 13–20. SciTePress.

[10] Hussain, I. and Islam, A.U. (2023). Research Direction Toward IoT-Based Machine Learning-Driven Health Monitoring Systems: A Survey. *In: Computational Vision and Bio-Inspired Computing: Proceedings of ICCVBIC 2022* (pp. 541–55). Singapore: Springer Nature Singapore.

[11] Santos, M.S., Fred, A.L., Silva, H. and Lourenço, A. (Feb. 2013). Eigen heartbeats for user identification. *In: International Conference on Bio-inspired Systems and Signal Processing*, 2, 351–55. SciTePress.

[12] Krishnaveni, A., Shankar, R. and Duraisamy, S. (2019). A survey on nature inspired computing (NIC): Algorithms and challenges. *Global Journal of Computer Science and Technology: D Neural and Artificial Intelligence*, 19(3).

[13] Bitam, S., Zeadally, S. and Mellouk, A. (2016). Bio-inspired cybersecurity for wireless sensor networks. *IEEE Communications Magazine*, 54(6), 68–74.

[14] Saleem, K., Alabduljabbar, G.M., Alrowais, N., Al-Muhtadi, J., Imran, M. and Rodrigues, J.J. (2020). Bio-inspired network security for 5G-enabled IoT applications. *IEEE Access*, 8, 229152–229160.

[15] Al-Nader, I., Lasebae, A., Raheem, R. and Ekembe Ngondi, G. (2024). A Novel Bio-Inspired Bat Node Scheduling Algorithm for Dependable Safety-Critical Wireless Sensor Network Systems. *Sensors*, 24(6), 1928.

[16] Goswami, A.D., Bhavekar, G.S. and Chafle, P.V. (2023). Electrocardiogram signal classification using VGGNet: A neural network based classification model. *International Journal of Information Technology*, 15(1), 119–28.

[17] Maach, A., Mazoudi, E., Houssine, E., Elalami, J. and Elalami, N. (2024). An Ensemble Dynamic Model and Bio-Inspired Feature Selection Method-based Decision Support System for Predicting Multiple Organ Dysfunction Syndrome in the ICU. *International Journal of Advanced Computer Science & Applications*, 15(2).

[18] Młyńczak, M. and Cybulski, G. (Feb. 2017). Decomposition of the cardiac and respiratory components from impedance pneumography signals. *In: International Conference on Bio-inspired Systems and Signal Processing*, 5, 26–33. SCITEPRESS.

[19] Lima, R., de Noronha Osório, D.F. and Gamboa, H. (Feb. 2019). Heart Rate Variability and Electrodermal Activity in Mental Stress Aloud: Predicting the Outcome. *In: Biosignals* (pp. 42–51). SciTePress.

[20] Canento, F., Lourenço, A., Silva, H. and Fred, A. (Feb. 2013). On real time ECG segmentation algorithms for biometric applications. *In: International Conference on Bio-inspired Systems and Signal Processing*, 2, 228–35. SciTePress.

[21] Lima, B.M.R., Ramos, L.C.S., de Oliveira, T.E.A., da Fonseca, V.P. and Petriu, E.M. (2019). Heart rate detection using a multimodal tactile sensor and a z-score based peak detection algorithm. *CMBES Proceedings*, 42.

[22] Eleftherakis, G., Baxhaku, F. and Vasilescu, A. (Nov. 2022). Bio-inspired Adaptive Architecture for Wireless Sensor Networks. *In: Proceedings of the 26th Pan-Hellenic Conference on Informatics* (pp. 116–22).

[23] Alfeo, A.L., Barsocchi, P., Cimino, M.G., La Rosa, D., Palumbo, F. and Vaglini, G. (2018). Sleep behaviour assessment via smartwatch and stigmergic receptive fields. *Personal and Ubiquitous Computing*, 22, 227–43.

[24] Ashwini, A. and Murugan, S. (2020) Automatic Skin Tumour Segmentation Using Prioritized Patch Based Region: A Novel Comparative Technique. *IETE Journal of Research*, 66, 1–12.

[25] Sathyanarayana, S., Satzoda, R.K., Sathyanarayana, S. and Thambipillai, S. (2018). Vision-based patient monitoring: A comprehensive review of algorithms and technologies. *Journal of Ambient Intelligence and Humanized Computing*, 9, 225–51.

[26] Lima, B.M.R., de Oliveira, T.E.A., da Fonseca, V.P., Zhu, Q., Goubran, M., Groza, V.Z. and Petriu, E.M. (Jun. 2019). Heart rate detection using a miniaturized multimodal tactile sensor. *In: 2019 IEEE International Symposium on Medical Measurements and Applications (MeMeA)* (pp. 1–6). IEEE.

[27] Lima, B.M.R., de Oliveira, T.E.A., da Fonseca, V.P., Zhu, Q., Goubran, M., Groza, V.Z. and Petriu, E.M. (Jun. 2019). Heart rate detection using a miniaturized multimodal tactile sensor. *In: 2019 IEEE International Symposium on Medical Measurements and Applications (MeMeA)* (pp. 1–6). IEEE.

[28] Lourenço, A., Silva, H., Leite, P., Lourenço, R. and Fred, A.L. (2012, February). Real Time Electrocardiogram Segmentation for Finger-based ECG Biometrics. *In: Biosignals* (pp. 49–54).

[29] Javaid, Mohd, Abid Haleem, Ravi Pratap Singh and Rajiv Suman. (2023). 5G technology for healthcare: Features, serviceable pillars, and applications. *Intelligent Pharmacy*, $1(1)$, 2–10.

[30] Mahmud, M.S., Wang, H., Esfar-E-Alam, A.M. and Fang, H. (2017). A wireless health monitoring system using mobile phone accessories. *IEEE Internet of Things Journal*, $4(6)$, 2009–18.

[31] Zaunseder, S., Aipperspach, W. and Poll, R. (2010, January). Discrimination between Ischemic and Heart-rate Related ST-Episodes-Nonlinear Classification for an Online Capable Approach. *In: International Conference on Bio-inspired Systems and Signal Processing*, 2, 245-251. SCITEPRESS.

[32] Lourenço, A., Silva, H., Santos, D.P. and Fred, A. (Jan. 2011). Towards a finger based ECG biometric system. *In: International Conference on Bio-inspired Systems and Signal Processing*, 2, 348–53. SciTePress.

[33] Nguyen, L.N., Casado, C.Á., Cañellas, M.L., Mukherjee, A., Nguyen, N., Jayagopi, D.B. and López, M.B. (2024). Multi-objective Feature Selection in Remote Health Monitoring Applications. *arXiv preprint arXiv:2401.05538*.

[34] Sarmah, S.S. (2020). An efficient IoT-based patient monitoring and heart disease prediction system using deep learning modified neural network. *IEEE Access*, 8, 135784–135797.

[35] Balasubramaniam, S., Joe, C.V., Manthiramoorthy, C. and Kumar, K.S. (2024). Relief-based feature selection and Gradient Squirrel Search Algorithm enabled Deep Maxout Network for detection of heart disease. *Biomedical Signal Processing and Control*, 87, 105446.

[36] Subbiah, S.S. and Chinnappan, J. (2022). A review of bio-inspired computational intelligence algorithms in electricity load forecasting. *Smart Buildings Digitalization*, 169–92.

[37] Choudhury, A., Balasubramaniam, S., Kumar, A.P. and Kumar, S.N.P. (2023). PSSO: Political squirrel search optimizer-driven deep learning for severity level detection and classification of lung cancer. *International Journal of Information Technology & Decision Making*, 1–34.

6 Bio-Inspired Algorithms-based Machine Learning and Deep Learning Models for Covid-19 Diagnosis

S. Sheik Asraf,[1*] M. Subash,[1] P. Nagaraj,[2] V. Muneeswaran[3] and Christopher Samuel Raj Balraj[4]

Severe Acute Respiratory Syndrome Coronavirus 2 causes COVID-19, which leads to many health issues. Most individuals recovered from insignificant to modest infections deprived of needing supplementary care. However, a tiny proportion may require medical attention. COVID-19 can affect anyone at any age, and understanding the illness and its diagnosis is crucial for reducing its spread. Bio-inspired optimization algorithms utilize biology, evolution, and specific behaviours of real organisms to address optimization issues across various application domains. Machine learning (ML) remains a field that uses information and computational processes to enhance the accuracy of artificial intelligence (AI) by replicating human learning processes over time. Deep learning (DL) is an ML subfield that engages neural networks (NN) to feign the intricate executive processes of the brain of *Homo sapiens*. Bio-inspired methods based on ML models, like DT, RF, LR, NB, KNN, and SVM, may be useful in the COVID-19 diagnosis. Bio-inspired algorithms (BIAs), as well as autoencoders based on DL models, SOMs, DBNs, RBFNs, CNNs, LSTMs, RNNs, GANs, and MLPs, have significantly aided in the COVID-19 diagnosis. The difficulties and prospects of applying BIAs to DL and ML models for the diagnosis of COVID-19 will be covered in detail in this chapter.

1. Introduction

SARS-CoV-2 virus, which causes lung infections and serious disease, is the source of COVID-19. Most individuals convalesce from insignificant to modest infections without needing supplementary therapeutic consideration. A miniscule

---

[1] Department of Biotechnology, School of Bio, Chemical and Processing Engineering, Kalasalingam Academy of Research and Education (Deemed to be University), Anand Nagar, Krishnankoil, Tamil Nadu, India.

[2] Department of Computer Science and Engineering, School of Computing, Kalasalingam Academy of Research and Education (Deemed to be University), Anand Nagar, Krishnankoil, Tamil Nadu, India.

[3] Department of Electronics and Communication Engineering, School of Electronics, Electrical and Biomedical Technology, Kalasalingam Academy of Research and Education (Deemed to be University), Anand Nagar, Krishnankoil, Tamil Nadu, India.

[4] International College of the Cayman Islands, Grand Cayman, Cayman Islands.

* Corresponding author: ssasraf@gmail.com and s.sheikasraf@klu.ac.in

percentage, nevertheless, might need medical care, especially in the elderly and those with underlying medical issues. Anyone at any age can contract COVID-19, and defence and containment of the virus depend on an awareness of the disease and its diagnosis. Bio-inspired optimization algorithms are techniques that draw inspiration from biology, evolution, and particular behaviours of real organisms to solve optimization issues in a range of application domains. Within the fields of computer science and artificial intelligence (AI), machine learning (ML) focuses on leveraging data and algorithms to replicate human learning processes in AI systems, hence improving their accuracy over time.

Deep learning (DL) is a branch of ML that imitates the complicated administrative processes of the brain of *H. sapiens* using multifaceted neural networks (NN). Bio-inspired methods based on ML models, like DT, RF, LR, NB, KNN, and SVM may be useful in the COVID-19 diagnosis. BIAs as well as autoencoders based on DL models, SOMs, DBNs, RBFNs, CNNs, LSTMs, RNNs, GANs, and MLPs have significantly aided in the diagnosis of COVID-19. This chapter delves into the challenges and potentials of incorporating Bio-Inspired algorithms (BIAs) into DL and ML models for the diagnosis of COVID-19.

2. COVID-19: A Worldwide Contagion

World Health Organization has classified the COVID-19 as a pandemic due to its high death toll and widespread SARS-CoV-2 spread [Figure 1] [1].

Over the past half-century, numerous viruses have surfaced, impacting various regions and nations; nonetheless, COVID-19 is one of the most widely dispersed global viruses [2]. Around the world, several countries are retorting to the COVID-19 contagion in various ways. Countries like China have experienced a lag in identification and response, overtaxing local health systems in the process. But in some other nations, effective containment procedures have meant that comparatively few cases have been documented since the pandemics began [3]. It has come to light that the COVID-19 outbreak is far more extensive and persistent than many first thought. There is still much to discover about the massive toll the epidemic has had on all patients, COVID-19 positive and negative, even after it has been going on for four years [4].

WHO classified COVID-19 as a pandemic [5]. While life expectancy has risen a few months annually in several countries over the past few decades, new data indicates that the COVID-19 pandemic will cause these trends to abruptly cease in many different countries [6]. The sole method of treatment, despite the accumulation of a substantial amount of scientific data, is the therapeutic management of COVID-19 via supportive care [7]. The world is in a state of flux. The COVID-19 epidemic may have a very high human cost. The pandemic necessitates taking numerous steps, including testing, treatment, and prevention [8]. The COVID-19 pandemic has highlighted the potential harm of emerging infectious disorders globally [9]. Researchers have rapidly gathered information on viral entry, dominant mutations, transmission routes, diagnostic targets, therapeutic

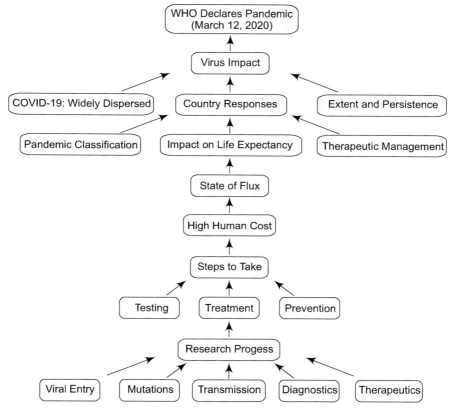

Fig. 1 Covid-19: A worldwide contagion.

targets, drug molecules, cross-neutralizing antibodies, and vaccine candidates for COVID-19 prevention [10].

3. Bio-Inspired Algorithms: An overview

BIAs are needed to quickly handle exceedingly complex problems [Figure 2]. This is particularly true when working with issues that have changing constraints, incomplete or inaccurate information, dynamic problem definitions, and constrained processing power. BIAs include NN, evolutionary algorithm [EA], bacterial foraging optimization algorithm [BFOA], cuckoo search optimization algorithm [CSOA], firefly optimization algorithm [FFOA], shuffled frog leaping algorithm [SFLA], bat algorithm [BA], flower pollination algorithm [FPA] and artificial plant optimization algorithm [APOA] [11]. BIAs use computer architectures that are modelled after natural phenomena or biosystems. These tactics provide sufficient information to develop high-performance computing methods and intelligent paradigms that can handle intricate formulations [12]. The four types of BIAs are ecology-based, swarm intelligence-based, multi-objective, and evolutionary-based [13]. BIAs are useful techniques for optimization. Since the current BIAs can solve the challenges, the most effective and ideal way would be to use an algorithm based on sentient animals such as humans, chimpanzees, or dolphins [14]. BIAs can effectively tackle multi-dimensional nonlinear issues, such as those generally encountered in biosignal investigation [15].

Finding sound, workable solutions to combinatorial optimization problems in reality is challenging because these problems frequently have ambiguous parameters, dynamic limits, heterogeneous solution representations, and precedence constraints. Randomized techniques, like BIAs, can be used to quickly solve incomprehensible combinatorial problems. BIAs employ naturalistic operators to address a range of problems [16]. They imitate certain essential elements of the neo-Darwinian evolutionary process [17]. Researchers are motivated to seek and create practical techniques for locating and optimizing the solutions to complicated optimization problems through BIAs due to the growing complexity of real-life challenges [18]. BIAs are inspired by the swarm behaviours of various animal groups, including fish schools, sheep herds, bee colonies, and bird flocks. These groups, along with insects such as bees, ants, and mosquitoes, often demonstrate remarkable abilities to solve intricate issues that appear to be much beyond their reach [19].

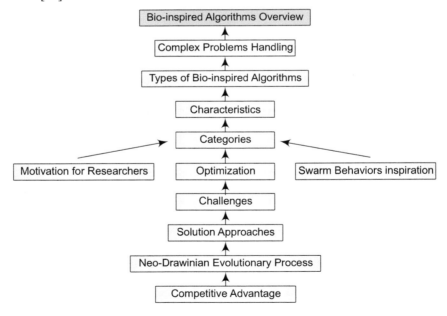

Fig. 2 Bio-Inspired Algorithms: An outline.

BIAs draw inspiration from biological processes found in nature to compete with competitor approaches of today. Complex scientific and technical problems can be solved as best they can be when ML techniques are combined with an algorithm that draws inspiration from biology [20].

4. Machine Learning: An Overview

ML [Figure 3] acquires data from its environment [21]. New learning theories and algorithms, as well as the ongoing spread of inexpensive computing and internet data, have all contributed to recent developments in ML [22].

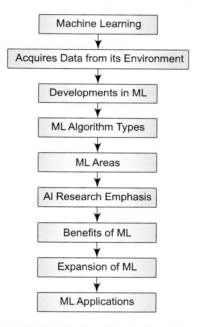

Fig. 3 Machine Learning: An Overview.

The primary benefit of ML is that it can operate autonomously once they figure out what to do with the data [23]. Common ML algorithm types include supervised [SV], unsupervised [US], semi-supervised [SS], reinforcement [RF], transduction [TD], and learning to learn [LTL] [24]. The main emphasis of AI research is ML [25]. ML can be divided into four main areas: (i) learning ensembles of classifiers to increase classification accuracy; (ii) scaling SV learning algorithms; (iii) reinforcement learning; and (iv) learning sophisticated stochastic models [26]. ML allows computers to mimic human behaviour, generating learning tools for future use from conversations and actions [27]. Over the past 50 years, ML has expanded due to computer engineers' curiosity and a neglected statistical discipline. It has created learning algorithms for computer vision, and speech recognition, and generated fundamental statistical-computational theories, boosting the data mining industry by uncovering hidden patterns [28]. Without explicit instructions, ML gathers broad principles from observed cases [29]. ML involves two aspects: a computer system that can perform classification and prediction tasks, and a heavily automated process that minimizes human involvement. The goal is to reduce human biases and improve algorithm performance and selection [30].

5. Deep Learning: An Overview

DL techniques in computational models [Figure 4] improve performance in fields like drug discovery and genomics, enhancing speech recognition, visual object recognition, and object detection [31].

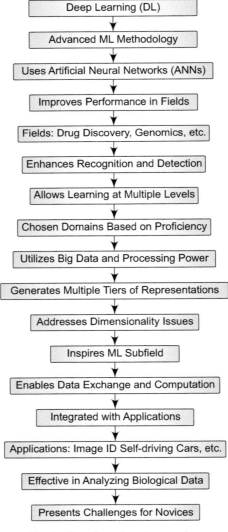

Fig. 4 Deep Learning: An overview.

DL is an advanced ML methodology that performs better than existing approaches by allowing models to learn features at several levels and progressively from unstructured input [32]. DL application domains are chosen based on the authors' proficiency, including computer vision, speech recognition, multimodal processing, information retrieval, and natural language processing [33]. DL, an ML branch, utilizes artificial neural networks (ANNs) to model sophisticated data concepts, gaining popularity because of its skill to leverage big data volumes and processing power [34]. DL, a more advanced method than traditional ML, is increasingly being utilized in academic research due to its practicality [35].

DL is an ML technique that automatically generates multiple tiers of representations of the underlying distribution of data [36]. DL uses a two-stage learning strategy to extract robust features from data, addressing the issue of dimensionality in shallow systems like the support vector machine (SVM) [37]. ANNs, which use synthetic neurons and synapses that resemble human brains, are the source of inspiration for the ML subfield recognized as DL. These NNs enable data exchange and computation by matching input, output, node, and interconnections [38]. DL draws interest from researchers because it improves predictive capability in computer devices with massive data and improved algorithms. ML is integrated with applications including image identification, object detection, self-driving cars, drug development, and disease diagnosis [39]. DL, a popular AI technique, is effective in analysing and categorizing biological data, but it presents significant challenges for those unfamiliar with it [40].

6. Applications of Bio-Inspired Algorithms-based ML Models for COVID-19 Diagnosis

BIAs [Figure 5] based on ML models, like DT, RF, LR, NB, KNN, and SVM are applied in the COVID-19 diagnosis process (Table 1).

Table 1 Bio-Inspired Algorithms-based ML models for COVID-19 diagnosis.

S. No.	Bio-Inspired Algorithms-based Machine Learning Models	References
1.	LR, SVM, ANN, KNN, K-MEANS, RF, BOOST, LDA	[41]
2.	SVM, XG-BOOST	[42]
3.	SVM	[44]
4.	NN, RF, BOOST, LR, SVM	[45]
5.	SVM, RF	[47]
6.	SVM, ANN, KNN	[48]
7.	XG-BOOST	[49]
8.	IBk, MLP, NBC, SVM	[50]

SVM is the furthermost extensively used ML method for the diagnosis of COVID-19 [41]. ML techniques can significantly aid in COVID-19 diagnosis by dispensing X-ray images of the chest [42]. ML can support the identification of COVID-19 patients, especially when Xray pictures of the chest are necessary [43]. Most ML algorithms used in the diagnosis of COVID-19 are SV learning techniques [44]. Recently, five ML algorithms were applied to an arbitrary model of 70% of COVID-19 patients. The algorithms' performance was then assessed using 30% of newly collected, unseen COVID-19 data [45].

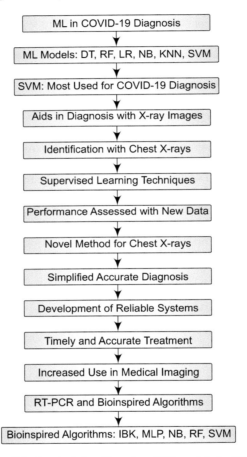

Fig. 5 Applications of Bio-Inspired algorithms-based ML models for COVID-19 diagnosis.

A novel ML method has been proposed for studying x-ray pictures of chests of COVID-19 patients [46]. ML techniques have significantly simplified the accurate diagnosis of COVID-19 in X-ray pictures of the chest [47]. ML techniques, including SVM, ANN, and KNN, can be used to develop reliable COVID-19 diagnosis systems, enabling timely and accurate treatment and patient management [48]. ML is being increasingly utilized for the diagnosis of COVID-19 using medical imaging [49]. RT-PCR has been successfully used for diagnosis of COVID-19 using five bio-inspired ML algorithms: IBk, MLP, NB, RF, and SVM [50].

Bio-Inspired Algorithms-based Machine Learning and Deep Learning Models for Covid-19 Diagnosis | 115

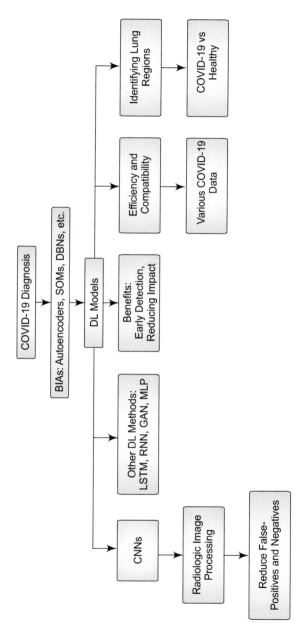

Fig. 6 Applications of Bio-Inspired algorithms-based DL models for COVID-19 diagnosis.

7. Applications of Bio-Inspired Algorithms-based DL Models for COVID-19 Diagnosis

COVID-19 diagnosis has greatly benefited from BIAs, such as autoencoders based on DL models, SOMs, DBNs, RBFNs, CNNs, LSTMs, RNNs, GANs, and MLPs (Figure 6; Table 2).

Table 2   Bio-Inspired algorithms-based DL models for COVID-19 diagnosis.

S. No.	Bio-Inspired Algorithms-based Deep Learning Models	References
1.	CNN, LSTM, GAN	[51]
2.	CNN, LSTM, GAN	[52]
3.	CNN, GAN	[53]
4.	CNN	[55]
5.	CNN, LSTM, RNN, GAN	[56]
6.	SOM, DBN, RBFN, CNN, LSTM, RNN, GAN, and MLP	[57]

Advanced computational methods like DL can aid in early COVID-19 patient detection, potentially reducing the virus's impact [51]. Convolutional neural networks (CNNs) are the furthermost frequently utilized DL architecture for diagnosing and classifying COVID-19 symptoms from X-ray pictures of the chest [52].

DL is being utilized to reduce false-positive and negative errors in COVID-19 radiologic image processing, thereby enabling secure, rapid, and cost-effective diagnostic services for patients [53]. DL techniques utilizing AI have been extensively utilized for the COVID-19 diagnosis [54]. DL techniques are continuously evolving, becoming more efficient and compatible with various types of COVID-19 data and diagnosis research [55]. Regional DL approaches are being used to identify lung regions infested by COVID-19, classifying them into COVID-19 and healthy individuals [56]. DL methods like Extreme Learning Machines (ELM), long short-term memory (LSTM), and generational adversarial networks (GANs) have been proven effective in diagnosing COVID-19 [57].

8. Challenges and Future Prospects of Bio-Inspired Algorithms-based ML and DL Models for COVID-19 Diagnosis

The laboratory identification of infections presents several difficulties [58]. RT-qPCR techniques used to diagnose COVID-19 have varying sensitivity and specificity, but some protocols have produced questionable test results, highlighting potential difficulties [59]. The entire analytical procedure for COVID-19 diagnosis, including sample gathering, treatment, viral ribonucleic acid amplification (RT-PCR), recognition, medical sensitivity, and specificity authentication, presents challenges [60]. The capacity to distinguish COVID-19 from unrelated viral pneumonia, the availability of public datasets, the cleanliness of the dataset, and the challenge of addressing issues from several perspectives are all obstacles [61] (Figure 7).

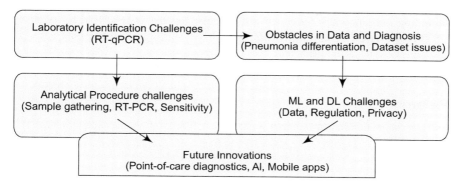

Fig. 7 Challenges and future prospects of Bio-Inspired algorithms-based ML and DL models for COVID-19 diagnosis.

ML and DL must overcome obstacles like regulation, lack of large-scale training data, noisy data, expertise in computer science and medicine, data privacy, incorrect structural data, early diagnosis using medical imaging, screening, triaging, finding therapies, risk assessments, and medical resource planning [62]. Future work will need to address new ML issues for the diagnosis of COVID-19 based on body fluid testing. In the future, point-of-care diagnostics will become more common due to the integration of lateral flow assays, AI, and state-of-the-art molecular diagnostics. This will be particularly valid in the case that worldwide pandemics such as COVID-19 occur [63]. Mobile apps that use a range of visual data and clinical symptoms will be crucial for prompt diagnosis during pandemics in the future [64].

AI models' ability to adapt to virus changes underscores their potential as a crucial technology for enhancing global health infrastructure [65] adaptability during pandemics and other epidemics [66-68].

Conclusion

SARS-CoV-2 virus causes lung infections and other serious disorders and is the source of COVID-19. After mild to moderate diseases, most patients recover without the need for further care. Only a very tiny portion, though, especially in the elderly and those with underlying medical issues, may need medical attention. COVID-19 can infect people of any age, and understanding the disease and how to diagnose it is essential to both preventing and controlling the virus. Bio-inspired optimization algorithms are techniques that use biological principles, evolutionary dynamics, and particular behaviours of real-world organisms as inspiration to solve optimization problems in a range of application domains.

ML is the study of how to use data and algorithms to simulate human learning processes in AI, hence improving AI accuracy over time. DL is a subfield of ML that uses multidimensional NNs to feign the intricate administrative processes of the brain of *Homo sapiens*. Bio-inspired methods based on ML models, like DT, RF, LR, NB, KNN, and SVM, may be useful for COVID-19 diagnosis. BIAs, including autoencoders based on DL models, SOMs, DBNs, RBFNs, CNNs, LSTMs, RNNs, GANs, and MLPs, have been significant in the diagnosis of COVID-19. The difficulties and opportunities of combining BIAs with DL and ML models for the diagnosis of COVID-19 were fully covered.

References

[1] Ciotti, M., Ciccozzi, M., Terrinoni, A., Jiang, W.C., Wang, C.B. and Bernardini, S. (2020). The COVID-19 pandemic. *Critical Reviews in Clinical Laboratory Sciences*, 57(6), 365–88.

[2] Suryasa, I.W., Rodríguez-Gámez, M. and Koldoris, T. (2021). The COVID-19 pandemic. *International Journal of Health Sciences*, 5(2).

[3] Khanna, R.C., Cicinelli, M.V., Gilbert, S.S., Honavar, S.G. and Murthy, G.V. (2020). COVID-19 pandemic: Lessons learned and future directions. *Indian Journal of Ophthalmology*, 68(5), 703–10.

[4] Myers, L.C. and Liu, V.X. (2022). The COVID-19 pandemic strikes again and again and again. *JAMA Network Open*, 5(3), e221760–e221760.

[5] Spinelli, A. and Pellino, G. (2020). COVID-19 pandemic: Perspectives on an unfolding crisis. *Journal of British Surgery*, 107(7), 785–87.

[6] Burdorf, A., Porru, F. and Rugulies, R. (2021). The COVID-19 pandemic. *Scandinavian Journal of Work, Environment and Health*, 47(4), 245–47.

[7] Mishra, S.K. and Tripathi, T. (2021). One year update on the COVID-19 pandemic: Where are we now? *Acta Tropica*, 214, 105778.

[8] Tabish, S.A. (2020). COVID-19 pandemic: Emerging perspectives and future trends. *Journal of Public Health Research*, 9(1).

[9] Balkhair, A.A. (2020). COVID-19 pandemic: A new chapter in the history of infectious diseases. *Oman Medical Journal*, 35(2), e123.

[10] Kumar, A., Singh, R., Kaur, J., Pandey, S., Sharma, V., Thakur, L., ... and Kumar, N. (2021). Wuhan to world: The COVID-19 pandemic. *Frontiers in Cellular and Infection Microbiology*, 11, 596201.

[11] Kar, A.K. (2016). Bio-inspired computing: A review of algorithms and scope of applications. *Expert Systems with Applications*, 59, 20–32.

[12] Cuevas, E., Oliva, D. and Osuna, V. (2020). Bio-inspired algorithms and Bio-systems. *Mathematical Biosciences and Engineering*, 17(3), 2400–2402.

[13] Fan, X., Sayers, W., Zhang, S., Han, Z., Ren, L. and Chizari, H. (2020). Review and classification of bio-inspired algorithms and their applications. *Journal of Bionic Engineering*, 17, 611–31.

[14] Pazhaniraja, N., Paul, P.V., Roja, G., Shanmugapriya, K. and Sonali, B. (Mar. 2017). A study on recent bio-inspired optimization algorithms. *In*: 2017 *Fourth International Conference on Signal Processing, Communication, and Networking* (*ICSCN*) (pp. 1–6). IEEE.

[15] Wario, F., Avalos, O. and Gálvez, J. (2022). Bio-inspired algorithms. *In*: *Biosignal Processing and Classification Using Computational Learning and Intelligence* (pp. 225–48). Academic Press.

[16] Assimi, H. (2023). *Application of Bio-inspired Algorithms to Selected Real-World Problems* (Doctoral dissertation). University of Adelaide.

[17] Wagner, M. (2013). *Theory and Applications of Bio-inspired Algorithms*. (Doctoral dissertation). University of Adelaide.

[18] Almufti, S., Marqas, R. and Ashqi, V. (2019). Taxonomy of bio-inspired optimization algorithms. *Journal of Advanced Computer Science & Technology*, 8(2), 23.

[19] Duan, H., Li, P., Li, P. and Duan, H. (2014). Bio-inspired computation algorithms. *In: Bio-inspired Computation in Unmanned Aerial Vehicles*, 35–69. Springer Link.

[20] Boopalan, K., Shanmuganathan, C., Lokeshwaran, K. and Balaji, T. (2022). A Short Overview on Various Bio-Inspired Algorithms. Machine Learning in Information and Communication Technology. *Proceedings of ICICT 2021, SMIT*, 295–301.

[21] El Naqa, I. and Murphy, M.J. (2015). *What is Machine Learning?* (pp. 3–11). Springer International Publishing.

[22] Jordan, M.I. and Mitchell, T.M. (2015). Machine learning: Trends, perspectives, and prospects. *Science*, 349(6245), 255–60.

[23] Mahesh, B. (2020). Machine learning algorithms: A review. *International Journal of Science and Research (IJSR)*. [Internet], 9(1), 381–86.

[24] Ayodele, T.O. (2010). Types of machine learning algorithms. Chapter 3, *In*: Y. Zhang (Ed.) *New Advances in Machine Learning*, (pp. 19–48). InTechOpen.

[25] Wang, H., Ma, C. and Zhou, L. (2009, December). A brief review of machine learning and its application. *In: 2009 International Conference on Information Engineering and Computer Science* (pp. 1–4). IEEE.

[26] Dietterich, T.G. (1997). Machine-learning research. *AI Magazine*, 18(4), 97–136.

[27] Alzubi, J., Nayyar, A. and Kumar, A. (Nov. 2018). Machine learning from theory to algorithms: An overview. *In: Journal of Physics: Conference Series, 1142*, 012012. IOP Publishing.

[28] Mitchell, T.M. (2006). The discipline of machine learning (Vol. 9, p. 3). Pittsburgh: Carnegie Mellon University, School of Computer Science, Machine Learning Department.

[29] Bzdok, D., Krzywinski, M. and Altman, N. (2017). Machine learning: A primer. *Nature Methods*, 14(12), 1119.

[30] Tarca, A.L., Carey, V.J., Chen, X.W., Romero, R. and Drăghici, S. (2007). Machine learning and its applications to biology. *PLoS Computational Biology*, 3(6), e116.

[31] LeCun, Y., Bengio, Y. and Hinton, G. (2015). Deep learning. *Nature*, 521(7553), 436–44.

[32] Mathew, A., Amudha, P. and Sivakumari, S. (2021). Deep learning techniques: An overview. *Advanced Machine Learning Technologies and Applications: Proceedings of AMLTA 2020*, 599–608.

[33] Deng, L. and Yu, D. (2014). Deep learning: Methods and applications. *Foundations and Trends® in Signal Processing*, 7(3–4), 197–387.

[34] Hao, X., Zhang, G. and Ma, S. (2016). Deep learning. *International Journal of Semantic Computing*, 10(03), 417–439.

[35] Du, X., Cai, Y., Wang, S. and Zhang, L. (Nov. 2016). Overview of deep learning. *In: 2016 31st Youth Academic Annual Conference of Chinese Association of Automation (YAC)* (pp. 159–64). IEEE.

[36] Lauzon, F.Q. (Jul. 2012). An introduction to deep learning. *In: 2012 11th International Conference on Information Science, Signal Processing, and their Applications (ISSPA)* (pp. 1438–39). IEEE.

[37] Arnold, L., Rebecchi, S., Chevallier, S. and Paugam-Moisy, H. (Apr. 2011). An introduction to deep learning. *In: European Symposium on Artificial Neural Networks (ESANN)*, Bruges. *1*, 477–88.

[38] Kim, H. (2022). Deep learning. *In: Artificial Intelligence for 6G* (pp. 247–303). Cham: Springer International Publishing.

[39] Khan, M., Jan, B., Farman, H., Ahmad, J., Farman, H. and Jan, Z. (2019). Deep learning methods and applications. *In: Deep Learning: Convergence to Big Data Analytics*, 31–42. Spinger Link.

[40] Webb, S. (2018). Deep learning for biology. *Nature, 554*(7693), 555–57.

[41] Alyasseri, Z.A.A., Al-Betar, M.A., Doush, I.A., Awadallah, M.A., Abasi, A.K., Makhadmeh, S.N., ... and Zitar, R.A. (2022). Review on COVID-19 diagnosis models based on machine learning and deep learning approaches. *Expert Systems, 39*(3), e12759.

[42] Mondal, M.R.H., Bharati, S. and Podder, P. (2021). Diagnosis of COVID-19 using machine learning and deep learning: A review. *Current Medical Imaging, 17*(12), 1403–18.

[43] Dabbagh, R., Jamal, A., Temsah, M.H., Masud, J.H.B., Titi, M., Amer, Y., ... and Hneiny, L. (2021). Machine learning models for predicting diagnosis or prognosis of COVID-19: A systematic review. *Computer Methods and Programs in Biomedicine, 205*, 105993.

[44] Alballa, N. and Al-Turaiki, I. (2021). Machine learning approaches in COVID-19 diagnosis, mortality, and severity risk prediction: A review. *Informatics in Medicine Unlocked, 24*, 100564.

[45] de Moraes Batista, A.F., Miraglia, J.L., Rizzi Donato, T.H. and Porto Chiavegatto Filho, A.D. (2020). COVID-19 diagnosis prediction in emergency care patients: A machine learning approach. *MedRxiv, 2020*(04).

[46] Elaziz, M.A., Hosny, K.M., Salah, A., Darwish, M.M., Lu, S. and Sahlol, A.T. (2020). New machine learning method for image-based diagnosis of COVID-19. *PloS One, 15*(6), e0235187.

[47] Mohammad-Rahimi, H., Nadimi, M., Ghalyanchi-Langeroudi, A., Taheri, M. and Ghafouri-Fard, S. (2021). Application of machine learning in diagnosis of COVID-19 through X-ray and CT images: A scoping review. *Frontiers in Cardiovascular Medicine, 8*, 638011.

[48] Salman, A.O. and Geman, O. (2023). Evaluating three machine learning classification methods for effective COVID-19 diagnosis. *International Journal of Mathematics, Statistics, and Computer Science, 1*, 1–14.

[49] Moura, L.V.D., Mattjie, C., Dartora, C.M., Barros, R.C. and Marques da Silva, A.M. (2022). Explainable machine learning for COVID-19 pneumonia classification with texture-based features extraction in chest radiography. *Frontiers in Digital Health, 3*, 662343.

[50] Gomes, J.C., Masood, A.I., Silva, L.H.D.S., da Cruz Ferreira, J.R.B., Freire Junior, A.A., Rocha, A.L.D.S., ... AND Dos Santos, W.P. (2021). COVID-19 diagnosis by combining RT-PCR and pseudo-convolutional machines to characterize virus sequences. *Scientific Reports, 11*(1), 11545.

[51] Siddiqui, S., Arifeen, M., Hopgood, A., Good, A., Gegov, A., Hossain, E., ... and Masum, S. (2022). Deep learning models for the diagnosis and screening of COVID-19: A systematic review. *SN Computer Science, 3*(5), 397.

[52] Ghaderzadeh, M. and Asadi, F. (2021). Deep learning in the detection and diagnosis of COVID-19 using radiology modalities: A systematic review. *Journal of Healthcare Engineering, 2021*.

[53] Aslani, S. and Jacob, J. (2023). Utilisation of deep learning for COVID-19 diagnosis. *Clinical Radiology, 78*(2), 150–57.

[54] Capuozzo, S. and Sansone, C. (Sep. 2023). A Systematic Review of Multimodal Deep Learning Approaches for COVID-19 Diagnosis. *In: International Conference on Image Analysis and Processing* (pp. 140–51). Cham: Springer Nature Switzerland.

[55] Bhuyan, H.K., Chakraborty, C., Shelke, Y. abd Pani, S.K. (2022). COVID-19 diagnosis system by deep learning approaches. *Expert Systems, 39*(3), e12776.

[56] Jamshidi, M., Lalbakhsh, A., Talla, J., Peroutka, Z., Hadjilooei, F., Lalbakhsh, P., ... and Mohyuddin, W. (2020). Artificial intelligence and COVID-19: Deep learning approaches for diagnosis and treatment. *IEEE Access, 8*, 109581–109595.

[57] Heidari, A., Navimipour, N.J., Unal, M. and Toumaj, S. (2022). The COVID-19 epidemic analysis and diagnosis using deep learning: A systematic literature review and future directions. *Computers in Biology and Medicine, 141*, 105141.

[58] Tang, Y.W., Schmitz, J.E., Persing, D.H. and Stratton, C.W. (May, 2020). Laboratory diagnosis of COVID-19: Current issues and challenges. *Journal of Clinical Microbiology, 58*(6), e00512. doi:10.1128/CM00512-20.

[59] Sule, W.F. and Oluwayelu, D.O. (2020). Real-time RT-PCR for COVID-19 diagnosis: Challenges and Prospects. *The Pan African Medical Journal, 35*(Suppl 2).

[60] Feng, W., Newbigging, A.M., Le, C., Pang, B., Peng, H., Cao, Y., ... and Le, X.C. (2020). Molecular diagnosis of COVID-19: Challenges and Research Needs. *Analytical Chemistry, 92*(15), 10196–10209.

[61] Alaufi, R., Kalkatawi, M. and Abukhodair, F. (2024). Challenges of deep learning diagnosis for COVID-19 from chest imaging. *Multimedia Tools and Applications, 83*(5), 14337–61.

[62] Alafif, T., Tehame, A.M., Bajaba, S., Barnawi, A. and Zia, S. (2021). Machine and deep learning towards COVID-19 diagnosis and treatment: Survey, challenges, and future directions. *International Journal of Environmental Research and Public Health, 18*(3), 1117.

[63] Sharma, A., Balda, S., Apreja, M., Kataria, K., Capalash, N. and Sharma, P. (2021). COVID-19 diagnosis: Current and future techniques. *International Journal of Biological Macromolecules, 193*, 1835–44.

[64] Gheisari, M., Ghaderzadeh, M., Li, H., Taami, T., Fernández-Campusano, C., Sadeghsalehi, H. and Afzaal Abbasi, A. (2024). Mobile Apps for COVID-19 Detection and Diagnosis for Future Pandemic Control: Multidimensional Systematic Review. *JMIR mHealth and uHealth, 12*, e44406.

[65] Balasubramaniam, S., Satheesh Kumar, K., Kavitha, V., Prasanth, A. and Sivakumar, T.A. (2022). Feature selection and dwarf mongoose optimization enabled deep learning for heart disease detection. *Computational Intelligence and Neuroscience, 2022*(1), 2819378.

[66] Muthumeenakshi, R., Singh, C., Sapkale, P.V. and Mukhedkar, M.M. (2022). An Efficient and Secure Authentication Approach in VANET using Location and Signature-based Services. *Adhoc & Sensor Wireless Networks, 53*.

[67] Muneeswaran, V., Nagaraj, P., Sai, K.P., Kumar, E.A. and Chanakya, S.R. (Aug. 2021.) Enhanced image compression using fractal and tree seed-bio-inspired algorithm. *In: 2021 Second International Conference on Electronics and Sustainable Communication Systems (ICESC)* (pp. 1125–30). IEEE.

[68] Kim, J., Choi, Y.S., Lee, Y.J., Yeo, S.G., Kim, K.W., Kim, M.S., ... and Lee, J. (2024). Limitations of the Cough Sound-based COVID-19 Diagnosis Artificial Intelligence Model and its Future Direction: Longitudinal Observation Study. *Journal of Medical Internet Research, 26*, e51640.

7 Bio-Inspired Intelligence in Early Cancer Detection
A Machine Learning Approach

Ashwini A.,[1*] Balasubramaniam S.[2] and Sundaravadivazhagan B.[3]

Severe Acute Respiratory Syndrome Coronavirus 2 causes COVID-19, which leads Scientists have been encouraged by the need for finding better methods of early cancer detection to explore these root principles of bio-inspired intelligence and machine learning. This chapter focuses on the applications of these two fields – the use of bio-inspired algorithms for improving the early detection of cancer. Bio-inspired intelligence in early cancer diagnosis is defined as taking cues from biological systems and techniques to develop new strategies for early detection of cancer related conditions. This multi-disciplinary approach uses biology, computer science, and engineering to solve the complex challenge of early detection of cancer when treatment is most successful. It begins by introducing the fundamental aspects of bio-inspired intelligence and how these concepts are incorporated in machine learning systems to identify cancer. The chapter focus on swarm intelligence for data clustering, modeling of tumor growth, and medical image applications. Therefore, bio-inspired intelligence will most probably offer inspiration for developing new strategies and techniques as well as algorithms for the early detection of cancer. The scientists, by leveraging on the natural laws governing the biological systems, have the chance to commission the enhancement of the efficacy of the cancer diagnostic which will lead to increased patient outcomes and survival rates.

1. Introduction to Cancer Diagnosis

One of the most important tasks in oncology is cancer diagnosis which focuses on the identification and characterization of malignant tumors. Early identification and accurate assessment of cancer are crucial for treatment and successful patient

---

[1] Department of Electronics and Communication Engineering, Vel Tech Rangarajan Dr. Sagunthala R&D Institute of Science and Technology, Avadi, Chennai, Tamilnadu, India.

[2] School of Computer Science and Engineering, Kerala University of Digital Sciences, Innovation and Technology (Formerly IIITM-K), Digital University Kerala, Thiruvananthapuram, Kerala, India.

[3] Department of Information Technology, University of Technology and Applied Science-AL Mussanah, Oman.

* Corresponding author: a.ashwinivel@gmail.com

management. There are various methods used in cancer diagnosis; they include imaging tests, histopathology, molecular biology, and computational approaches. All these techniques are essential in establishing whether or not a person has cancer, the type of cancer, and the stage of cancer, which is helpful for cancer treatments and prognoses. Historically, the identification of cancer has been primarily based on medical imaging methods, including X-ray, CT, MRI, and ultrasound. These methods help clinicians to see internal images and spot any abnormal masses or lesions. After the questionable area is identified, a biopsy is usually taken, and a pathologist later analyzes the sampled tissue using a microscope [1]. Microscopic examination of tissue samples is still the most reliable way to make cancer diagnosis and it gives much information about the structure of the tumor tissue.

Today, the rapid development of molecular biology methods has profoundly changed cancer diagnostics. Molecular tests for cancer include PCR, NGS, liquid biopsy, which identify genetic alterations, epigenetic markers, or circulating tumor DNA in blood. These molecular diagnostic tools also offer the hope of early cancer detection at a stage when it is not detectable in any imaging studies as well as additional information on the nature and type of tumor under study due to the information about tumors at the genetic and molecular level. This is very important in the area of personalized medicine because this information allows the recognition of the idea of having individual treatment on cancer's characteristics in each patient.

The use of machine learning (ML) and artificial intelligence (AI) in cancer diagnosis is the next frontier in cancer diagnosis in the use of developing AI and ML in diagnosis which would ensure to improve the precision and effectiveness of diagnosis of cancer. ML algorithms are able to search any medical information such as scans, pathology slides and information regarding aberrations to find cancer [2]. One of them is bio-inspired intelligence which exploits mechanisms gained from biological systems to enhance the performance of these algorithms. Through the stimulation of neuronal processes in the brain, evolutionary computation, and artificial immune systems, bio-inspired AI models can provide increased diagnostic accuracy and support early cancer detection and prognosis for improved clinical outcomes and mortality rates.

2. Evolutionary Algorithms in Feature Selection

Evolutionary algorithms (EAs) are one of the types of bio-inspired computational techniques using the principles of natural evolution as a model for problem solving, in the context of feature selection for early cancer detection. In general, EAs have significant applications in feature selection for early cancer detection as they demonstrate a great potential in enhancing the efficiency and accuracy of tumor detection of machine learning (ML) models by selecting the most important features from a pool of features [3]. Here's a detailed explanation of how evolutionary algorithms are applied to feature selection.

2.1 Initialization

This involves generating an initial population of potential solutions referred to as chromosomes or individuals. Each of the chromosome stands for a part of the feature set. Such subsets can be chosen randomly or by some heuristic criteria [4]. For example, in the dataset that has hundreds of features, each chromosome can be presented as a binary vector in which '1' means that the feature is chosen and '0' means that it is not.

2.2 Fitness Evaluation

The next step is to find the fitness of the individual in the population. Accuracy is the fitness of the particular feature set chosen in a classification or prediction problem. This usually entails utilizing the chosen features to train an ML algorithm and then determining how well it works on a validation set. Popular fitness functions for evaluation purposes are accuracy, precision, recall, F1 score, or some combination of these. A high fitness score implies that the given chromosome is associated with a high-performing model for the features chosen.

2.3 Selection

Selection is the process of replacing the old generation with a new one that is derived from the existing population. This step is based on the fitness scores, with better fitter having a higher probability of selection. Suitable methods include roulette wheel selection, tournament selection, or rank-based selection [5]. The aim is to guarantee that good solutions get passed down to the succeeding generation without getting stuck in a local optima due to lack of diversity.

2.4 Crossover (Recombination)

Crossover is another genetic operator that refers to the process of combining the features of two parent individuals to form an offspring. This process is supposed to imitate biological reproduction and would attempt to create a new individual with characteristics from both individuals involved in the reproduction process [6]. Typical examples of crossover operators are single-point crossover, multi-point crossover, and uniform crossover. For example, in single-point crossover, a random point on the parent chromosomes is chosen, and the subsequences following this point are exchanged between two parents, generating two offspring.

2.5 Mutation

Mutation involves introducing random alterations on individual chromosomes to ensure diversity in the population. This step aims at improving the search space and making sure that it does not get trapped in local optima. In the case of the feature selection problem, mutation can be defined as a process of changing one bit of the binary vector, that is, substituting a '1' with a '0', or vice versa [7]. The mutation rate which describes when a given mutation occurs is usually low so that the general form of the good solutions is not destroyed but new variations can be tested.

2.6 Replacement

The replacement process follows crossover and mutation where a decision is made on the evaluation of the new generated individuals as to whether they will form part of the next generation. This step can involve replacing the entire population with the new individuals or a blend of the best individuals from both the current and new populations. Such strategies like elitism where a specific number of the 'fittest' individuals are transferred to the next generation are employed to prevent the algorithm from losing the 'best' solutions [8].

2.7 Termination

The evolutionary process proceeds through the sequence of fitness evaluation, selection, crossover, mutation, and replacement till a stopping condition is satisfied. Typical stopping conditions include reaching a fixed number of generations, reaching a targeted fitness for the population, or failing to see any increase in fitness for a certain number of generations.

3. Genetic Programming (GP) for Model Optimization

GP is an important evolutionary algorithm that is used to describe a computer program optimization based on the genetic algorithms (GAs). GP works on populations of computer programs that usually have tree representation as opposed to GAs which work with parameter vectors of fixed length [9]. Such programs can carry out specified activities or address specific issues; therefore, GP is useful in diverse applications including modeling for optimizing early cancer detection.

3.1 Foundations and Representation

GP is a type of evolutionary algorithm in which solutions are evolved over time through a process that resembles natural selection. The individual or elemental unit of GP is a computer program. These programs are usually depicted in the form of trees where various nodes stand for functions or operations (for instance)—variables, mathematical functions, logical operators, and leaves—represent inputs/variables. This tree-based representation is general since it can represent many different computational structures and solutions [10]. Random permutation is commonly used to generate the first population of all possible programs. Each program is one of the possible solutions of the problem and diversification of the initial population gives a wide field for the evolutionary algorithms to search.

3.2 Fitness Evaluation

The fitness of each program in the population is a critical component in GP. Cross validation is the process of fitness evaluation where each program is run on a training set and the performance is recorded. In the context of cancer detection, a program's strength could be defined as the efficiency with which the program is classifying the samples as cancerous or non-cancerous. Fitness functions can also include other performance parameters like precision, recall, F1 score, or computational speed.

Fitness evaluation serves two main purposes: It offers a framework for classifying programs in terms of their fitness, and it determines the choice of programs to be copied based on their fitness [11]. This performance-based selection is crucial to the evolutionary process as it ensures the effective spread of favorable traits throughout the population.

3.3 Genetic Operations: Selection, Crossover, and Mutation

Genetic operations are the means by which GP progresses the population through subsequent generations.

Selection

Selection deals with the process where individuals are picked from the existing population to reproduce the next generation. Methods like roulette wheel selection, tournament selection, or the rank-based selection are employed to stochastically include higher-fitness individuals in the next population without eliminating diversity completely.

Crossover (Recombination)

Crossover is a reproduction strategy in which parts of two parent programs are mixed together. Crossover in GP mainly involves swapping of sub-trees from each of the parents. For instance, a subtree of one parent performing a particular function or a decision block may be replaced by another subtree from a different parent to thus give rise to new combinations of operations and inputs [12]. This recombination can generate offspring with better traits from their parents and it can be used to generate better solutions.

Mutation

Mutation entails the creation of random alterations to individual programs so as to keep diversity and search for new regions of the solution space. Recombination/ mutation in GP might include changing a node in the tree, e.g., it includes substituting one operator for another (for example, replacing the addition operator with a multiplication operator), and introducing new nodes or removing already existing ones. These random changes ensure that the population does not become trapped on sub-optimal local solutions too early and promotes the search for diverse solutions [13].

3.4 Iterative Evolution and Termination

The above events of selection, crossover, and mutation are repeated for several generations. Each generation is a set of population that changes with time as expected enhancement in the fitness of the population as better programs are produced and the weaker programs are omitted [14]. This process is repeated until a certain stopping condition is fulfilled, which may be a predefined number of iterations, a certain computational time, or sufficiently high fitness values for the entire population.

4. Biological System Modeling for Tumor Growth Prediction

Mathematical modeling of tumors for the diagnosis of growing tumors and cancer prognosis deals with the application of mathematical, computational, and biological techniques to describe the processes of cancer development. These models assist in forecasting the developments of tumors, their possibilities of metastasizing, and their responses to medications.

4.1 Introduction to Biological System Modeling

Biological system modeling is a computational approach that seeks to define biological systems using models that can computationally describe the behavior of these systems. In cancer research, these models are primarily aimed at studying aspects of tumor development and malignant behavior and involve mimicking the effects of cancer cells on their tissue environments [15]. It hopes to accurately simulate tumor progression and determine the emergence of opportunities for diagnosis and treatment.

4.2 Types of Models

There are several types of models used for tumor growth prediction, each with its unique strengths and applications:

4.2.1 Mechanistic Models

The mechanistic models in pharmacodynamics depend on the biological processes governing tumor growth. These models apply mathematical equations to define the rate of occurrence of cellular events, including the proliferation, death (apoptosis), and formation of blood vessels (angiogenesis). For example: Many of the tumor-cell population dynamics are described using Ordinary Differential Equations (ODEs) which represent time evolutions of the cell populations. Partial differential equations (PDEs) take into consideration both positional and temporal variations and describe the dynamics of how tumors move over space and their growth over time.

4.2.2 Phenomenological Models

Phenomenological models are more data-oriented; they simply describe the observed quantitative relationships without necessarily outlining the formal processes that cause the observations. These models can be used to forecast information where there is a significant amount of historical data [16]. Examples include: *Statistical Models*: These employ regression methods to determine if there are measurable relationships between factors like the rate of tumor growth and the patient's age or the size of the tumor at the time of diagnosis or the presence of certain genetic markers. *Machine Learning Models*: ML represents mathematical techniques such as neural networks and decision trees that can model massive datasets aimed at extrapolating tumor behavior and patient responses.

4.2.3 Hybrid Models

The third strategy is to use hybrid models, which integrate mechanistic and phenomenological theories in a way that enables the benefits of each to be exploited. They also combine specific biological mechanisms with statistical techniques to produce more realistic forecasts.

4.3 Key Components of Tumor Growth Models

Important aspects of tumor growth comprise several essential biological mechanisms that characterize the process of cancer progression [17]. Such variables include cellular proliferation- the rate in which the tumor cells divide, angiogenesis—the formation of new blood vessels for the tumor to acquire nutrients and oxygen and finally various microenvironment interactions involved, which include the effects of the tumor on the surrounding tissue and vice versa, the immune response and the extracellular matrix around the tumor.

4.3.1 Cellular Proliferation

This component represents the differentiation of the cancer cells used in the growth. Some of the factors that could be used include the genetic mutation, nutrients, and the signaling pathways in the cell that could promote cell proliferation. The equations represent various dynamics for how the number of cancer cells depends on time [18].

4.3.2 Angiogenesis

Tumor angiogenesis is essential in the growth of tumors because it helps in the provision of basic substances and oxygen to the tumors. Angiogenic factors such as

VEGF (vascular endothelial growth factor) and their implications in blood vessel development are sometimes included in the model.

4.3.3 Microenvironment Interactions

Tumor tissues are highly dynamic and are characterized by the recruitment of various immune cells as well as stromal cells and deposition of the extracellular matrix. Such models include these interactions to predict how the tumor 'shapes' the environment and how this transformed environment influences the growth of the tumor.

4.3.4 Invasion and Metastasis

Sophisticated systems reproduce the stages of invasion (cancer cells spreading to surrounding tissue) and metastasis (disease dissemination in the body). These processes include the simulation of cell locomotion, the action of enzymes on the extra-cellular matrix, and the trafficking of cells through the blood stream.

4.3.5 Treatment Response

The impact of current treatments such as Chemotherapy, Radiation, and targeted therapies must be factored in [19]. Models model how these treatments influence the viability, development rate, and development of potential immune mechanisms in tumor cells. But the concrete models in addition often have much more explicit descriptions of the process of invasion/micro metastasis—how cancer cells move from one part of the body to another – and of therapeutic response that is how tumor cells perceive chemotherapy and radiation. It is necessary to mention that the models of tumor growth are effective because they include all these components and create a full working system for tumor simulation.

4.4 Mathematical and Computational Techniques

The Mathematical and Computational Methods for Bio-Inspired Cancer Diagnosis is presented as a new class of bio-clinical cancer diagnosis that uses principals of biology and computer science for making digital predictions through making use of mathematical models that can be thought of in the way computers do it [20]. This includes the equations that model mathematical representations of the growth and development of a tumor using differential equations, the cell-agent model with interactions of certain cells with their environments, and the cellular automata model for grid-based chemical and biological systems computations. Neuro nets and support vector machines (SVMs) are also used to address large datasets to obtain the difference between the features that can characterize the presence of cancer.

4.4.1 Differential Equations

Differential equations ODEs and PDEs are employed to describe continuous changes in some parameters such as the number of tumor cells and the concentration of nutrients. They have more accuracy and specificity essential for modeling biological systems.

4.4.2 Agent-Based Models (ABMs)

ABMs are computational models that generate emergent patterns at the population level by reproducing cell behaviors based on individual cells' actions and intercellular interactions. Each cell applies clear principles and observing their interaction enables one to notice emerging growth mechanisms [21].

4.4.3 Cellular Automata

Cellular automata are based on the idea that a periodic structure is employed with each of the cells of the structure capable of existing in a specified state such as healthy, cancerous, and necrotic. Each cell has a state that is dependent on predefined rules driven from adjacent cells to mimic local interaction and growth.

4.4.4 Machine Learning

Unsupervised ML approaches, namely, neural networks, SVMs, and ensembles can be utilized to improve the model [22]. These models are able to notice complex patterns from big datasets which can act as a good complement to mechanistic approaches.

5. Algorithmic Procedure for Anomaly Detection

A technique suggesting the implementation of collective behaviors of decentralized systems for the surveillance of cardiac system of human body as this is modeled on the behavior of real social insect colonies found in nature for the creation of a more efficient process is a novel approach. Figure 1 shows the processing flow of bio-inspired algorithms.

6. Bio-inspired Optimization for Hyperparameters

Anomaly detection-based bio-inspired cancer diagnosis based on immunological algorithms develops from the observation that the biological immune system possesses the capability to distinguish the difference between the targets or self-objects, and subject or non-self-entities to identify and eliminate pathogens or abnormal cells. These algorithms capture the Adaptive and Innate immune responses and uses Negative selection, Clonal selection, and Immune network theory to identify the anomalies in biological data [23]. The aim here is to be

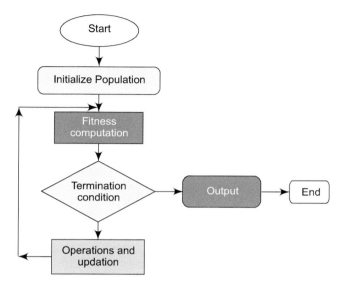

Fig. 1 Process flow of bio-inspired optimization.

able to predict outliers that do not belong, and in the case of diagnosing cancer is able to predict the existence of certain cellular or molecular patterns that suggest cancerous cells are growing in the body.

6.1 Negative Selection Algorithm

The negative selection algorithm is a well-known immunological technique for anomaly detection. It is grounded on the process of T-cell development in the thymus T-cells that exhibit high affinity to self-antigens that are eliminated so that mature T-cells that can recognize non-self-antigens are obtained. In computational terms, this means producing a set of detectors which characterizes normal behavior. These detectors are then exposed to self-samples, and those that give a response similar to the self-samples are eliminated. The rest detectors that fail to identify the self-samples are useful for detecting anomalies. It is used in cancer diagnosis to flag abnormal patterns observed in a patient's data, for example, abnormally high gene expressions or imaging a pattern that might suggest the presence of tumors.

6.2 Clonal Selection Algorithm

Immunological Clonal selection is another approach with inspiration from the adaptive immune response where B-cells that interact with antigens are allowed to multiply and undergo hyper mutation in an effort to raise the affinity of a cell to the antigen. When translated computationally, it involves creating a population of possible solutions (antibodies) that have to be exposed to a set of data (antigens). Antibodies which recognize abnormalities or malformations (known as antigens) are chosen for propagation and undergo alteration or modifications to create different versions [24]. It is an iterative optimization which is important in improving the system's capability to recognize anomalies peculiar to the system. In cancer diagnosis, clonal selection algorithms can dynamically enhance their identification skills by repeatedly learning new patterns from new data and this is in line with enhanced detection skills of cancer cells.

6.3 Artificial Immune Networks

Artificial immune networks consist of a graph of relations between different immune cells and the responses of these cells to antigens which are the pathogens and the relations that form dynamic evolving detector networks. These networks comprise of vertices which represent different detectors (immune cells) and edges which may show the interaction between the different detectors. The network learns by analogy to the immune system through mechanisms that include suppression and stimulation, but preserves a diverse pool of detectors helpful in recognizing a wide range of anomalies. As far as cancer diagnosis is concerned and can find use in integrating diverse biological datasets, e.g., of integrating numerous data sources (genetic, proteomic, and imaging) to build a multidimensional, fault-tolerant, and learning system that can successfully identify more elusive and sophisticated derivatives of abnormality potentially associated with cancer.

7. Adaptive Cancer Diagnosis Learning Algorithms

Cancer diagnosis are computational approaches that are based on imitation of natural processes existing in living organisms for identifying, classifying, and predicting the incidence of cancer cells [25]. Rather, these algorithms are designed in such a way that they learn and modify with time and experience as it happens in living organisms in a given environment, in this case cancer diagnosis. A brief overview of applications of the main types of such algorithms for cancer diagnosis is discussed.

7.1 Introduction to Adaptive Bio-inspired Algorithms

Bio-inspired adaptive algorithms in engineering are based on different processes in nature including evolution, immune systems, and brain activity. These algorithms are accompanied by the following features: they can learn from data, they can exploit new information, and they can increase the performance of the algorithm in time [26, 27].

7.2 Types of Adaptive Bio-inspired Algorithms

In cancer diagnosis, these algorithms need to work out well with multidimensional medical data to detect features and abnormalities that are relevant to the cancer.

7.2.1 Genetic Algorithms (GAs)

GAs borrow their principles from a study of nature and the process of evolution. As they operate, they develop a set of candidate solutions to the problem by employing operations of selection, crossover, and mutation [28–30]. To discriminate cancerous tissues, GAs can be applied to choose the relevant features, set model variables, or generate classification strategies. They work by repeatedly selecting the best solution and 'breeding' new populations of solutions until satisfactory solutions are obtained—a process which finds and optimizes or approximates optimal solutions for complex diagnostic problems.

7.2.2 Genetic Programming (GP)

GP is another variation of GAs in which solutions are computer programs or models instead of fixed-length character strings. GP works with tree structures representing computational models and improves programs by choosing, merging, and changing them. For cancer diagnosis, GP may use descriptive capabilities to develop predictive models that combine multiple types of inputs, e.g., big data: consist of massive amounts of structured/semi-structured/unstructured information, such as genomic, proteomic, imaging to generate precise and/or interpretable forecasting rules.

7.2.3 Artificial Immune Systems (AIS)

The AIS are modeled after the human immune system which is capable of identifying foreign substances in the body and neutralizing them. AIS algorithms are applied in forecasting or detecting anomalies and/or novel patterns in data; for instance, negative selection algorithm or clonal selection algorithm. AIS can also be applied in cancer diagnosis in that it pinpoints abnormal data in medical records that could possibly suggest cancer. Such systems go through changes on a regular basis and also learn from new sets of data that enhance detection skills.

7.2.4 Neural Networks and Deep Learning

Artificial neural networks (ANNs) along with their derivatives including convonutional neural networks (CNNs) and recurrent neural networks (RNNs) are based on the human brain and its mechanism of working. These networks are made up of neurons that are arranged in layers and handle the information accordingly [31]. Multilayered deep learning models can be used in the identification of complex patterns and features in massive datasets. Modern CNNs are effective at analyzing medical images for cancer diagnostics, while RNNs are suitable for time-series data, including data from patient monitoring.

7.2.5 Swarm Intelligence Algorithms

Particle Swarm Optimization (PSO) and Ant Colony Optimization (ACO) are two examples of swarm intelligence algorithms which are based on the behavior of particles of various social organism like bird, fish, or ant. The latter are algorithms which improve solutions by mimicking the flocking and swarming behavior and communication of these organisms. In cancer diagnostics, he swarm intelligence algorithms help in searching for the best solution from the vast dataset that helps optimize the diagnostic models, feature selection, and treatment planning.

7.3 Key Components and Mechanisms

Learning and Adaptation

Evolutionary ML techniques process patterns in an iterative manner where data is used to test parameter and structure modifications of the algorithms. It entails training with datasets that have been used in the past to detect a pattern and then testing with other datasets to verify and improve the models [32]. The adaptation mechanism undertakes to maintain the algorithms relevant in the presence of new data or altered data conditions.

Feature Selection and Dimensionality Reduction

The dimension of medical data is usually very high in cancer diagnosis; hence, feature selection is crucial. Some of these techniques borrow from nature with bio-inspired algorithms like genetic evolution, swarm behavior, and neural network pruning used to discard noise and de-noise the data to obtain relevant features for better results in the models. This process increases the interpretability and efficiency of diagnostic models. Table 1 shows the different dimensionality reduction techniques used in bio-inspired optimization procedure.

Table 1 Various dimensionality reduction techniques.

Types	Merits	Search method	Effectiveness
Wrapper Method	Classifier interaction and feature selection	Deterministic	Superior with high efficiency
Feature Extraction	High discriminating power	PCA, ICA	Used in hybrid algorithm
Filter Method	Autonomous and high speed calculation	Univariate, Multivariate	Quicker
Embedded Method	Low overfitting values	Integrated and Simplified model	Computations are less expensive
Hybrid Method	Combination of various feature selection and extraction	In-depth search method	Complexity

Robustness and Generalization

Advantages of bio-inspired algorithms include a capability to work well with robust and generalized data. This is attained through such mechanisms like mutation and crossover in GAs that provide diversification to prevent overfitting. Other algorithms such as the neural networks and deep learning models employ regularization mechanisms and dropout layers to retain the generalization abilities.

7.4 Applications in Cancer Diagnosis

Early Detection and Screening

Modern heuristic bio-mimicking methods are used in the pre-clinical cancer diagnosis. Such algorithms can look at imaging results, compare them with genetic information, and even check the levels of certain biomarkers to spot the first signs of cancer before people experience any symptoms. This type of detections at the earlier stage improves the efficacy of treatment as well as the chances of survival of the patient.

Personalized Medicine

This can be solved through adaptive algorithms which are developed to alter the models to fit the individual attributes of the patient [33]. These algorithms are able to combine the data of genomics, the data of proteins, and clinical data to determine the most suitable drug for a particular patient using their individual genetic and biological markers.

Prognosis and Risk Assessment

ML involves use of the bio-inspired adaptive algorithms for predicting the progress and outcome of disease and for Cancer Risk Estimation. These models try to forecast the trends of patients in the future based on the past patients and also attempt to identify patterns of diseases and patient revisit behaviors and survival rates. This is important because the clinicians are the people who will be responsible for making decisions about the care of the patient and treatment as well as follow-ups and continuing care.

Treatment Response Prediction

Making accurate forecasts on how a patient is going to respond to various treatments is another critical use [34]. Swarm computational intelligence databases process personalized information and predicts individual reactions to chemotherapy, radiation, and biologic drug therapies to optimize treatments and reduce toxicity.

8. Hybrid Bio-inspired Approaches

Bio-inspired hybrid methods for cancer diagnosis are combinations of fundamental biochemical and biological concepts from different sources of biological systems and computational algorithms to improve the performance of diagnosis. These approaches involve hybridization of various algorithms that are used for example in genetic algorithms, AIS and neural networks; the main idea behind such hybridization is that it would improve performance on detection and classification of the cancerous growths via elimination of weaknesses of individual approaches. Through utilizing the underlying biology and versatility of living beings hybrid methods have great potential in modeling the dynamic and complex nature of cancer for enhanced diagnosing results.

One of the common hybrid applications in cancer diagnosis includes using the GAs with the ML classifiers like SVMs or decision trees. GAs are applied to the tasks of determining feature subsets, model coefficients, or classification conditions based on repeatedly improving a set of potential solutions through a selection, crossover, and mutation process. Meanwhile, other algorithms, like SVMs or decision trees, apply the selected features to fit efficient classification models according to the training data [35]. This approach combining GAs for feature selection and ML for classification by building a diagnostic model is a hybrid approach because it combines GAs for solving feature selection problems with machine learning for classification problem and it guarantees that the resulting model requires a minimal number of features but has a high predictive performance.

A second type of merged bio-inspired strategies involves the use of AIS in combination with more 'conventional' ML techniques for cancer classification. AIS algorithms attempt to replicate the human immune system's capacity to detect deviations from normalcy and use AIS algorithms to pattern find and eventually find patterns associated with cancer in large medical datasets. When combining AIS with ML algorithms, the result can be an ML model enhanced with anomaly detection capabilities or an AIS model that gains the classification power of ML and the generalization ability of ensemble methods with the random forests algorithm. This combination of features makes the system robust and able to accurately detect cancer in various datasets based on unique and efficiently discriminating between normal and abnormal patterns [36].

9. Challenges and Future Directions

Challenges and opportunities reveals that future development of bio-inspired cancer diagnosis will be an intricate process that reflects the complicated nature of both biological systems and computational methods [37].

9.1 Data Integration and Heterogeneity

The first issue in bio-inspired cancer diagnosis is that of data integration where data from all types of biology such as genomic, proteomic, imaging, and clinical needs to be unified. These data sources tend to manifest high degrees of heterogeneity and present a challenge to integrating them into models that comprehensively describe cancer biology. Future efforts will include the research and advancement into means on how heterogeneous data sets can be integrated and harmonized to provide a better and more accurate diagnosis of cancer cases.

9.2 Interpretability and Explainability

Even though bio-inspired algorithms may reach a high level of accuracy in cancer diagnosis, they have a crucial limitation: these models are not very explainable and interpretable. Clinicians need lucid and comprehensible models that translate to the biological foundation of diagnosis. An area of future work will involve the creation of approaches for decision-justification to support the clinician by explaining the decisions of bio-inspired models, and developing the clinician's trust in them.

9.3 Robustness and Generalization

The generalization and stability of the models inspired by bio-organisms for cancer diagnosis should be guaranteed for their industrial applications. Such models need to work in population subgroups, in various healthcare systems, with different quality and quantity of data available. Future work will include finding ways to effectively tune bio-inspired models to improve their robustness and generalization abilities using techniques for data augmentation, transfer learning, and model regularization.

9.4 Ethical and Regulatory Considerations

The development of bio-inspired cancer diagnosis technologies to date makes the discussion of ethical and regulatory issues relevant. These types of technologies pose significant ethical and legal concerns, including patient privacy, informed consent, and algorithmic bias, which must be properly managed and regulated to avoid or minimize the potential harm from AI and ML's misuse and misapplication. Future study work will shape in creating an ethical standard and laws or regulations that put value to the growth and quality of bio-inspired cancer diagnosis models for the coming years.

9.5 Clinical Validation and Translation

Finally, clinical validation of the testing procedure and demonstrating its clinical implementation in bio-inspired cancer diagnosis is crucial for its success. Well-designed and randomized control trials must be conducted to assess the accuracy and efficacy of these models in clinical practice to establish the models contribution to patient outcomes, clinical decisions, and healthcare. Future works will include the large-scale clinical trials to further elucidate diagnostic performance and clinical utility of bio-inspired cancer diagnosis models toward broader application in clinical decision support.

Nano bio-cancer technology is a new field that can be used to detect and treat cancer and has great potential for the future. But, there are still some critical barriers that need to be overcome to achieve this potential fully. These challenges include data integration, interpretability, robustness, ethical, and clinical validation; therefore, addressing these problems will allow the researchers to leverage the most promising bio-inspired approaches in cancer diagnosis.

Conclusion

Bio-inspired design has several distinct advantages in the detection and classification of cancerous cells and in prognosis of cancer growth. However, problems like data heterogeneity, interpretability, and regulation, among others, continue to hinder progress in this area as researchers and health organizations strive towards enhancing the accuracy of cancer diagnosis and achieving more personalized and accessible approaches. More advancements in data interoperability, model explainability, clinical verification, and ethical management will enable bio-inspired cancer diagnosis to radically transform clinical cancer care by predicting improved cancer patient outcomes and more efficiently guiding clinical decision-making.

References

[1] Ghoniem, R.M. (2020). A novel bio-inspired deep learning approach for liver cancer diagnosis. *Information, 11*(2), 80.

[2] Singh, N.K., Gupta, R. and Sahu, S. (2023). Bio-inspired swarm-intelligent with machine learning framework for prediction and classification of lung cancer. *Multidisciplinary Science Journal, 5*.

[3] A.R. Akkar, H. and A. Salman, S. (2020). Detection of biomedical images by using bio-inspired artificial intelligent. *Engineering and Technology Journal, 38*(2A), 255–64.

[4] Al-Tawil, M., Mahafzah, B.A., Al Tawil, A. and Aljarah, I. (2023). Bio-inspired machine learning approach to Type 2 Diabetes Detection. *Symmetry, 15*(3), 764.

[5] González-Patiño, D., Villuendas-Rey, Y., Argüelles-Cruz, A.J. and Karray, F. (2019). A novel bio-inspired method for early diagnosis of breast cancer through mammographic image analysis. *Applied Sciences, 9*(21), 4492.

[6] Sharma, M., Gupta, S., Sharma, P. and Gupta, D. (2019). Bio-inspired algorithms for diagnosis of breast cancer. *International Journal of Innovative Computing and Applications, 10*(3–4), 164–74.

[7] Mohamed, T.I., Ezugwu, A.E., Fonou-Dombeu, J.V., Ikotun, A.M. and Mohammed, M. (2023). A bio-inspired convolution neural network architecture for automatic breast cancer detection and classification using RNA-seq gene expression data. *Scientific Reports, 13*(1), 14644.

[8] Bhoi, A.K., Mallick, P.K., Liu, C.M. and Balas, V.E. (Eds.). (2021). *Bio-inspired Neurocomputing* (Vol. 310). Berlin/Heidelberg, Germany: Springer.

[9] Firdous, M., Sharma, S. and Mahajan, A. (Jun. 2023). Breast Cancer Detection from Mammograms using Deep Learning and Bio-inspired Optimization Algorithm. *In: International Conference on Machine Learning, Deep Learning, and Computational Intelligence for Wireless Communication* (pp. 361–73). Cham: Springer Nature Switzerland.

[10] Rundo, F., Banna, G.L. and Conoci, S. (2019). Bio-inspired deep-CNN pipeline for skin cancer early diagnosis. *Computation, 7*(3), 44.

[11] Gonçalves, C.B., Souza, J.R. and Fernandes, H. (2022). CNN architecture optimization using bio-inspired algorithms for breast cancer detection in infrared images. *Computers in Biology and Medicine, 142*, 105205.

[12] Ahmed, A., Ali, M. and Selim, M. (2019). Bio-inspired based techniques for thermogram breast cancer classification. *International Journal of Intelligent Engineering and Systems, 12*(2), 114–24.

Bio-Inspired Intelligence in Early Cancer Detection | 139

[13] Aljahdali, S.H. and El-Telbany, M.E. (Dec. 2009). Bio-inspired machine learning in microarray gene selection and cancer classification. *In: 2009 IEEE International Symposium on Signal Processing and Information Technology (ISSPIT)* (pp. 339–43). IEEE.

[14] Salma, M.U. (Oct. 2015). BAT-ELM: A bio-inspired model for prediction of breast cancer data. *In: 2015 International Conference on Applied and Theoretical Computing and Communication Technology (iCATccT–* (pp. 501–506). IEEE.

[15] Vijh, S., Gaurav, P. and Pandey, H.M. (2023). Hybrid bio-inspired algorithm and convolutional neural network for automatic lung tumor detection. *Neural Computing and Applications, 35*(33), 23711–724.

[16] Shah, H., Chiroma, H., Herawan, T., Ghazali, R. and Tairan, N. (2019). An efficient bio-inspired bees' colony for breast cancer prediction. *In: Proceedings of the International Conference on Data Engineering 2015 (DaEng-2015)* (pp. 597–608). Springer Singapore.

[17] Sayed, G.I., Soliman, M. and Hassanien, A.E. (2016). Bio-inspired swarm techniques for thermogram breast cancer detection. *In: N. Dey, V. Bhatija & Aboul. E. Hassanein (Eds.), Medical Imaging in Clinical Applications: Algorithmic and Computer-Based Approaches,* 487–506. Springer Link.

[18] Rundo, F., Banna, G.L., Spampinato, C. and Conoci, S. (2021). Bio-Inspired Physiological Signal (s) and Medical Image (s) Neural Processing Systems Based on Deep Learning and Mathematical Modeling for Implementing Bio-Engineering Applications in Medical and Industrial Fields. *Frontiers in Neuroinformatics, 15*, 763699.

[19] Silva, M.B., Narloch, P.H., Dorn, M. and Broin, P.Ó. (Jun. 2021.) Optimization of Cancer Status Prediction Pipelines using Bio-Inspired Computing. *In: 2021 IEEE Congress on Evolutionary Computation (CEC)* (pp. 442–49). IEEE.

[20] Zenbout, I., Bouramoul, A., Meshoul, S. and Amrane, M. (2023). Efficient bioinspired feature selection and machine learning based framework using omics data and biological knowledge data bases in cancer clinical endpoint prediction. *IEEE Access, 11*, 2674–99.

[21] Munish Khanna, Singh, L.K. and Garg, H. (2024). A novel approach for human diseases prediction using nature inspired computing and machine learning approach. *Multimedia Tools and Applications, 83*(6), 17773–809.

[22] Jeevitha, J. and Sangeetha, V. (Apr. 2023.) Exploration on Breast Cancer Prediction and Recurrence Diagnosis Using Bio-Inspired Algorithms. *In: International Conference on Soft Computing for Security Applications* (pp. 593–607). Singapore: Springer Nature Singapore.

[23] Gautam, A. and Chouhan, U. (2021). Bio-inspired approaches for classification of benign and malignant tumor of the skin. *International Journal of Bioinformatics Research and Applications, 17*(5), 424–33.

[24] Ashwini, A. and Murugan, S. (2020). Automatic Skin Tumor Segmentation using Prioritized Patch Based Region: A Novel Comparative Technique. *IETE Journal of Research, 66*, 1–12.

[25] Houssein, E.H., Oliva, D., Samee, N.A., Mahmoud, N.F. and Emam, M.M. (2023). Liver Cancer Algorithm: A novel bio-inspired optimizer. *Computers in Biology and Medicine, 165*, 107389.

[26] De Albuquerque, V.H. C., Gupta, D., De Falco, I., Sannino, G. and Bouguila, N. (2020). Special issue on Bio-inspired optimization techniques for Biomedical Data Analysis: Methods and applications. *Applied Soft Computing, 95*, 106672.

[27] AlShamlan, H. and AlMazrua, H. (2024). Enhancing Cancer Classification through a Hybrid Bio-Inspired Evolutionary Algorithm for Biomarker Gene Selection. *Computers, Materials & Continua, 79*(1).

[28] Hatamlou, A. (2017). A hybrid bio-inspired algorithm and its application. *Applied Intelligence, 47*(4), 1059–67.

[29] Yu, W., Kang, H., Sun, G., Liang, S. and Li, J. (2022). Bio-inspired feature selection in brain disease detection via an improved sparrow search algorithm. *IEEE Transactions on Instrumentation and Measurement, 72*, 1–15.

[30] Mahmud, M.S., Wang, H., Esfar-E-Alam, A.M. and Fang, H. (2017). A wireless health monitoring system using mobile phone accessories. *IEEE Internet of Things Journal, 4*(6), 2009–18.

[31] Kalaiselvi, P. and Anusuya, S. (2022). Design of Bio-Inspired Algorithm for Optimizing the Feature Selection Prepared for Classification in Liver Tumor Detection. *Indian Journal of Computer Science and Engineering, 13*(4), 1185–96.

[32] Anousouya Devi, M., Ravi, S., Vaishnavi, J. and Punitha, S. (2016). Bio-inspired Model Classification of Squamous Cell Carcinoma in Cervical Cancer using SVM. *In: Intelligent Systems Technologies and Applications 2016* (pp. 585–96). Springer International Publishing.

[33] Pasha, S.J. and Mohamed, E.S. (Sept. 2019). Bio-inspired ensemble feature selection (BEFS) model with machine learning and data mining algorithms for disease risk prediction. *In: 2019 5th International Conference on Computing, Communication, Control, and Automation (ICCUBEA)* (pp. 1–6). IEEE.

[34] Pasha, S.J. and Mohamed, E.S. (Sept. 2019). Bio-inspired ensemble feature selection (BEFS) model with machine learning and data mining algorithms for disease risk prediction. *In: 2019 5th International Conference on Computing, Communication, Control, and Automation (ICCUBEA)* (pp. 1–6). IEEE.

[35] Balasubramaniam, S., Syed, M.H., More, N.S. and Polepally, V. (2023). Deep learning-based power prediction aware charge scheduling approach in cloud-based electric vehicular network. *Engineering Applications of Artificial Intelligence, 121*, 105869.

[36] Balasubramaniam, S. and Kumar, K.S. (2022). Fractional Feedback Political Optimizer with Prioritization-Based Charge Scheduling in Cloud-Assisted Electric Vehicular Network. *Ad Hoc & Sensor Wireless Networks, 52*(3–4), 173–98.

[37] Alshamlan, H.M., Badr, G.H. and Alohali, Y.A. (2014). The performance of bio-inspired evolutionary gene selection methods for cancer classification using microarray dataset. *International Journal of Bioscience, Biochemistry, and Bioinformatics, 4*(3), 166.

8 Bio-Inspired Algorithms in Machine Learning and Deep Learning for Diabetes Diagnosis

S. Aathilakshmi,[1*] Balasubramaniam S.[2] and Ayodeji Olalekan Salau[3]

Bio-inspired algorithms in machine learning and deep learning for Diabetic diagnosis are important as diabetes affects millions of individuals throughout the globe and is the leading cause of blindness in persons of working age. This highlights the critical need of a trustworthy retinal screening method. Recently, with the use of effective Image Processing technology, Deep Learning algorithms have shown promise for application in population diagnosis and classification. In this research, the proposed system used a Conventional Neural Network as part of a deep learning approach to rapidly detect diabetes in newly recorded medical images. Classifiers well-suited to many different classification tasks may be mined from data. Main objective of this research is to solve the challenge of detecting diabetes and Glaucoma in retinal pictures, using feed-forward neural network. The suggested approach significantly improves the speed and accuracy of illness detection over conventional techniques due to its much greater rate of complete classification. When a self-trained model is used, such as Alexnet, extensive testing may assist improve accuracy. As a result, the suggested approach vastly enhances the speed and precision of diabetes recognition. The results show a classification accuracy of 99.61%, sensitivity of 98.65%, and specificity of 98.60%.

1. Introduction

Diabetic diagnosis is important as diabetes causes severe vision loss and is a global health crisis. About a third of the roughly 285 million persons who have diabetes mellitus globally also have diabetic symptoms. Diabetics develop an eye condition over time as a consequence of having diabetes; another one-third of persons in this group encounter the more severe kind of diabetic symptoms called vision-threatening diabetic retinopathy. High blood glucose levels call for a different issue in diabetic diagnosis, like it will affect the retina, leading to Diabetic diagnosis [1].

---

[1] Department of ECE, Chennai Institute of Technology.
[2] School of Computer Science and Engineering, Kerala University of Digital Sciences, Innovation and Technology (Formerly IIITM-K), Digital University Kerala, Thiruvananthapuram, Kerala, India.
[3] Department of Electrical and Computer Engineering, Afe Babalola University, Nigeria.
Email: ayodejisalau98@gmail.com
* Corresponding author: aathilakshmis@citchennai.net

Vision loss occurs when these tiny blood vessels are broken and the contents bleed onto the retina. This occurs when the retina, the light-sensitive area at the back of the eye, does not get enough oxygen and nutrients because blood vessels there have been damaged. A diabetic may initially have relatively little visual impairment [2].

The great bulk of research in this area makes use of fundus photographs, which are visual records of a person's current ocular condition. Determining whether or not diabetic symptoms are present in these fundus images requires segmentation of retinal blood vessels, lesions, and the diabetic itself [3].

Microaneurysms (MA), superficial retinal haemorrhages, exudates (Exs) (both soft and hard), intraretinal haemorrhages, and cotton-wool patches are all examples of lesions that may be utilised to determine the presence or absence of diabetic symptoms and their development [4]-[5]. To avoid irreversible vision loss or damage, an early Diabetic diagnosis is essential. Some individuals claim to have seen alterations, such as a diminished ability to read or concentrate on distant objects. These visual deviations might manifest in ways you wouldn't anticipate. As the disease progresses, blood vessels in the retina may start to bleed into the vitreous, the gel-like substance that fills the eye. In the last two decades, the prevalence of diabetes has increased Diabetic Automatically.

The World Health Organisation predicts this number will reach 700 million by 2045, making public health an increasingly pressing problem on a worldwide basis. Diabetics is caused by damage to the retina's blood vessels in the retina's underlying layer [6]. If neglected and left untreated for an extended period of time, it may have disastrous effects, including blindness. This emphasises the critical nature of finding a solution to this problem. However, some persons with Diabetic diagnosis may see dot-like or streaky patterns [7], which resemble a spider web. These spots may go away without treatment, but it's best to take care of them immediately. It's important to stop the bleeding since it may reoccur, become worse, or create scarring if the wound doesn't heal correctly if left untreated.

Non-proliferative and proliferative phases of Diabetic diagnosis are distinguished. Vision loss at this point is caused by fluid leakage inside the retinal blood vessels [8]. Because of the swelling and subsequent wetness of the retina, vision is impaired. Non-proliferative Diabetic diagnosis is characterised by microaneurysms (MAs), microhaemorrhages, and exudates (Exs). A leading global cause of blindness in diabetics is a matter of concern. Because of how common it is in developed countries, it is crucial for finding a way to detect, identify, and diagnose it quickly [9]. Nearly a third of the roughly 285 million people around the world who have diabetes mellitus show symptoms of diabetic, and another one-third of those people have a more severe manifestation of diabetic known as vision-threatening diabetics [10]. However, a significant challenge remains in successfully collecting actionable information from segmented images. Convolutional Neural Networks (CNNs) may be utilised to improve segmentation results when this is the case.

The use of a Hybrid Neural Network allowed for the classification of Diabetic diagnosis into several subtypes. In this study, the VGG network was employed

Bio-Inspired Algorithms in Machine Learning and Deep Learning for Diabetes Diagnosis | 143

for feature extraction to help build the recommended CNN-based model using a transfer learning mechanism inside the InceptionV3 framework to investigate a unique alternative approach. After that, the user employed a Support Vector Machine (SVM) to sort diabetic instances into groups.

An entirely automated method for classifying diabetic was first presented in the publication Automated Detection of diabetic [11]. This sorting task was accomplished using five distinct Transfer Learning models. These models achieved impressive levels of validation accuracy, with Exception (86.25%), Inception Res-Net V2 (96.25%), Mobile Net V2 (93.75%), Dense-Net 121 (81.25%), and NAS-Net Mobile (80.00%) performing best. Following that, the user advanced the idea of employing deep CNNs for automating the process [12]. This research made use of a transfer learning approach inspired by the DenseNet-121 structure. Mas, Exs, and haemorrhages were identified in the input pictures and utilised to detect DIABETIC; the preprocessing and augmentation methods performed to the image data were also outlined in the research to further increase the model's sensitivity. Results from the trained and validated version of the constructed classifier were encouraging. It achieved very high levels of accuracy throughout training (96.3%) and validation (94.9%). In addition, the model's quality was summarised by its 0.88 qua Diabetic weighted kappa score.

Diabetic diagnosis and Normal Retinal Image Classification through CNN and SVM propose employing CNN and SVM as a classification approach to distinguish between Diabetic diagnosis and normal retinal images [13]. At its heart, the method employs transfer learning to glean summary statistics from the last fully connected layer of a CNN. An SVM is used to categorise data once the features have been extracted. This method not only increases accuracy, but also Diabetic automatically reduces the processing time required for classification, all thanks to the combination of CNN with fine-tuning. The researchers put their method to the test on a set of retinal images from the Messidor database (n = 77 in base 12, and 70 in base 13). They discovered a remarkable degree of accuracy; 95.75% for base 12, and 95.24% for base 13. The recent researchers tried out a variety of transfer learning models, including VGG, Alex-Net, Inception, Google Net, Dense Net, and Res-Net [14].

In order to classify cases of Diabetic, the authors of [15] compared CNNs, Transformer-based networks, and multi-layered perceptrons (MLPs), three deep-learning architectures. The study included the use of much deep learning architecture such as Efficient Net, Res-Net, Swin-Transformer, Vision-Transformer (ViT), and MLP-Mixer. Models based on the transformer design were found to have the highest levels of accuracy among the options studied. This provides more evidence that transformer-based networks, like Swin-Transformer and Vision-Transformer, are superior when it comes to diabetic categorization. The DenseNet-121 model was employed to identify Diabetic in fundus images [16]. The proposed model was built to analyse retinal images that have already been processed, without the need for further feature improvement, and was designed to take advantage of the power of deep learning (DL) models based on the Dense-Net architecture in order to provide an automated diagnostic solution for the identification of Diabetic. To increase the accuracy of diabetic detection, the authors utilised basic preprocessing techniques on images with noise. The approach used by Saranya et al. showed some encouraging results. The model's superiority in diagnosing Diabetic diagnosis was shown by an accuracy of 0.83 and a precision of 0.99.

Using a previously trained model is a cutting-edge approach to diabetic classification. After that, we'll use an image classifier powered by a deep CNN. By beating baseline models despite having access to less training photos, this novel approach demonstrates its worth. Another research group [17] employed transfer learning to improve the diabetic detection accuracy of the EfficientNet-B0, EfficientNet-B4, and EfficientNet-B7 models used similar frameworks to group Diabetic into referable and possibly blinding categories. Area Under the Curve (AUC) values of 0.984 for referable diabetic (R-diabetic) and 0.990 for vision-threatening diabetic demonstrated superior classification performance for the novel network model on the Eye PACS dataset, indicating that the authors' proposed method is effective in detecting signs of Diabetic diagnosis on the APTOS 2019 dataset. The methods explain ability was improved with the help of a custom algorithm.

This study used the Efficient Net-B3 architecture [18], using ImageNet weights as the initialisation set. The completely connected layers were populated during training using data from the He initialisation. Experiments were conducted to prove that the Efficient Net model outperformed the gold standard data. Zhang, Z. looked at several different models, including the Efficient Net, Res-Net, Swin-Transformer, ViT, and the MLP-Mixer, and found that the devices having a basis in transformer design performed the best. In addition [19], the authors classified cases of DIABETIC in a different way. The ensemble model was built from three individual CNN models. This ensemble model was built on the principle of stack generalisation.

2. Related Work

Alex-Net, ResNet-50, and VGG-16 models were the ones most extensively explored. The authors empirically compared and contrasted the performance of 28 unique deep hybrid architectures. Cases of diabetic were classified using these frameworks into two categories: referable and non-referable [20]. Researchers compared end-to-end DL models to a three-class classification of fundus images (normal, glaucomatous, and diabetic eyes) [21]. For the purpose of diabetic classification, a wide variety of CNN models were used. Among them were MobileNetV2, DenseNet-121, InceptionV3, InceptionResNetV2, ResNet-50, and VGG-16. In their publication [22], the authors detail how they used the DenseNet-169 framework to develop an original CNN model. The model's performance was improved by adding a convolutional block attention module (CBAM).

The purpose of the revamped format is to streamline the process of classifying Diabetic-diagnosis severity. ResNet-101, a model reported in [23], was used to assign a severity rating to Diabetic and determine the likelihood of macular edema. The findings demonstrated that ResNet-101 was a more effective model than ResNet-50. This research [24] provided a heuristically constructed deep neural network for assessing the severity of diabetic. The authors' experiments demonstrated that the proposed network performed very well in diagnosing the presence of the disease. Mirroring and spinning the pictures were only two of the ways that the data collection was improved in this study [25] for grading Diabetic and it demonstrated promising results in differentiating between various degrees of severity associated with diabetic. These methods were used to complement the data already available. Overall, the accuracy of both approaches was high, at 94.4% and 88.8%, respectively. Existing automated algorithms for diabetic classification are commensurate with these levels of accuracy. One method for diagnosing diabetic relies on the original model's binary 'yes' or 'no' categorization. Fundus pictures are segmented into four distinct diabetic severity stages using the second model, which does a subtler job. To classify the seriousness of the originally presented, the Hinge Attention Network (HA-Net) model was used. Its effectiveness was boosted by integrating many attention tiers. A pretrained VGG-16 network was used to analyse the input images and generate the first spatial representations. Since overfitting occurs while using CNNs to categorise the seriousness of diabetics, [26] several regularisation strategies for this task were investigated. In their research, Diabetic copout regularisation was demonstrated to be effective in reducing overfitting and improving accuracy.

By using image processing and feature extraction techniques to complete fundus pictures, an automated method was developed in a prior study to identify diabetic. In the process of categorising the data, data mining methods were used. Preprocessing the images was the initial stage, followed by the determination of statistical, GLCM-based, and histogram-based measures. Inefficiently, this information was sent into an SVM classifier, which attempted to place the fundus image into a disease category such as diabetic. Retinal fundus photographs, however, were used to gauge the RNFL thickness in an effort to detect glaucoma. This approach is often used by ophthalmologists since it requires no invasive treatments. Taking photos in a manner that allows those with healthy and diseased retinas to see them is crucial. In circumstances like screening campaigns for people who do not have regular access to healthcare services, the portability and ease-of-use of the technology makes it important to healthcare practitioners [27–28].

3. Machine Learning-based Diabetic Diagnosis Method

The primary purpose of this research is to develop a CNN method for automatically identifying diabetic from digital fundus images and more accurately characterising its severity. Specifically, this research proposed a clinical picture order model for retinal fundus images for the diagnosis of Diabetic diagnosis. Focusing on the details extracted from retinal images by image processing techniques, this study accurately arranges retina-related diseases based on the extracted highlights. In order to identify diabetics from healthy individuals in retinal images, a CNN classifier is trained using highlight extraction. The suggested framework's rapid general characterisation will boost productivity and set the disease apart from previous models. To accurately identify diabetic with little effort, our proposed model employs Alex Net, a Self-prepared CNN architecture trained on a dataset of fundus images. Retinal Diabetic in, microaneurysms, glaucoma, and other eye diseases are all well represented in the database. First, the patient's retinal image is segmented to correspond with the Alex Net's information layer. Next, the brain network extracts features (using the HOG extractor), and finally the model is built up and ready to further arrange the Diabetic diagnosis. Figure 1 depicts the suggested architectural model, which includes the convolutional portion as well

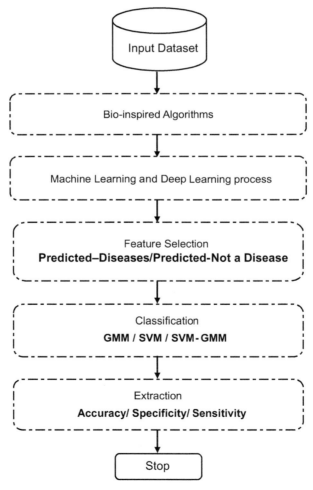

Fig. 1 Block diagram of the proposed functional system.

Bio-Inspired Algorithms in Machine Learning and Deep Learning for Diabetes Diagnosis | **147**

as FC4, FC5, and fc6+soft max. The final CNN layer is built such that distinct boundaries are assigned to each component of the image.

3.1 Graphical Analysis of Bio-Inspired Diabetic Diagnosis Method

Researchers have access to retina-related images and explanatory text detailing the severity of Diabetic diagnosis. The following are some of the most common exploration datasets that have been tested:

- Database of Electronic Ophthalmoscopy Images for Vessel Extraction.
- High-Goal Fundus Dataset, MESSIDOR Dataset, Retinopathy Online Test Dataset, and the Structured Investigation of the Retina Dataset.
- Datasets DIARETDB0 and DIARETDB1.

Alex Net's findings demonstrate that a massive, deep CNN can achieve world-record performance on a notoriously challenging dataset with just a somewhat complicated supervision. One year following Alex Net's release, all passages in the ImageNet competition opted to use the Convolutional Brain Organisation for the classification challenge. Alex Net was an early innovator in CNN, ushering in a new era of experimentation. After the release of so many significant learning packages, Alex Net's implementation is remarkably straightforward. The input dataset was collected from TensorFlow and forwarded to diabetic detection-based applications. The bio-inspired algorithm is used to optimize the workflow of the machine learning and deep learning with effective optimization algorithm. The machine learning steps involved feature extraction, classification, and resolution. To attain this way this research focused on mainly three different algorithms such as SVM in Machine Learning. The work flow of this system was shown in Figure 1 with the collection of different dataset. The confusion matrix between diseases and conditions that are really not diseases is shown in Table 1. Classification and grading results for photos with Diabetic diagnosis using the proposed technique, as well as results from using a standard CNN and a standard deep learning-based classifier trained on CNN characteristics.

Table 1   The confusion matrix of the actual disease and the actual not a disease.

Matrix Parameters	Actual-Disease	Actual-Not a Disease	Total
Bio-Inspired Authorization process	820	2	822
Bio Non-inspired process	6	592	598
Total	740	564	1304

Using CNN-extracted features, the author trained a separate GMM for each class. The number of elements is determined via trial and error. The suggested model was run in Python on a 32 GB RAM HP Z4 G4 workstation shown in Figure 2. The log-likelihood vectors from the class-specific GMMs are used to train the SVM classifier. Various SVM parameters have been selected for their empiricism in terms of performance.

For the best results, set C = 8 for the trade-off parameter and use a 0.8-width radial basis kernel. Classification Accuracy (CA) for the E-ophtha dataset using the bio-inspired algorithm in Machine and Deep learning process.

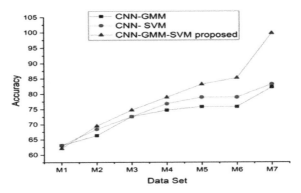

Fig. 2   Classification accuracy of the Bio-inspired machine learning method.

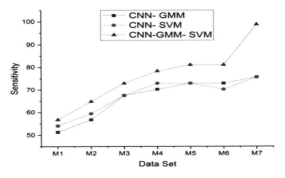

Fig. 3   Classification sensitivity of the Bio-inspired machine learning method.

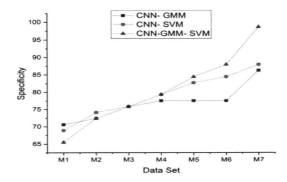

Fig. 4   Classification specificity of the Bio-inspired machine learning method.

Evaluation of Classification Efficiency Using the E-ophtha Dataset: Here have a look at how several models fared when asked to classify retinal pictures from the E-ophtha dataset. All the different models, including regular bio-inspired algorithm in Machine and Deep learning process, have been tested with the CNN features extracted at different layers (M1, M2, M7). Figure 4 shows the confusion matrix from the CNN-GMM model applied to the E-ophtha dataset with feature maps from different layers, and Figure 5 shows the confusion matrix from the same model applied to the same dataset.

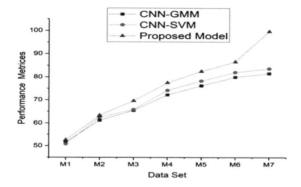

Fig. 5 Performance metrics of the Bio-inspired machine learning method.

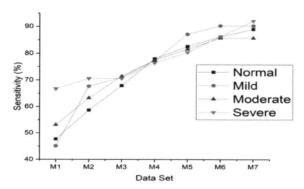

Fig. 6 Classification sensitivity of the Bio-inspired deep learning method.

In addition, the confusion matrix derived on the E-ophtha dataset for the categorisation of normal and impaired retinal pictures using different hierarchical features constructed on models such the bio-inspired algorithm in machine and deep learning process is shown in Figures 6 and 7. The confusion matrix derived from several models shows that the overlapping seen in the lower levels disappears as the number of layers in question increases. Classification specificity is improved by 3.2% in the bio-inspired algorithm in machine and deep learning process model

150 | Bio-inspired Algorithms in Machine Learning and Deep Learning for Disease Detection

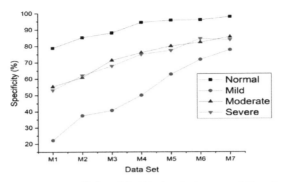

Fig. 7 Classification specificity of the Bio-inspired proposed Deep learning method.

shown in Tables 2 and 3, with a sensitivity and specificity of 81.0% and 89.6%, respectively, for the classification tasks shown. The classification accuracy of the bio-inspired algorithm in machine and deep learning process model is 4.6% high machine learning bio-inspired algorithm model. To demonstrate the efficacy of the proposed model, this research compared the results obtained by using the bio-inspired ML feature extraction with those obtained by employing an ML-based classifier and an SVM-based classifier. Additionally, an evaluation of a fully connected CNN using the aforementioned parameters yields an accuracy of 52.4%. The log-likelihood derived by bio-inspired algorithm in machine and deep

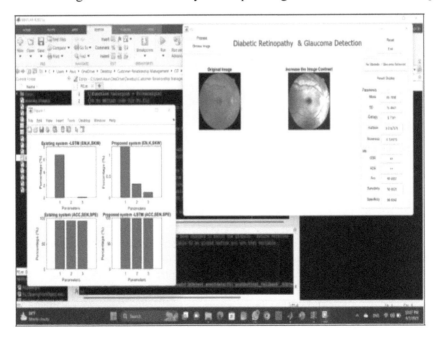

Fig. 8 Simulation results of the No diabetic simulation.

learning process, on the other hand, gives important and significant properties that are class-specific.

4. Multi-stage Analysis of Accuracy, Severity and Sensitivity on Messidor Data Set

4.1 Stages of Diabetic Output 0 = Nothing Happens

The result demonstrates No diabetic at Stage 0 using the present method's comparison settings. When applied to grading tasks, bio-inspired algorithm in machine and deep learning process with extracted hierarchical features at the M7 level achieves an overall accuracy of 89.1%. Figure 8 displays the classification accuracy achieved by the different models on the Messidor dataset for the different classes.

Table 2 Analysis of classification accuracy with different dataset model.

Models	Classification Accuracy (in%)			
	SVM	GMM	CNN	Bio-inspired Algorithm
M_1	45.0	63.1	63.1	62.1
M_2	45.0	66.3	68.4	69.5
M_3	45.0	72.6	72.6	74.7
M_4	45.0	74.7	76.8	78.9
M_5	45.0	75.8	78.9	83.1
M_6	45.0	75.8	78.9	85.2
M_7	45.0	82.1	83.1	99.69

Table 2 shows the analysis of classification accuracy with various models based on Convolution network based with various optimized algorithms like SVM, and so on. In Table 2, out of seven different models using three different bio-inspired algorithm and analysis; from the observation the last model produces more accuracy and resolution from the way of approach. Classification accuracy is most important to analyse the strategy of the proposed algorithm.

Table 3 Sensitivity and specificity analysis of different dataset models.

Models	Bio Sensitivity (in%)			Bio-Specificity (in%)		
	SVM	CNN	Bio- inspired algorithm	SVM	CNN	Bio- inspired algorithm
M_1	51.3	54.0	56.7	70.6	68.9	65.5
M_2	56.7	59.4	64.8	72.4	74.1	72.4
M_3	67.5	67.5	72.9	75.8	75.8	75.8

Contd.

M_4	70.2	72.9	78.3	77.5	79.3	79.3
M_5	72.9	72.9	81.0	77.5	82.7	84.4
M_6	72.9	70.2	81.0	77.5	84.4	87.9
M_7	**75.6**	**75.6**	**98.66**	**86.2**	**87.9**	**98.60**

Table 3 shows the sensitivity and specificity analysis with various models based on Convolution network with various optimized algorithms like SVM, and so on. In Table 3, out of seven different models using three different bio-inspired algorithm and analysis, from the observation the last model produces more accuracy and resolution from the way of approach. Sensitivity and specificity analysis is most important to analyse the strategy of the proposed algorithm.

Table 4 Sensitivity, Precision obtained Analysis of different Dataset models.

Models	Bio-Sensitivity (in %)				Bio-Precision (in %)			
	Normal	Mild	Moderate	Severe	Normal	Mild	Moderate	Severe
M_1	47.7	45.1	53.1	66.7	78.8	22.2	55.3	53.1
M_2	58.7	67.7	63.3	70.6	85.3	37.5	60.8	62.1
M_3	67.9	71.0	71.4	70.6	88.1	40.7	71.4	67.9
M_4	78.0	77.4	77.5	76.5	94.4	50.0	76.0	75.0
M_5	82.6	87.1	81.6	80.4	95.7	62.8	80.0	77.3
M_6	86.2	90.3	85.7	86.3	95.9	71.8	82.3	84.6
M_7	**89.0**	**90.3**	**85.7**	**92.1**	**97.9**	**77.7**	**85.7**	**83.9**

Table 4 shows the sensitivity, precision, and specificity analysis with various models based on Convolution network with various optimized algorithms like SVM, and so on. In this above listed out seven different models using three different bio-inspired algorithm and analysis, from the observation the last model produces more accuracy and resolution from the way of approach. Sensitivity and specificity analysis is most important to analyse the strategy of the proposed algorithm.

4.2 Diabetic Output Stages Mild Diabetic Output Stage 1

Different models were tested and compared shows in Figure 9, including the mild diabetic simulation. The experimental findings outperformed the results of regular ML and Deep Learning. Classification accuracy is at 86.2%, while grading accuracy is at 89.1%. When compared to ML and Deep Learning, a bio-inspired algorithm with ML produced superior results. In addition, we've expanded our efforts to make greater precision gains. Therefore, a feature-learning-based ensemble of classifiers using CNNs has been suggested for diabetic picture classification and grading.

Bio-Inspired Algorithms in Machine Learning and Deep Learning for Diabetes Diagnosis | 153

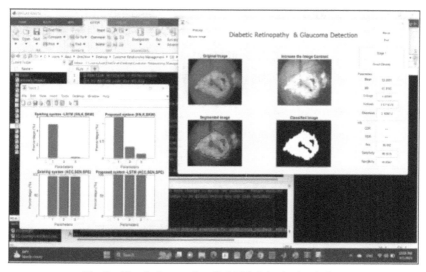

Fig. 9 Simulation results of a Mild diabetic simulation.

4.3 Stage 1: Diabetic Detection at Low Levels

Previous analysis shows the results of an examination of the ML and Deep Learning achieved by several models, including the bio-inspired ML and Deep Learning algorithm. In addition, result shows the mild diabetic simulation derived on the dataset for the grading tasks utilising different structural features constructed on models like ML, and Deep Learning-SVM. These findings demonstrate that using

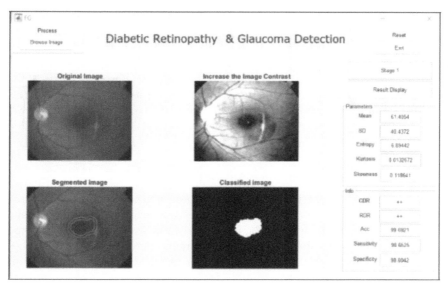

Fig. 10 Simulation results of a Mild diabetic simulation.

just traditional GMM is insufficient to generate a model with higher accuracy. Figure 10 shows the results of mild diabetic systems, theretofore log-likelihood has been included into the proposed model. Since the basic derived from GMMs supplies the important and relevant class-specific characteristics, the ML classifier constructed over the signal analysis vector space outperforms regular report.

4.4 Severe Storm Stage 2

Stage 2 comparison parameters per existing approach are shown in the result, indicating moderate diabetic.

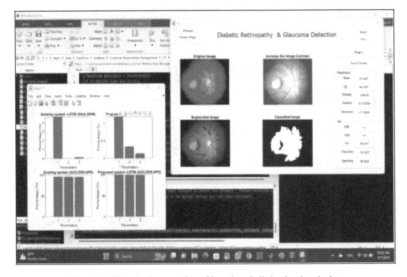

Fig. 11 Simulation results of low level diabetic simulation

Bio-inspired ML and Deep Learning were investigated in this suggested system for the classification and grading of retinopathy pictures. Both the E-ophtha and the Messidor databases were used in the experiments. Using the parameters P (Number of components in bio-inspired algorithm) = 6, supposed design = 88, various parameters = 6, r = 0.85, the ML model achieved 99.6% accuracy on the grading assignment.

4.5 Stage 3: Severe Dehydiabetication

Figure 12 shows the experimental results have proven to be better when compared with those of conventional ML. The accuracy obtained for classification and grading tasks are 86.2% and 89.1%, respectively. The results of the bio-inspired ML model were better than ML and Deep learning. Furthermore, our work has been extended to improve the accuracy even further. Hence, an ensemble of classifiers using CNN that use a feature learning-based approach for classification and grading of diabetic images has been proposed.

Bio-Inspired Algorithms in Machine Learning and Deep Learning for Diabetes Diagnosis | 155

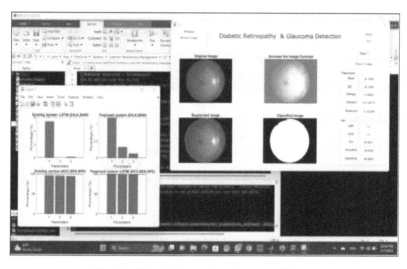

Fig. 12 Simulation results of a severe diabetic.

4.6 Stage 4: Proliferative Diabetic

When compared to ML and Deep Learning, the suggested model has been shown to perform better on classification and grading tasks. Specifically, when it comes to the grading job, the bio-inspired model is 5.4% more effective than the CNN-SVM model. Figure 13 shows the ML model to the Bio-inspired model; the latter is 7.5% more effective.

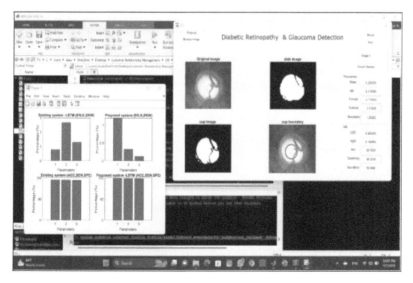

Fig. 13 Simulation results of Proliferative diabetic.

Conclusion

The proposed model makes use of Alex Net, a CNN architecture, to provide a state-of-the-art automated method for recognising retinal images affected by diabetes and glaucoma with little human interaction. It is difficult and error-prone to do periodic diabetic manually due to a lack of resources and reliable expert opinion. This technique may allow for more accurate and precise scanning of fundus images. The amount of work required from human beings decreases. In order to train the models, they required a larger dataset. This analysis showed the feasibility of training CNNs to detect Diabetic diagnosis in fundus images. Ophthalmologists may consult CNNs for a second opinion on a categorization problem. A more advanced set of algorithms may allow for a further increase in the capacity of aberrant photographs in a certain length of time. The new classifier is used for the purpose of image categorization. In the forthcoming work, we'll do a similar evaluation of newly released DL-based diabetic segmentation and lesion detection studies. Future improvements in networks and datasets may make real-time categorization from CNNs a useful tool for diabetic doctors.

References

[1] Dai, L., Wu, L.,Li, H., Cai, C., Qiang Wu, Hongyu Kong, Ruhan Liu, et al. (2021). A deep learning system for detecting Diabetic diagnosis across the disease spectrum, Nature communications, *12*, 3242.

[2] Karan, B.M., Little, K., Augustine, J., Stitt, A.W. and Curtis, T.M. (2023). Aldehyde Dehy Diabeticogenase and Aldo-Keto Reductase Enzymes: Basic Concepts and Emerging Roles in Diabetic diagnosis. *Antioxidants*, *12*, 1466.

[3] H. Naz, H., Nijhawan, R., Ahuja, N.J., Saba, T., Alamri, F.S. and Rehman, A. (2023). Micro-segmentation of retinal image lesions in Diabetic diagnosis using energy-based fuzzy C-Means clustering (EFM-FCM). *Microscopy Research and Technique*. doi:10.1002/jemt.24413.

[4] Krishnamoorthy, S., Weifeng, Y., Luo, J. and Ka, S. (2023). Diabetic y, GO-DBN: Gannet Optimized Deep Belief Network Based wavelet kernel ELM for Detection of Diabetic diagnosis. *Expert Systems with Application*, *229*, 120408.

[5] Akella, P.L. and Kumar, R. (2023). An advanced deep learning method to detect and classify Diabetic diagnosis based on colour fundus images. *Graefe's Archive for Clinical and Experimental Ophthalmology*. doi: 10.1007/s00417-023-06181-3.

[6] Hegde, N., Krishna, S. and Manvi, S.S. (2023). Diabetic Diagnosis System Based on Artificial Intelligence. *In: Human-Machine Interface Technology Advancements and Applications* (pp. 213–30). CRC Press.

[7] McGrath, O.E. and Aslam, T.M. (2022). Use of Imaging Technology to Assess the Effect of COVID-19 on Retinal Tissues: A Systematic Review. *Ophthalmology and Therapy*, *11*, 1017–30.

[8] Agarwal, S. and Bhat, A. (2023). A survey on recent developments in Diabetic diagnosis detection through integration of deep learning. *Multimedia Tools and Applications*, *82*, 17321–351.

[9] Usman, T.M., Yakub Kayode Saheed, Djitog Ignace and Augustine Nsang. (2023). Diabetic diagnosis detection using principal component analysis multi-label feature extraction and classification. *International Journal of Cognitive Computing in Engineering*, *4*, 78–88.

[10] Chan, L.K.Y., Lin, S.S., Chan, F. and Ng, D.S.C. (2023). Optimizing treatment for diabetic macular edema during cataract surgery. *Frontiers in Endocrinology*, *14*, 1106706.

Bio-Inspired Algorithms in Machine Learning and Deep Learning for Diabetes Diagnosis | 157

[11] Karthikeyan, R. and Alli, P. (2018). Feature selection and parameters optimization of support vector machines based on hybrid glowworm swarm optimization for classification of Diabetic diagnosis. *Journal of Medical Systems, 42*, 1–11.

[12] Sanjana, S., Shadin, N.S. and Farzana, M. (2021). Automated Diabetic diagnosis detection using transfer learning models. *In: 2021 5th International Conference on Electrical Engineering and Information Communication Technology (ICEEICT)*, IEEE. doi: 10.1109/ICEEICT53905.2021.9667793.

[13] S. Gayathri, S., Gopi, V.P. and Palanisamy, P. (2020). A lightweight CNN for Diabetic diagnosis classification from fundus images. *Biomedical Signal Processing and Control, 62*, 102115.

[14] Kim, H.E., Linan, A.C., Santhanam, N., Mahboubeh Jannesari, Mate E. Maros and Thomas Ganslandt. (2023). Transfer learning for medical image classification: A literature review. *BMC Medical Imaging, 22*, 69.

[15] Rêgo, S., Medeiros, M.D., Soares, F. and Soares, M.M. (2021). Screening for Diabetic diagnosis using an automated diagnostic system based on deep learning: Diagnostic accuracy assessment. *Ophthalmologica, 244*, 250–57.

[16] Alghamdi, H.S. (2022). Towards explainable deep neural networks for the automatic detection of Diabetic diagnosis. *Applied Sciences, 12*, 9435.

[17] Sebastian, A., Elharrouss, O., Maadeed, S.A. and Almaadeed, N. (2023). A Survey on Deep-Learning-Based Diabetic Diagnosis Classification. *Diagnostics, 13*, 345.

[18] Farag, M.M., Fouad, M. and Abdel-Hamid, A.T. (2022). Automatic Diabetic Diagnosis Severity Classification using the DenseNet and Convolutional Block Attention Module. *IEEE Access, 10*, 38299–308.

[19] Atwany, M.Z., Sahyoun, A.H. and Yaqub, M. (2022). Deep learning algorithms for Diabetic diagnosis classification: A survey. *IEEE Access, 10*, 28642–655.

[20] Bhatti, U.A., Huang, M., Wu, D., Zhang, Y., Mehmood, A. and Han, H. (2019). Recommendation system using feature extraction and pattern recognition in clinical care systems. *Enterprise Information Systems, 13*, 329–51.

[21] Bhatti, U.A., Zeeshan, Z., Nizamani, M.M., Bazai, S., Yu, Z. and Yuan, L. (2022). Assessing the change of ambient air quality patterns in Jiangsu Province of China pre-to post-COVID-19. *Chemosphere, 288*, 132569.

[22] Bora, A., Balasubramanian, S., Babenko, B., Virmani, S., Venugopalan, S., Mitani, A., de Oliveira Marinho, G., et al. (2021). Predicting the risk of developing Diabetic diagnosis using deep learning. *The Lancet Digital Health, 3*, e10–e19.

[23] Asia, A.O., Zhu, C.Z., Althubiti, S.A., Alimi, D.A., Xiao, Y.L., Ouyang, P.B. and Al-Qaness, M.A. (2022). Detection of Diabetic diagnosis in retinal fundus images using CNN classification models. *Electronics, 11*, 2740.

[24] Nielsen, K.B., Lautrup, M.L., Andersen, J.K., Savarimuthu, T.R. and Grauslund, J. (2019). Deep learning-based algorithms in screening of Diabetic diagnosis: A systematic review of diagnostic performance. *Ophthalmology Retina, 3*, 294–304.

[25] Balasubramaniam, S., Vijesh Joe, C., Sivakumar, T.A., Prasanth, A., Satheesh Kumar, K., Kavitha, V. and Dhanaraj, R.K. (2023). Optimization Enabled Deep Learning-Based DDoS Attack Detection in Cloud Computing. *International Journal of Intelligent Systems, 2023*(1), 2039217.

[26] Muthumeenakshi, R., Singh, C., Sapkale, P.V. and Mukhedkar, M.M. (2022). An Efficient and Secure Authentication Approach in VANET using Location and Signature-based Services. *Adhoc and Sensor Wireless Networks, 53*.

[27] Mo, J., Zhang, L. and Feng, Y. (2018). Exudate-based diabetic macular edema recognition in retinal images using cascaded deep residual networks. *Neurocomputing, 290*, 161–71.

[28] Zengchen, Y., Wang, K., Wan, Z., Xie, S. and Lv, Z. (2023). Popular deep learning algorithms for disease prediction: A review. *Cluster Computing, 26*, 1231–51.

9 | A Multi-Objective Optimized Bio-Inspired Deep Learning Framework for Autism Spectrum Disorder Diagnosis in Toddlers

K. Vijayalakshmi[1*] and Venkatesh Naganathan[2]

Bio-inspired optimized algorithms are stimulated by behaviours of living beings and physical principles that addresses problems across various application domains. A developmental disorder in the neurological system of a human is referred to be an Autism-Spectrum Disorder. It is considered based on communication difficulties, restricted and repetitive behaviours, rational thinking and societal responsibilities. Recognizing and handling it timely may reduce the risk and improve the condition when compared to the prior. To do such diagnosis, the current assessment can be too expensive which leads to the requirement of Deep learning models to be integrated with neuroimaging bio-inspired methods. A novel methodology is proposed in this chapter to detect autism by combining Artificial Neural Network with GridSearch optimization and Particle Swarm Optimization with Multi-Objective functionality. Particle Swarm is a bio-inspired technique which is metaheuristic by nature, applied for feature selection. The relative analysis based on evaluation of this proposed model is carried out further with various machine learning models using the classification metrics. The proposed model is built using pyswarm, sklearn, matplotlib, seaborn, and is unique due to its bio-inspired characteristics, achieving maximum model accuracy with a minimum number of attributes, indicating its potential for early treatment with mediation for better curability.

1. Introduction

Autism Syndrome Disorder (ASD) is a chronic ailment which has an emotional impact on a large proportion of the population. It also affects the physical appearance of the face and during the developmental phases its signs and indicators appear very often. It means that the symptoms can be clearly witnessed between two years from the time of birth. It has a multifaceted issue in its diagnostic process and necessitates specialized medical knowledge and instruments that rely on interpretive encoding of the child's remarks and opinions, discussions, and conversation with parents, and physically examining the case. As there are no specialized tests, such as blood tests or medical exams for ASD, diagnosing it becomes a difficult task. Doctors collect a child's developmental history and behavioural patterns from the

---

[1] School of Computer Science and Applications, REVA University, Bangalore, Karnataka, India.
[2] Senior Consultant cum Professor, Amity Global Institute, Singapore.
* Corresponding author: vgkrishna20@gmail.com

various assessment tools like neurological tests, the "Autism Diagnostic Interview-Revised (ADI-R)", the "Autism Diagnostic Observation-Schedule (ADOS)", and the "Childhood Autism Rating-Scale (CARS)". Even though there is no cure for autism, doctors provide behavioural therapies that aid in the child's gradual improvement. Multilayered machine learning (ML) techniques offer exceptional capabilities in handling intricate classification tasks by meticulously examining intricate patterns and relationships concealed within extensive datasets. The use of multilayered ML techniques can greatly improve manual analysis and diagnosis systems. Convolutional Neural Networks (CNNs) algorithm is used in the facial expression detection to identify facial expressions and Artificial Neural Networks (ANNs) algorithm is used for prediction in the questionnaire system.

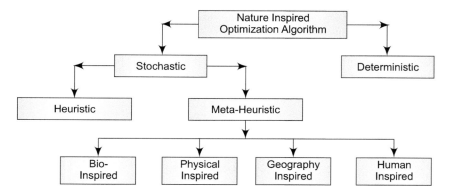

Fig. 1 Types of Nature-Inspired Algorithms.

Bio-inspired computational models draw stimulation through the biological systems. It is due to the fact that the human brain and nervous systems can readily tackle highly complexed computational problems with high quality solutions. The work is aimed to create a supportive system that assists doctors in dealing with complications while also providing children and families with access to practical diagnosis assessment. As a result, the proposed chapter employs multilayered optimized Deep learning (DL) techniques to create a low-cost automated system with better autism diagnosis.

The chapter covers the various bio-inspired algorithms and their applications in the healthcare domain for disease prediction. It covers the background study to analyse the need to address this topic of interest for disease detection. A novel algorithm is proposed to detect the ASD, especially in toddlers combining DL algorithms with well-known bio-inspired algorithms like particle swarm optimization (PSO) for feature selection and classification that are metaheuristic by nature. This study demonstrates the effectiveness of using Bio-inspired deep learning techniques for ASD prediction. It highlights the significance and importance of timely identifying the cause and intervention which is the need of an hour. It is addressed to include both the conceptual along with the algorithmic details of the approach to make the readers to understand and learn it better. The content presented in this chapter will be useful for both academicians and IT professionals, such as those who are interested in Artificial intelligence (AI), ML, Bio-inspired or Nature-inspired, classification and optimization techniques. It provides a comparative and rigorous analysis of the convergence of the proposed algorithm. It includes tables, illustrations, and figures to provide the reader's understanding on the proposed work. The multi-objective optimizations combined with bio-inspired metaheuristic algorithms offer a more promising approach to solve complex real-world problems efficiently.

1.1 Overview of Bio-Inspired Metaheuristic Algorithm

By making use of the capable, contributing and competent strategies identified in nature, the Bio-inspired algorithms offer innovative solutions for a variety of real-world applications. The following section introduces the basic principles of bio-inspired algorithms and their variants to the reader to understand their wider scope in the field of research.

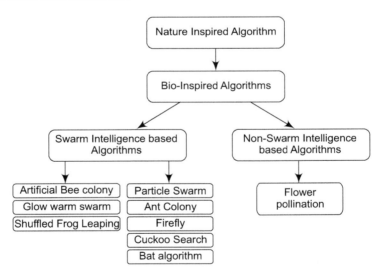

Fig. 2 Types of Bio-Inspired Algorithms.

1.1.1 Bio-Inspired Algorithms

Bio-inspired metaheuristic methods are optimization algorithms that draw inspiration from natural phenomena or biological systems to develop strategies for efficient problem-solving. These techniques are very often used for highly complexed problems and where the conventional ideas to determine optimal solutions may be difficult. Based on the different biological phenomena, bio-inspired algorithm variants exist as listed below:

- *Genetic Algorithms (GA)*: This is the most well-known bio-inspired metaheuristic algorithm that is based on the natural selection and genetics process. It is to evolve the candidate solutions using mutation, selection, and crossover to seek for optimal/near optimal solutions.
- *Particle Swarm Optimization (PSO)*: This is a metaheuristic-cum-population-based technique derived by the social manners of bird flocking or fish schooling. In PSO, based on its neighbours and experience, a cluster of sub-solutions is determined as the particles move around the search space for the best solution.
- *Ant Colony Optimization (ACO)*: This is defined from the foraging nature of ants that involves modelling. It is based on how ants communicate amongst themselves using pheromones and also finds its shortest route for its feed. It is used widely for combinatorial-based optimization problems.
- *Artificial Bee Colony (ABC) Algorithm*: This is inspired by the foraging behaviour of honeybees to seek the strategy for food resources such as local search and global search to optimize numerical functions.
- *Simulated Annealing (SA)*: This imitates the annealing process in metallurgy where a material is heated and then slowly cooled for it to approach a low-energy state. It is used to optimize problems by allowing the algorithm to take in worse solutions with a certain chance to escape local optima.
- *Genetic Bee Colony Algorithm*: It combines the principles of both genetic and bees behaviour to provide better solutions with more efficient.
- *Fish Swarm Algorithm*: It mimics the behaviour of a fish shoaling in order to fix the better and right solution for the complex problems.
- *Cat Swarm Optimization*: It is influenced through the hunting nature of cats to provide optimized solution using swarm intelligence approach.
- *Whale Optimization Algorithm*: It is influenced based on the bubble net hunting activities of the humpback whales for optimization.
- *Artificial Algae Algorithm*: It is inspired from the growth and the movement patterns of large clusters of algae to attain optimization solution.
- *Elephant Search Algorithm*: This obtains optimized solution based on the herding behaviour of elephants.
- *Cuckoo Search Optimization Algorithm*: It optimizes the solution using a search process combining with the nature of brood parasitism behaviour of cuckoo birds.
- *Moth Flame Optimization*: This is based on the optimization of solution using a moth's behaviour of navigation towards light sources.
- *Grey Wolf Optimization Algorithm*: The optimization process uses the societal and chasing nature of grey-wolves.

1.2 Optimization in Bio-Inspired Metaheuristic Algorithms

Bio-inspired metaheuristic optimization algorithms require highly computational strategies inspired by the natural processes and behaviours to unravel intricate problems with optimality. These algorithms imitate the behaviour of living

162 | Bio-inspired Algorithms in Machine Learning and Deep Learning for Disease Detection

organisms and natural phenomena to search from the space to find solutions for the way out of the problem. By analysing the principles observed in nature, such as evolution, swarm intelligence or animal behaviours, bio-inspired metaheuristic algorithms can efficiently explore solutions and find near-optimal solutions for various types of optimization problems. Hence, they useful for solving complex optimization problems where traditional methods might struggle due to high dimensionality, nonlinearity, or the presence of noisy objective functions.

1.2.1 Metaheuristic Optimization Algorithms

The bio-inspired algorithms are metaheuristic that provide an effective mechanism to address wisely on optimization related problems by using nature's process and its functionalities. It basically explores in widespread search space for solutions of optimality to address more than one objective. Due to this ability, it can handle various complex problems and sustain the diversity in their solutions. As per the timelines, these techniques effectively demonstrate the NP—hard problems in determining the near optimal solutions. These algorithms are basically defined through its capability to both local and global searches and finally get convergence to its end optimal solution.

1.2.2 Multi-Objective Optimization (MOO)

MOO is a method of satisfying more than one functional objective whose aim is to determine the better optimization solution from the search space. The bio-inspired algorithms score their significance due to their MOO ability and solve many crucial complexed problems by considering multiple objectives to find an optimal or near optimal solution. Few bio-inspired techniques that are basically defined with MOO characteristics are given below:

- ***Evolutionary Multi-objective optimization (EMO)*:** It uses population-related mechanism with various strategies to specifically address multiple objectives.
- ***Non-Dominated Sorting Genetic Algorithm (NSGA-II)*:** It is non-dominating and uses sorting that maintain a variety of solutions and compromise on objectives with conflicts.
- ***PSO for MOO (PSO-MOO)/ACO for MOO (ACO-MOO)*:** These are the techniques which already are defined in previous the section 1.1.1 that use the characteristics of swarm and ant to effectively perform with a single objective, whereas this technique additionally handles MOO to determine the set of outcomes that are not dominated ones.

All these algorithms which are nature-inspired with multifunctional objectives and can be used in various domain fields of expertise as image recognition and processing, banking and finance, robotics and engineering design, healthcare, and scientific research, etc.

Their versatility, robustness, and ability to handle complex optimization problems make them great valuable tools for researchers and practitioners seeking efficient solutions to the real-world challenges that need to be solved.

1.2.3 Applications and Advantages

Bio-inspired algorithms have found their broad spectrum of applications in various fields due to their ability to efficiently solve any complex problem requiring an optimized solution. Some common applications include:

- ***Engineering Design Optimization***: In engineering, bio-inspired algorithms are put to use in optimization of design, structural analysis, control systems, and other engineering tasks. These algorithms can assist in finding optimal solutions to complex engineering problems that may be tedious to solve using orthodox methods. Optimizing designs with multiple conflicting objectives as cost, performance, and reliability.
- ***Robotics and NLP***: Bio-inspired algorithms are used in natural language processing (NLP) for chores as analysis of text, sentiment, machine translation, and speech recognition. These algorithms greatly improve the accuracy and efficiency of language processing systems.
- ***Cybersecurity***: In cybersecurity applications, bio-inspired algorithms are utilized for the detection of any intrusion, malware analysis, and network security. These algorithms help an organization protect their digital assets and dodge the cyber threats effectively.
- ***Time-Series Analysis***: Bio-inspired algorithms are applied in time-series analysis for predicting future trends, recognizing patterns, anomaly detection, and data mining. They can help analysts derive valuable insights from their time-dependent datasets.
- ***Recommender Systems***: Bio-inspired algorithms play a role in creating recommender systems that are extensively applied in the domain of e-commerce and social-media platforms, along with service of streaming. These techniques, in turn, provide better personalized suggestions or recommendations based on the user's preference to improve the end-user experience and exposure.
- ***Financial Forecasting***: Bio-inspired algorithms are used in business and management for tasks such as process optimization, allocation of resources, and decision-making. These forecasting algorithms greatly assist businesses in the reduction of cost, increase in the efficiency, and overall performance. They are specifically used for tasks like optimization of portfolio, risk management, algorithmic trading, and fraud detection. These algorithms can effectively aid in financial institutions in making clear decisions and manage risks effectively, especially portfolio optimization, while considering risk and return as competing objectives.
- ***Bioinformatics and Healthcare***: Bio-inspired algorithms find their applications in healthcare for medical image analysis, diagnosis of a disease, treatment planning, and drug discovery. These algorithms can contribute in the sectors of personalized medicine and healthcare.

The advantages of Bio-inspired algorithms for Multi-objective optimization are:

- ***Robustness***: Bio-inspired algorithms exhibit robustness in handling complex optimization problems which include multiple conflicting objectives.
- ***Diversity***: These algorithms promote diversity amongst the solutions, which helps in exploring a wide range of trade-off solutions on the Pareto front.
- ***Adaptability***: Bio-inspired algorithms can adapt to dynamic environments and changing problem situations effectively.
- ***Parallelism***: Many bio-inspired algorithms can be parallelized easily, allowing them to efficiently explore the solution spaces.

2. Background of the Study: Experiential Investigation of Bio-Inspired Algorithms for Disease Detection in Statistical Perspective

Omar, K.S. et al. (2019) [1] proposed a prediction model for ASD using ML methods with mobile app deployment for autism people of any age. It is a hybrid model comprising of RandomForest (RF) - CART and RandomForest-ID3 which is applied on AQ1-10 and 250 real datasets. The model delivers improved results in terms of accuracy, specificity, sensitivity, precision, and FPR for both kinds of datasets. Alsaade, F.W. et al. (2022) [2] proposed a system for ASD detection using deep learning techniques like CNN with transfer-learning and the flask framework. Three pre-trained models, Xception, VGG19, and NASNETMobile, were used to classify 2,940 face images collected from Kaggle. The Xception model contributed high performance compared to other models.

Rabbi, M.F. et al. (2021) [3] focused on detecting autism in children using Multilayered Perceptron (MLP), RF, Gradient Boosting Machine (GBM), AdaBoost (AB), and CNN where CNN achieved the highest accuracy of 92.31%. Wei, W. et al. (2019) [4] proposed a new model for predicting saliency in images for children with ASD based on CNN and used multilevel features to generate three attention maps, which are then combined to produce the predicted saliency map. Li, B. et al. (2019) [5] introduced an ML system to classify ASD using facial attributes like emotions, expressions, actions, etc. to train CNN. Experimental results show improvement in the model's performance on various metrics for ASD classification with an improvement of about 7%. Popescu, A.L. et al. (2020) [6] proposed the deployment of a mobile app using ML techniques for multiclass image classification that predicts emotional state based on children's (between 2–5 years old with autism) drawings. The application uses Firebase and has been proven to be robust, providing an accuracy of 80.6% in identifying emotional states.

Karuppasamy, S.G. et al. (2022) [7] used AI (artificial intelligence) specifically DL algorithms to diagnose ASD using neuroimaging-based approaches that provide information on anatomy and activity of brain, which can aid in identifying ASD. The work uses CNN to detect ASD patients from a huge collection of data that has the patterns of the brain for identifying the region of interest (ROI) using feature extraction techniques and achieved 95% accuracy. Baranwal, A. et al. (2020) [8]

analysed a dataset for screening ASD in adults, children, and adolescents using ML algorithms such as ANN, RF, Logistic-Regression (LR), Decision-Tree (DT), and Support-Vector Machines (SVMs) which obtained accuracy of 80%, 88%, 92%, 80%, 76% for adult dataset, and accuracy of 82%, 82.2%, 90%, 90.3%, 96%, 95% for child dataset.

Tao, Y. et al. (2019) [9] proposed SP-ASDNet, a DNN that combines CNNs and LSTM (long short-term memory) networks for the classification of an observer who has ASD or is typically developed based on their scan path of a given image. The model achieved an accuracy of 74.22% for validation. Maria Sofia et al. (2022) [10] proposed a cost-effective system for autism diagnosis in children using automatic and analytic tools that includes a questionnaire tool based on ADI-R for parents/caregivers to provide developmental history and an observatory system based on ADOS to analyse autistic patients' behaviours like eye movements and facial expressions. Ali, N. A.et al. (2020) [11] developed a Dl model using CNN with six layers for autism detection by using a dataset of 20 individuals from King Abdulaziz University, Saudi Arabia which achieved an accuracy of 80%, Raj, S. et al. (2020) [12] attempts to detect ASD using various ML and DL techniques and evaluates their performance on three nonclinical datasets: child, adolescents, and adult. The results show that CNN performed well compared to a conventional SVM achieving an accuracy of 98.3% for the ASD Child dataset after handling missing values.

Islam, S. et al. (2020) [13] proposed a model to diagnose autism in children at an age less one year through the set of questionnaires. The dataset collected from 'Q-CHAT' and 'AQ' tools applied on SVM, RF, Naive Bayes (NB), and KNN (K-Nearest Neighbour) predicted with an accuracy of 83%, 93%, 89%, and 98% for toddlers. Hashemi, J. et al. (2021) [14] proposed and validates computer vision methods that automatically relate the behaviours for the identification of risk markers of ASD early. It is applied to video recordings from a mobile device's front camera while the child watches movie stimuli designed to elicit such behaviours. Vakadkar, K. et al. (2021) [15] conducted a study to investigate the application of ML techniques to complement the conventional methods used to diagnose ASD. It applied SVM, RF, NB, LR, and KNN to a dataset to construct predictive models and found that LR provided the highest accuracy.

Singh, A. et al. (2021) [16] aimed to improve the ASD diagnosis by using ML models to identify significant indicators of autism in toddlers. The study used an ASD dataset and designed an NN (neural network) and RF classifier with feature selection.

Hossain, M.D. et al. (2021) [17] focused on automating the ASD diagnostic using ML techniques on ASD datasets of 'toddlers, children, adolescents, and adults'. It is to identify the most significant traits and best-performing classifier and feature selection techniques and found that the MLP classifier outperformed by achieving accuracy of 100% with a minimal contributing features for all four datasets. Hammood, W.A. et. al. (2017) [18] provides a comprehensive overview of bio-inspired optimization algorithms, focusing on those derived from natural phenomena such as DE, Ffly, PSO, ABC, and Bat with its limitations and challenges (dependency on parameter tuning, balancing exploration, and exploitation phases) and suggested the ongoing advancements and hybrid approaches.

Jakšić, Z. et. al. (2023) [19] provides a wide-ranging overview of bio-inspired optimization algorithms in microelectronics and nanophotonics by exploring various heuristic and metaheuristic approaches. Mujawar, S. et. al. [20] (2022) performed a wide-range of review in bio-inspired optimization algorithms applied to medical disease classification, focusing on heart disease, neurological disorders, cancer, lung cancer, and COVID-19. It highlights the application of various algorithms such as GA, PSO, CNN comparing their outcome in terms of accuracy and computational complexity. It addresses the variability in performance of different algorithms across various diseases and signal types, making it difficult to generalize results and integrate LSTM and GRU (gated recurrent unit) with bio-inspired models to enhance classification accuracy and address these limitations.

Yadav, M.K. et. al. (2022) [21] explores the integration of ML and bio-inspired algorithms to improve the early diagnosis of liver diseases using ultrasound imaging. It addresses the strength, challenges, and limitations of diagnostics through computer-assisted tools and techniques. It addresses the inherent difficulty in detecting liver disease at an early stage due to the organ's ability to appear healthy despite significant damage. The proposed methodology, involving preprocessing, feature extraction, and advanced classification algorithms, aims to address these issues but requires extensive validation and refinement.

Haque, N.I. et. al. (2021) [22] outlines the BIOCAD framework, a digital healthcare system utilizing ML models for classification of disease and detection of anomaly and evaluates the work using bio-inspired optimization algorithms, particularly the WO, GWO, and FO methods, on three distinct medical datasets. While the WO algorithm shows promising outcomes as FScores with 0.89 to 1.0, several limitations and challenges are evident. The framework's performance on imbalanced datasets, such as the Parkinson dataset, is hampered by high false-negative rates, indicating a challenge in generalizing across different medical conditions.

Giampaglia, D. et. al.'s (2012) [23] paper introduces a unique computerized approach for categorizing cells in "fluorescence microscopy images" using a classifier-based approach on bio-inspired information that relies on the dispersal of divergence within the cell images. The method demonstrates high classification precision of over 96% on the HEp-2 Cells dataset. S Lohi, S.A. et. al. (2023) [24] presents an innovative disease detection in crop and yield prediction model utilizing multi-featured bio-inspired representation of feature with ensemble classifier. The model addresses the complexity and the computational overhead in the integration of diverse classifiers such as SVM, MLP, LR, DT, and NB and GA-based feature selection, while optimizing feature variance.

Digumarthi, J. et. al. (2022) [25] underscores the critical need for advanced predictive methods to address cardiovascular diseases (CVDs), emphasizing the prospective of bio-inspired optimization algorithms in enhancing the prediction of classification of heart diseases, particularly arrhythmias. Using Cuckoo Search, BAT, and Modified Salp Swarm Optimization, the research demonstrates significant improvements in diagnostic accuracy. Bhargava, R. et. al. (2022) [26] present a thorough exploration of the application of the Ant Lion Optimizer (ALO) metaheuristic technique to address the ELD (economic load dispatch) issues in power system to reduce cost involved in fuel while satisfying various constraints.

Pham, T.H. et. al. (2023) [27] have done the systematic literature review for valuable insights into the application of bio-inspired algorithms for feature selection addressing publication bias and the variability in research methodologies and evaluation metrics across the included studies. Trojovský, P. et. al. (2022) [28] introduce a novel metaheuristic algorithm, STO (symbol-timing offset) influenced by the hunting cum fighting behaviours of Siberian tigers. It primarily focuses on the algorithm's performance on optimization tasks but lacks a comprehensive analysis of its scalability to handle larger and more complex problem spaces. It addresses noisy or uncertain objective functions of STP (Spanning Tree Protocol) to enhance its credibility and applicability as a viable optimization tool in practical settings.

Givi, H. et. al. (2023) [29] present an innovative metaheuristic algorithm, Red Panda Optimization (RPO), inspired by the searching cum climbing behaviours of red pandas. It addresses the scalability of RPO performance on extremely high-dimensional optimization problems and robustness and adaptability across diverse problem landscapes. Yang, Q. et. al. (2018) [30] explore the usage of unmanned aerial vehicles (UAVs) for efficient monitoring of critical infrastructures through optimal flight path planning mechanisms using bio-inspired algorithms presents promising avenues for enhancing data collection from WSN (weighted sum model). It addresses the complexity of deriving the optimal UAV flight path amidst various environmental factors such as prohibited airspace, geographical conditions, and sensor deployment statistics, which are NP-hard problems. Jain, A. et. al. (2023) [31] briefed in the paper a technique for the early diagnosis using ML with bio-inspired algorithms like Bat and firefly.

3. Autism Diagnosis using Bio-Inspired Metaheurisitc Optimization Algorithms for Feature Selection

Today, due to the development in the growth of innovations in algorithmic reach, it is very significant and important to attract the industry through its contributions. As discussed in the previous section, these bio-inspired algorithms are learnt and derived from the natural phenomena and biological process. They have the ability to solve multiple complex problems to determine optimal solutions from the set of search space of solutions. Due to this, they can address challenges of any kind in various domains of applications which include the very sensitive healthcare related issues like disease diagnosis, image processing, computer-aided counselling, etc. In this context, the diagnosis of autism carried through these natural influenced algorithms can commendably improve its ML predictive models' performance.

Bio-inspired Algorithms in Machine Learning and Deep Learning for Disease Detection

These techniques provide the assurance of achieving the optimal solution for the autism related diagnostic complex problems [32–33].

The most popular bio-inspired optimization algorithm is PSO that has a number of particles through which it determines the potential solution. Usually the larger number of particles will increase the probability of finding of a quality solution. But at the same time, the complexity exists in terms of its computational overheads. So there must be a trade-off between search efficiency and computational cost [34]. PSO requires the following aspects of parameters to search for an optimal solution:

- Particle position
- Velocity update
- Social and cognitive learning
- Swarm topology

The simple steps of PSO comprises of the following:

- Determine the movement of the particles in the swarm by specifying the position of the particle in the search space.
- Determine the velocity of the particle using the below equation:

$$vel(t+1) = w * vel(t) + c1 * rand\,(0,1) * (Pbest(t) - pos(t))$$
$$+ c2 * rand(0,1) * (Gbest(t) - pos(t)) \qquad ...(1)$$

where, w is the inertia weight, a constant determines the quantity of particle's previous velocity moved to the next iteration; $c1$, $c2$ are the acceleration constant that determines how much the particles influenced by the Gbest and Pbest solutions; rand $(0,1)$ – random function generates the randomness between 0 and 1 in the particle movement and initializes velocity to zero.

- Determine the new position of the particle based on its velocity using the equation:

$$pos(t+1) = pos(t) + vel(t+1) \qquad ...(2)$$

- Apart from these, the algorithm considers few constraints to restrict the particle to move far away or get stuck in same local optima from its search space for the solution. It specifies the limits of maximum velocity.
- Hence the particle movement is based on the combination of the current position and the velocity of the particle along with the personal best and the global best solutions.
- By fine tuning the parameters w and $c1$, $c2$, the behaviour of the particle can be improved and the performance of the algorithm also can be increased.

3.1 Data Profile

The PSO and ACO bio-inspired algorithms can enhance the accuracy of DL models to predict ASD. The data and the algorithms are the major key resources for the prediction of autism using bio-inspired algorithms. Data-profiling is the process of analysing and examining the data sources at different parts of integrity to know its structure, quality, and content. The purpose of data-profiling is to identify patterns, inconsistencies, and anomalies in the data, and to assess its accuracy and completeness. To analyse the data, the data-profiling techniques can be done using data visualization such as box plots, heat maps, etc.

3.1.1 Autism Behavioural Dataset

The ASD Behavioural dataset is used to perform the prediction in Toddler Autism as of July, 2018. The dataset is provided by Thabtah, University of California available at Kaggle.com, and is an open source for all ML techniques. This dataset can be utilized for study environment collected from the ASD Tests screening app [4]. The dataset contains 18 attributes including the class variable and 1,054 cases or records. The 18 attributes are the descriptive features, and the dependent feature is the class label for ASD traits (Yes/No), means toddler has ASD or not. In addition, the parents, the caregiver, and the medical personnel each answered the 10 questions which are A1–A10 and responses to the Q-CHAT question are chosen as "0" or "1" in the dataset. Most of the data in this case is of the Boolean or binary variety, which is suitable for classifier computation. Apart from these, the dataset consists of numerical and categorical attributes that need to be scaled and converted before they can be used in classifiers to try out the best possible outcomes. The attributes (A1–10) and its mapping corresponding to the 'Q-Chat-10' questionnaires as listed in Table 1.

Table 1 Details of variables mapping to the Q-Chat-10 screening methods.

Attributes	*Corresponding Q-chat-10-Toddlers Questionnaires*
A1 –10 (Screening on response, eye contact, communication, vocabulary, starring, understand and console, etc.,)	Respond when someone calls by name?
	Keep eye contact?
	Express the wish when they want something?
	Point interest to others for sharing?
	Pretend to act?
	Follows your way through?
	Signs of warmth to keep others comfort when they are upset?
	First word spoken?
	Use any basic body signals?
	Stare at nothing without any purpose?

The values will be gathered using the Q-CHAT questionnaires and the total of these question values is reflected by the Q-Chat 10 score. Finally, the score which is greater than 3 indicates that the toddler has a significant risk of developing ASD symptoms [8], else with 3 or less indicates that there are no evident ASD features. The complete dataset description is provided in Table 2 that describes the unique characteristics of each toddler that may be used to determine which variables will influence the occurrence of ASD.

Table 2 Features with its descriptions.

Feature	Type	Description
A1–10: QA	Binary	Code generated based on the screening method used
Age	Numerical	Age in months – Toddlers
Score by Q-chat-10	Numerical	<=3: no ASD traits > 3: ASD traits
Sex	Categorical	Male: Female
Ethnicity	Categorical	Ethnicities
Born with jaundice	Boolean	Jaundice Symptoms
Family member with ASD history	Boolean	Family History/Genetical
Who is completing the test?	Categorical	Parent, self, caregiver, medical staff, clinician, etc.
Why have you taken the screening?	Categorical	Use input textbox
Class variable	Categorical	Yes: ASD traits No : No ASD traits

3.1.2 Data Preprocessing

Originally, the dataset that consists of 1,054 observations and 18 characteristics (with target variable) includes categorical, continuous, and binary variables. The data preprocessing is very much required to provide quality data to the training model by removing noise and bias out of it. Depending on the number and nature, missing values are identified and handled in the dataset either by imputing them with the mean or median value or removing the missing values. It is required to identify the contributing features through the feature selection techniques. Also the categorical data must be converted to numerical as machine learning algorithms performs well with numerical data. The preprocessing once completed, the data will be ready and suitable for training and analysis [35–36]. The following preprocessing steps will be followed before developing any ML model.

- **Handling Duplicates:** Duplicate entries in the dataset are identified and removed.
- **Handling Outliers:** Outliers in the dataset are identified and handled either by removing them or capping their values at a predetermined threshold.
- **Label Encoding (LE):** Non-numerical variables like sex, jaundice, family_ mem_with_ASD, and class/ASD_Traits are converted to numerical (binary- 0/1) format using label encoding technique.
- **One-hot Encoding [15]:** LE is not effective for those when there are more than two values/classes and hence one-hot encoding is employed for multiclass features like 'Ethnicity' to avoid hierarchical ranking.

- **Feature Decomposition:** Categorical attributes with multiple categories are identified for which one hot encoding is not feasible, hence feature composition technique is used to group different categories into a single category.
- **Feature Engineering:** When all characteristics in a dataset are employed, classification accuracy may suffer [10]. Furthermore, having fewer characteristics minimizes the time and memory consumption that are needed to fit the model. Hence, rank the attributes to determine the subset of most significant attributes from the given dataset that results in the maximum accuracy.

3.2 Data Visualization Techniques

Various data visualization techniques are used in Autism prediction using behavioural data to analyse and present the data in a meaningful way [37]. Here are some techniques for data visualization that can be referred for feature importance:

- *Heat Maps***:** It is used to show coefficient correlations between attributes of behavioural data; reducing data dimensionality can be used to visualize data patterns by colour-coding different values. The Heat map given in the Figures 3

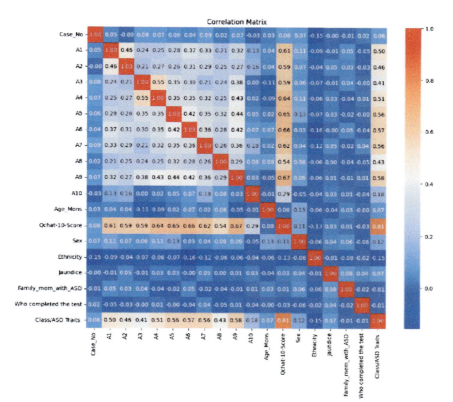

Fig. 3 Correlation Matrix.

172 | Bio-inspired Algorithms in Machine Learning and Deep Learning for Disease Detection

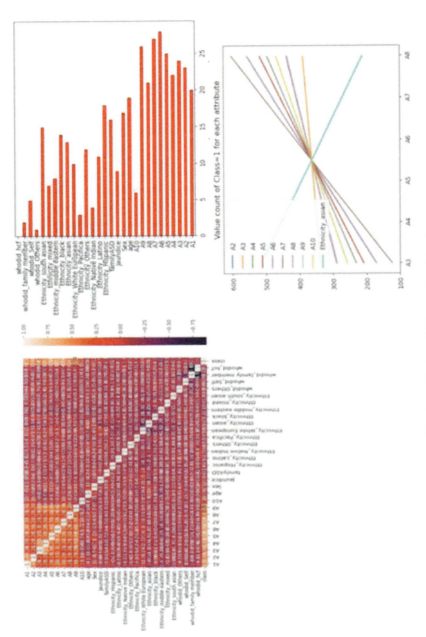

Fig. 4 (a) Heatmap (b) Bar chart (c) Line chart.

and 4a perform feature engineering and aids to reduce data dimensionality by removing highly correlated variables.

- **Bar Charts**: They are commonly used in data analysis and visualization to compare different categories and their values. To predict autism, a bar chart can be used to display the frequency or prevalence of certain behaviours or symptoms associated with autism across different groups.

The bar chart in Figure 4(b) explains the importance of various attributes considered in the dataset which are calculated using the Fisher score. It helps in eliminating attributes from the dataset which have less importance and to reduce data dimensionality. Also, by using the bar chart the distribution of ages of the individuals in the ASD group can be represented as in Figures 5a and b. The plot explains by having age on the x-axis and the number of individuals on the y-axis in understanding how the ages of the toddlers are spread across the dataset.

- **Line Charts**: These represent the data to be displayed in terms of coordinates linked by a line. They are used frequently to demonstrate the trends and changes in data over time. The developmental trajectory of certain autism-related behaviour from the dataset as shown in Figure 4c.
- **Box Plot**: It provides a summary of the central tendency and spread of the 'Qchat-10-Score' for each sex, including the median, quartiles, and potential outliers as in Figure 5c. It helps in understanding if there are any notable differences in the Qchat-10 scores between males and females.
- **Count Plot**: It provides a graphical assessment of the number of cases for each ethnicity, divided by the presence (or absence) of ASD traits as shown in Figure 5d. This helps in identifying if certain ethnicities have a higher or lower count of ASD traits within the dataset.
- **Point Plot**: It is useful to visualize the mean values and confidence intervals, highlighting trends and differences between groups over a continuous variable like age as in Figure 5e.

4. Bio-Inspired ANN-GSOM with PSO

Behavioural models use data on behaviour such as societal interaction, communication skills, and repetitive or tiresome behaviours to identify the outlines and characteristics that are associated with autism. This section introduces the novel algorithm to detect autism in Toddlers behavioural dataset using ANN validated utilizing GridSearch and feature selection operating PSO with multiple objective functionality [38].

4.1 Methodology

The comprehensive workflow to build the proposed model to classify autism spectrum disorder traits in toddlers is depicted in Figure 6 as a framework. The behavioral dataset is gathered from the online data source kaggle and it is read into Pandas DataFrame. ANN-GSOM model is built using a multilayered neural

174 | Bio-inspired Algorithms in Machine Learning and Deep Learning for Disease Detection

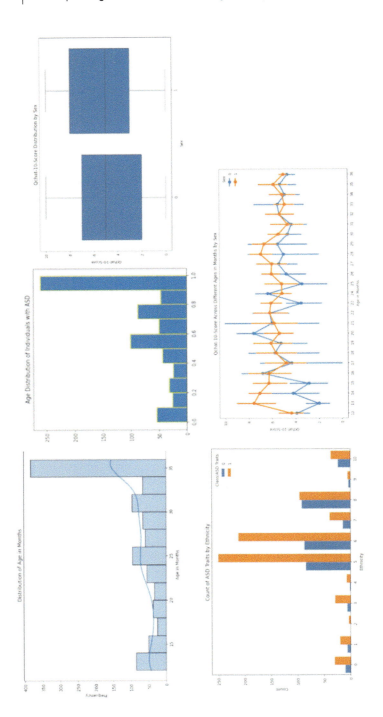

Fig. 5 Distribution of (a) 'Age_Mons' of toddlers in months, (b) Age of individuals with ASD, (c) 'Qchat-10-Score' between male and female toddlers, (d) count of toddlers with and without ASD traits across different ethnicities, (e) 'Qchat-10-Score' changes with age, separated by sex.

network on a behavioural training dataset, ANN is designed to learn hierarchical representations of data, which can be particularly useful for identifying complex patterns in autism prediction data. The ANN framework is also fit to build on the same training data using Rectified Linear Activation Function (RELU) and Binary Cross-Entropy loss function. In order to enhance its performance, it is made to train on 30 epochs which helps in reducing the error and loss. Further, to assess the model, it is evaluated on test data which ensure its generalization by avoiding overfitting or underfitting.

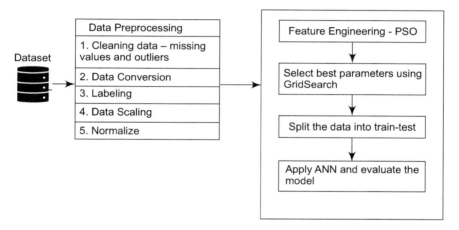

Fig. 6 Work Flow of ANN-GSOM with PSO.

An effective technique to fine tune the best fit parameters in supervised models to avoid underfit or overfit is the grid search. Using PSO, the bio-inspired algorithm, it is able to identify the relevant features of importance from the data. These features once applied on the model with the best fit parameters using GridSearch helps the model to improve the performance particularly in healthcare domain. The objective of this proposed idea is to build a DL pipeline to classify ASD traits in toddlers using a dataset of various features, including demographic information, behavioural assessments, and test scores. It is the intersection of healthcare and AI integrating with bio-inspired algorithms to demonstrate how ML and DL models can enhance diagnostic processes.

4.2 Algorithmic Procedure to Build ANN-GSOM with PSO

The algorithm comprises of preprocessing, visualizing data, performing feature selection using PSO, determine the best parameters using Grid Search optimization, and model building and evaluation. The functionality of PSO converts the 'features' array into a Boolean array to select the features from the feature matrix 'X'. Splits the selected features ('X_selected', as in Figure 7) and the target variable ('y') into train_ test sets using a '80:20' split ratio.

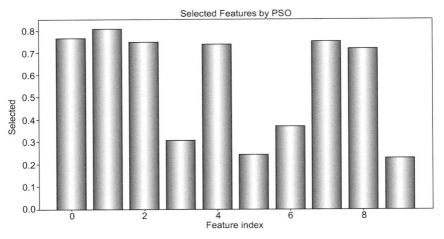

Fig. 7 Feature selection using PSO.

It initializes an MLPClassifier (a type of ANN) with a maximum of 1,000 iterations and a random state of 42. A parameter grid is defined, specifying various hyperparameters for the MLPClassifier that includes hidden_layer_sizes, activation, solver, alpha and learning_rate that describes the different configurations and activation function of hidden layers, weight optimization, L2 regularization parameter, and learning rate schedule for weight updates. The GridSearch with cross validation (GridSearchCV) is used to accomplish an extensive search among the specified hyperparameter grid with five folds (cv = 5). To increase the speed on computation, the search is parallelized with n_jobs = –1 to utilize multiple CPU cores. The best parameters are identified based on the highest average cross-validated score on the completion of the search process. On fitting ANN on the trained observations, the target case can be predicted by the assessment of the model on unknown new observations. Finally, evaluate the model by calculating its accuracy score of the forecasts.

To do so, install the pyswarm library for PSO and import all the necessary libraries. To develop the model, following are the important steps to follow:

- Import Libraries (numpy, pandas, sklearn [model_selection, preprocessing, metrics etc.], train_test_split, GridSearchCV, LabelEncoder, StandardScaler, MLPClassifier, accuracy_score, pso, classification_report, confusion_matrix, matplotlib, seaborn)
- Load the necessary behavioural autism Dataset for Toddler.
- Preprocess the data: Clean the data by checking for missing values and duplications, visualize the data that ensures for feature selection and model training.
- Transform the categorical data into numerical using label encoding technique.
- Feature Scaling using StandardScalar technique.

- Define the objective function of PSO (Bio-inspired algorithm) for feature selection that contributes the prediction of ASD with better measures.
- 'objective_function (features, X, y) where features is a list or array of binary values indicating which features to select, 'X' is the feature matrix containing all features and 'y' is the target variable or labels.
- Fine-tune the parameters of ANN model by applying the parameter grid of ANN using GridSearch based Optimization.
- Using train_test_split function with ratio [80:20], divide the given data into train and test.
- Build the ANN classification based model on best fit parameters on the selected features from the bio-inspired algorithms to train the models effectively.
- Assess and validate the optimized model on unseen data to ensure the model generalization.
  - Evaluate the framework on the unseen observations and measure its performance of ASD prediction task using metrics of classification.
  - Relate its performance with other ML frameworks: "SVM, RF, DT, and LR".

Overall, by leveraging bio-inspired algorithms for feature selection and combining them with various DL techniques, it is aimed to enhance the accuracy of ASD prediction models using genomic and subjective characteristic. Also, applying metaheuristic optimization algorithms inspired by biological processes offers a more promising avenue for enhancing autism diagnosis procedures. By applying these innovative approaches in these models which act as support systems for healthcare professionals, it helps them to potentially and effectively personalize their experience on their ASD diagnoses.

4.3 Results and Discussions

The evaluation of the model helps to determine its quality by using the confusion matrix which is generally used to define the outcomes of a classification process. It is represented in the table format that summarizes the actual count of right and wrong predictions given by a classifier in binary classification situations. The parameters that represent the class (output) are true-negative, true-positive, false-negative, and false-positive. A user might assess the accuracy by visualizing the confusion matrix and analysing the diagonal values to count the number of correct classifications.

- *True-Positive (TP):* is the number actually had ASD and accurately anticipated that the person had ASD.
- *True-Negative (TN):* is the count of ASD-not and accurately anticipated that he or she did not have ASD.
- *False-Positive (FP):* is the measure of ASD-not, but it is wrongly anticipated that the individual does referred as Type-1 error.
- *False-Negative (FN):* is the count of having ASD, but wrongly anticipated that the individual did not have ASD referred as a Type 2 error.

Figure 8 depicts the ANN-GSOM with PSO model's confusion matrix in which the individual is observed with ASD or not.

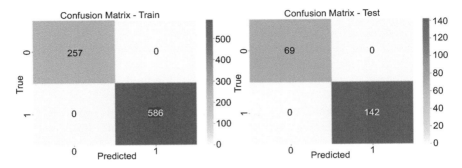

Fig. 8 Confusion Matrix.

The metrics used to assess the model performance are Precision, Accuracy, F1 Score, and Recall and is defined as below:
- *Accuracy*: refers to how near the measured value is to the standard value and is the proportion of the total number of correct forecasts.

$$\text{Accuracy} = \frac{TP + TN}{TP + FP + TN + FN} \quad \ldots(3)$$

- *Precision*: denotes the measure of quality of positive predictions.

$$\text{Precision} = \frac{TP}{TP + FP} \quad (4)$$

- *Recall (Sensitivity)*: indicates the measure of quantity that defines how many of the true positives a model catches from the total positive samples and it is referred as TPR.

$$\text{Recall} = \frac{TP}{TP + FN} \quad \ldots(5)$$

- *F1 Score*: counts both false negatives and false positives and produces a weighted average. In most cases, it is more valuable than precision due it's harmonic mean.

$$F1 - \text{Score} = 2X \frac{\text{Precision} \times \text{Recall}}{\text{Precision} + \text{Recall}} \quad \ldots(6)$$

The classification report (Figure 9) provides the precision, recall, and F1 score curves for a binary classifier. The *F*1 score curve is a harmonic mean of accuracy and recall that balances both measurements.

```
Classification Report (Train):
              precision    recall  f1-score   support

           0       1.00      1.00      1.00       257
           1       1.00      1.00      1.00       586

    accuracy                           1.00       843
   macro avg       1.00      1.00      1.00       843
weighted avg       1.00      1.00      1.00       843


Classification Report (Test):
              precision    recall  f1-score   support

           0       1.00      1.00      1.00        69
           1       1.00      1.00      1.00       142

    accuracy                           1.00       211
   macro avg       1.00      1.00      1.00       211
weighted avg       1.00      1.00      1.00       211
```

Fig. 9 Classification Report.

The tradeoff between the precision and the recall is captured by the F1-score which achieves its maximum value when accuracy and recall are balanced.

Table 3 Comparison of ANN- PSO with other models.

Algorithm	Accuracy	Precision	Recall	F1-Score
SVM	100	100	100	100
Logistic Regression	100	100	100	100
Decision Tree	93.83	97.29	94.11	95.68
Random Forest	98.43	98.32	99.34	98.70
ANN -GSOM	100	100	100	100
ANN- PSO	100	100	100	100

The results after optimizing the model achieved an accuracy of 100%, a precision of 100%, a recall of 100%, and an F1score of 100%. Additionally, the performance of the proposed model was compared to the performance of the other models, and the results showed that it is outperformed the other models in terms of accuracy and other metrics (Table 3). The work aims to maximize the model's performance on the given dataset by ensuring robustness and generalization capability. It is evident from the evaluation of the model that the objective of the work is achieved with minimum features that in turn reduces the memory resource and increase the computational effectiveness.

Conclusion with Future Enhancements

ASD is a neurodevelopmental disorder that can be detected as early as the age of two. The lack of cost-effective diagnostic tools keeps families of autistic children from seeking diagnosis and treatment becomes difficult. Their behavioural aspects can be greatly improved if diagnosed early and developed effective tools makes it simpler and more accessible to everyone to easily predict whether a child is autistic or not. Integration of this tool with Clinical Practice can assist clinicians in early diagnosis and monitoring of ASD.

The domain of this project is highly impactful, aiming to leverage optimized Bio-inspired ANN algorithm with best parameter using GridSearch cross validation is to improve the early diagnosis of ASD in toddlers. The entire workflow covers from the data loading, preprocessing, ANN training with feature selection using PSO, and model optimization using GridSearch, and evaluation and visualization of results. The results of the proposed model are unique compared with other ML models (SVM, LR, and ANN-GSOM) because of its bio-inspired multi-objective functionality. The interpretability of this model states that it achieved maximizing the model accuracy with minimizing the number of attributes which indicates its potential for early diagnosis and intervention. In future, other bio-inspired optimization techniques can be applied to diagnose autism on behavioural aspects and as well as facial image dataset of toddlers.

Acknowledgements

I acknowledge sincerely with immense gratitude to all who supported and motivated to complete this chapter.

References

[1] Omar, K.S., Mondal, P., Khan, N.S., Rizvi, M.R.K. and Islam, M.N. (Feb. 2019). A machine learning approach to predict autism spectrum disorder. *In: 2019 International Conference on Electrical, Computer, and Communication Engineering (ECCE)* (pp. 1–6). IEEE.

[2] Alsaade, F.W. and Alzahrani, M.S. (Feb. 2022). Classification and detection of autism spectrum disorder based on deep learning algorithms. *Computational Intelligence and Neuroscience, 2022.*

[3] Rabbi, M.F., Hasan, S.M., Champa, A.I. and Zaman, M.A. (Feb. 2021). A convolutional neural network model for early-stage detection of autism spectrum disorder. *In: 2021 International Conference on Information and Communication Technology for Sustainable Development (ICICT4SD)* (pp. 110–14). IEEE.

[4] Wei, W., Liu, Z., Huang, L., Nebout, A. and Le Meur, O. (Jul. 2019). Saliency prediction via multi-level features and deep supervision for children with autism spectrum disorder. *In: 2019 IEEE International Conference on Multimedia and Expo Workshops (ICMEW)* (pp. 621–24). IEEE.

[5] Li, B., Mehta, S., Aneja, D., Foster, C., Ventola, P., Shic, F. and Shapiro, L. (Sept. 2019). A facial affect analysis system for autism spectrum disorder. *In: 2019 IEEE International Conference on Image Processing (ICIP)* (pp. 4549–53). IEEE.

[6] Popescu, A.L. and Popescu, N. (Oct. 2020). Machine learning-based solution for predicting the affective state of children with autism. *In: 2020 International Conference on e-Health and Bioengineering (EHB)* (pp. 1–4). IEEE.

[7] Karuppasamy, S.G., Muralitharan, D., Gowr, S., Arumugam, S.R., Devi, E.A. and Maharajan, K. (Apr. 2022). Prediction of autism spectrum disorder using convolution neural network. *In: 2022 6th International Conference on Trends in Electronics and Informatics (ICOEI)* (pp. 1096–1100). IEEE.

[8] Baranwal, A. and Vanitha, M. (Feb. 2020). Autistic spectrum disorder screening: Prediction with machine learning models. *In: 2020 International Conference on Emerging Trends in Information Technology and Engineering (IC-ETITE)* (pp. 1–7). IEEE.

[9] Tao, Y. and Shyu, M.L. (Jul. 2019). SP-ASDNet: CNN-LSTM-based ASD classification model using observer scanpaths. *In: 2019 IEEE International Conference on Multimedia and Expo Workshops (ICMEW)* (pp. 641–46). IEEE.

[10] Maria Sofia, S., Mohanan, N. and Jomiya Joju, C. (2022). Autism diagnosis tool using machine learning. *Int. J. Eng. Res. Technol. (IJERT)*, *11*(04).

[11] Ali, N.A., Syafeeza, A.R., Jaafar, A.S., Alif, M.K.M.F. and Ali, N.A. (2020). Autism spectrum disorder classification on electroencephalogram signal using deep learning algorithm. *IAES International Journal of Artificial Intelligence*, *9*(1), 91–99.

[12] Raj, S. and Masood, S. (2020). Analysis and detection of autism spectrum disorder using machine learning techniques. *Procedia Computer Science*, *167*, 994–1004.

[13] Islam, S., Akter, T., Zakir, S., Sabreen, S. and Hossain, M.I. (Dec. 2020). Autism spectrum disorder detection in toddlers for early diagnosis using machine learning. *In: 2020 IEEE Asia-Pacific Conference on Computer Science and Data Engineering (CSDE)* (pp. 1–6). IEEE.

[14] Hashemi, J., Dawson, G., Carpenter, K.L., Campbell, K., Qiu, Q., Espinosa, S. and Sapiro, G. (2021). Computer Vision Analysis for Quantification of Autism Risk Behaviours. *IEEE Transactions on Affective Computing*, *12*(01), 215–26.

[15] Vakadkar, K., Purkayastha, D. and Krishnan, D. (2021). Detection of autism spectrum disorder in children using machine learning techniques. *SN Computer Science*, *2*, 1–9.

[16] Singh, A., Farooqui, Z., Sattler, B., Usua, U. and Helde, M. (2021). Using machine learning optimization to predict autism in toddlers. *In: Proc. Int. Conf. Ind. Eng. Oper. Manag* (pp. 6920–31).

[17] Hossain, M.D., Kabir, M.A., Anwar, A. and Islam, M.Z. (2021). Detecting autism spectrum disorder using machine learning techniques: An experimental analysis on toddler, child, adolescent, and adult datasets. *Health Information Science and Systems*, *9*, 1–13.

[18] Hammood, W.A., Zamil, K.Z. and Ali, A.M. (Jan. 2017). A Review of bio-inspired algorithm. *In: Conference: (SOFTEC Asia 2017)*, at Kuala Lumpur Convention Centre (Vol. 12).

[19] Jakšić, Z., Devi, S., Jakšić, O. and Guha, K. (2023). A comprehensive review of Bio-Inspired optimization algorithms including applications in microelectronics and nanophotonics. *Biomimetics*, *8*(3), 278.

[20] Mujawar, S. and Gupta, J. (Mar. 2022). A Statistical Perspective for Empirical Analysis of Bio-Inspired Algorithms for Medical Disease Detection. *In: 2022 International Conference on Emerging Smart Computing and Informatics (ESCI)* (pp. 1–7). IEEE.

[21] Yadav, M.K., Singh, A. and Singh, A. (Dec. 2022). A study on the Application of Bio-Inspired Algorithms in the Diagnosis of Efficient Ultrasound Liver Images. *In: 2022 5th International Conference on Contemporary Computing and Informatics (IC3I)* (pp. 1301–1307). IEEE.

[22] Haque, N.I., Khalil, A.A., Rahman, M.A., Amini, M.H. and Ahamed, S.I. (Sept. 2021). Biocad: Bio-inspired optimization for classification and anomaly detection in digital healthcare systems. *In: 2021 IEEE International Conference on Digital Health (ICDH)* (pp. 48–58). IEEE.

[23] Giampaglia, D., Barlaud, M., Piro, P., Nock, R. and Pourcher, T. (Nov. 2012). Classification of biological cells using Bio-inspired descriptors. *In: Proceedings of the 21st International Conference on Pattern Recognition (ICPR2012)* (pp. 3353–57). IEEE.

[24] S Lohi, S.A. and Bhatt, C. (Feb. 2023). Design of a Crop Disease Detection Model using Multi-parametric Bio-inspired Feature Representation and Ensemble Classification. *In: 2023 4th International Conference on Innovative Trends in Information Technology (ICITIIT)* (pp. 1–6). IEEE.

[25] Digumarthi, J., Gayathri, V.M. and Pitchai, R. (Apr. 2022). Early Prediction of Cardiac Arrhythmia using Novel Bio-inspired Algorithms. *In: 2022 8th International Conference on Smart Structures and Systems (ICSSS)* (pp. 01–04). IEEE.

[26] Bhargava, R., Dixit, M., Gupta, I., Prasad, T.N., Muthu, R. and Naidu, R.C. (Dec. 2022). A Bio-inspired Metaheuristic Optimization Approach for Economic Load Dispatch. *In: 2022 7th*

International Conference on Environment Friendly Energies and Applications (EFEA) (pp. 1–6). IEEE.

[27] Pham, T.H. and Raahemi, B. (2023). Bio-inspired feature selection algorithms with their applications: A systematic literature review. *IEEE Access, 11.*

[28] Trojovský, P., Dehghani, M. and Hanuš, P. (2022). Siberian tiger optimization: A new Bio-inspired metaheuristic algorithm for solving engineering optimization problems. *IEEE Access, 10*, 132396–132431.

[29] Givi, H., Dehghani, M. and Hubálovský, Š. (2023). Red panda optimization algorithm: An effective bio-inspired metaheuristic algorithm for solving engineering optimization problems. *IEEE Access, PP*(99), 01–01.

[30] Yang, Q. and Yoo, S.J. (2018). Optimal UAV path planning: Sensing data acquisition over IoT sensor networks using multi-objective bio-inspired algorithms. *IEEE Access, 6*, 13671–684.

[31] Jain, A. and Singhal, A. (Nov. 2023). Utilizing Metaheuristic Machine Learning Techniques for Early Diabetes Detection. *In: 2023 Second International Conference on Informatics (ICI)* (pp. 1–6). IEEE.

[32] Vijayalakshmi, K., Dhanamalar, M., Lepakshi, V.A. and Jamtsho, S. (2024). Smart Checkpoint Management System for Automatic Number Plate Recognition in Bhutan Vehicles using OCR Technique. *SN Computer Science, 5*(5), 579.

[33] Vijayalakshmi, K. and Vinayakamurthy, M. (Oct. 2020). A hybrid recommender system using multi-classifier regression model for autism detection. *In: 2020 International Conference on Smart Technologies in Computing, Electrical, and Electronics (ICSTCEE)* (pp. 139–44). IEEE.

[34] Prekshith, C.R. and Vijayalakshmi, K. (2024). Decoding Covid-19: Harnessing CNN Models for Chest X-Ray Classification. *EPRA International Journal of Multidisciplinary Research (IJMR), 10*(5), 551–57.

[35] Balasubramaniam, S., Kadry, S. and Kumar, K.S. (2024). Osprey Gannet optimization enabled CNN-based Transfer learning for optic disc detection and cardiovascular risk prediction using retinal fundus images. *Biomedical Signal Processing and Control, 93*, 106177.

[36] Kadry, S., Dhanaraj, R.K., K, S.K. and Manthiramoorthy, C. (2024). Res-Unet based blood vessel segmentation and cardiovascular disease prediction using chronological chef-based optimization algorithm based deep residual network from retinal fundus images. *Multimedia Tools and Applications*, 1–30.

[37] Harshitha, E.S. and Vijayalakshmi, K. (2024). Deployment of Enhanced Deep Learning Model with the Best Estimators on Optimizers and Activation Functions for Healthcare in Web Application. *EPRA International Journal of Multidisciplinary Research (IJMR), 10*(5), 75–82.

[38] Fathima, N., Vijayalakshmi, K., Patel, I.S. and Matthew, B.B. (Nov. 2023). Diabetes Prognosis: A Supervised Learning Approach. *In: 2023 2nd International Conference on Ambient Intelligence in Health Care (ICAIHC)* (pp. 01–06). IEEE.

10 | Bio-Inspired Algorithms using Machine Learning and Deep Learning for Social Phobia Treatment

Abinaya M.,[1] Vadivu G.,[2] Balasubramaniam S.[3] and Sundaravadivazhagan B.[4]

Social phobia, sometimes called social anxiety disorder, has a significant role in the domain of mental health and the challenges are the irrational fear or the behavior of avoidance of any particular situation. Two different treatments followed traditionally, cognitive-behavioural therapy and pharmacotherapy, are efficacy in the mental health domain, some of the interventions are needed for social phobia. This chapter delves into the combination of bio-inspired algorithms along with Machine Learning and the Deep Learning techniques for social phobia optimization. Natural systems produce the need for computational intelligence and bio-inspired algorithms and they offer new innovative solutions for the treatment and the challenges for the phobic people and the long-term medication people. In this chapter, the clinical perspectives of social phobia and the challenges are highlighted in the potential of bio-inspired optimization algorithms in personalization of treatment, approaches of machine learning for the prediction of therapy, and deep learning architectures to enhance the curatives and engagement. Future gaps and directions are discussed in the bio-inspired algorithms for social phobia treatment. Through the practical case studies, this chapter helps social phobic students to come up with mental issues.

1. Introduction

1.1 Clinical Perspectives and Treatment Challenges

Social phobia is the fear of social situations or circumstances that make people fear and make the fear irrational [1]. People with more social phobia have avoidance and stress because of the social phobic situation, which ruins their day-to-day activity

---

[1,2] Department of Data Science and Business Systems SRM Institute of Science and Technology, Kattankulathur, Chennai-603203.

[3] School of Computer Science and Engineering, Kerala University of Digital Sciences, Innovation and Technology (Formerly IIITM-K), Digital University Kerala, Thiruvananthapuram, Kerala, India.

[4] Department of Information Technology, University of Technology and Applied Science-AL Mussanah, Oman.

* Corresponding author: am0150@srmist.edu.in

and makes life chaotic. A lot of research is needed to analyse the implications and the interventions of social phobia [2].

Social phobia has the following symptoms and the characterization: self-fear, fear of criticism, avoiding social events like going to parties, events, etc., and the various physical changes in the body such as palpitation, diffusion of oxygen, and the like [3]. These occur due to different reasons like going to public meetings, during a public speech, and many more. The development of this particular situation is due to divergent characteristics like biological changes, psychological changes, and different characters [4]. Some traditional methods help to resolve this, but there are a lot more to rectify this issue and the following parameters are checked [5].

1.2 Conventional Treatment Methods

For the effective treatment of social phobia, cognitive-behavioural therapy (CBT) is widely considered as the prominent way. CBT always concentrates on capturing a particular pattern of behaviour and focusing on the particular data related to social anxiety [6]. In this method, the person is exposed to the environment they fear and the situation. With the systematic systems they are exposed to the same environment and by the individual in a more regulated manner [7].

Pharmacotherapy is selective in serotonin reuptake inhibitors (SSRIs) and serotonin-norepinephrine reuptake inhibitors (SNRIs), which are frequently used by social phobic students [8]. These medications are taken by the individual to calm down the person and to talk to the students in real time. Sometimes the medications will not produce the exact report result as that of the other individual. Pharmacotherapy is not the exact medication for all social phobic individuals [9].

1.3 Importance of Tailored Interventions

Even though the interventions are effective in the traditional method, a lot of intermediations are needed [10]. The social phobia manifestations and the nature are the combination of variations, and the treatment outcomes are the effective way, and the implications are the effective one [11].

The interventions for social phobia are the different aspects and the treatment is dependent on the intensity level, duration of social phobia, and the delivery format. Clinicians produce the best treatment and enhancement according to the severity of symptoms, conditions of the scombroid, preferences of the patient, and the history of treatment [12].

The progress of technology like telemedicine services, and data teleportation gives the necessary data related to social phobia. Applications of mobile phones, simulations of virtual reality, and community support offer adaptable and conventional methods of treatment and for therapeutic, self-interventions according to the user data and the particular situation of the data used [13].

In the forthcoming sections, we will discuss the new novel solutions and the best methods and techniques to deal with social phobia and the interventions of this data are incorporated with the new novel Bio-Inspired Algorithms, Deep Learning, and Machine Learning methods. The main motto of this book is to combine the multi-disciplinary and produce effective treatment for people with social phobic people [14].

2. Algorithms for Optimization Inspired by Biology

For effective treatment, the method like the hybrid one is used and combined with the best optimal algorithms and solutions to produce the data in a more effectual manner for the treatment of individuals with social phobia [15].

2.1 Evolutionary Computation for Personalized Treatment

The principles of natural selection and genetics draw the computational efficiency and the techniques in a biological system to treat social phobia. By applying various techniques like mutation, selection, and crossover, each and every concept of genetic algorithms provides a more prominent and important technique. This is the process that replicates the natural process that is taking place biologically [16].

This particular section deals with genetic algorithms and how they are connected with biological systems [17]. There are plenty of applications with the help of genetic algorithms like the exposure of construction hierarchies, dosages of medication, and therapy session scheduling. The goal of this method is to reduce the effect and the treatment of experience undergone during the therapeutic interventions [18]. *Case Studies*: A genetic algorithm is used to give the preferences of people with social phobia and the interventions are produced in the area related to the domain with the use of best optimal solutions of genetic algorithms [19].

2.2 Utilizing Swarm Intelligence for the Development of Adaptive Therapy Planning

Swarm colony optimization is an algorithm that is derived by other algorithms like bird flocks, ant colony optimization algorithm, and particle swarm optimization (PSO). These algorithms are run in a novel solution that the spaces and the solution are known, the treatment plans are adjusted, and the response from the patient are known dynamically.

The decision-making and the utilization are the collective behaviours of swarm particle optimization for the development of swarm particle optimization algorithm. This particular algorithm plays an effective role in the optimization and utilization of data and their behaviour [20].

The help of ant colonies and the particle swarm can be used for the treatment of social phobia. These are possible by the treatment and the real-time adjustment of data based on the response and the feedback of the patient and the response obtained from the trajectories [21].

The combination of clinical decision support and the integration of this swarm optimization is used in the planning of treatment and decision-making. This makes the system more efficient and the outcome treatment [22].

2.3 Hybrid Algorithms for Optimizing Treatment Parameters

Various techniques and algorithms are combined and the computation algorithms like computation evolutionary, local search methods, and the constraints of the individual and the advantages are capitalized by the hybrid algorithm for increasing the efficiency, reliability, and efficiency of the treatment optimization and for the treatment of social phobia [23]. Figure 1 shows Particle Swarm Optimization (PSO) Algorithm for Adaptive Therapy Planning in Social Phobia Treatment.

2.3.1 Hybrid Algorithms

Hybrid algorithms are useful in facing large complex data and the optimization algorithm is used in the effective treatment of data and the efficacy is shown in the data.

Optimizing Treatment Parameters: This method is best suitable for the social phobia treatment and for the best novel solution, and to get the new data more optimally and the treatment in a superior way [24].

This chapter shows the efficacy of using these hybrid algorithms and their effectiveness in a more unique way and the treatment of social phobia is discussed later in this section. This combine provides a more effective and optimal solution [25].

3. Methods of Machine Learning

3.1 Models for Predicting Outcomes Using Supervised Learning

3.1.1 Predicting Treatment Outcomes using Machine Learning Approaches

Supervised Learning methods are very crucial in predicting the outcome of the treatment in giving therapy for social phobia. The data and the label are achieved by knowing the pattern, recognizing it, and the treatment response. There are various supervised algorithms like decision trees, support vector machines, logistic regression, and many more for using guidance in the outcome of treatment and also in the decision-making in clinical settings [26].

3.1.2 Supervised Learning

This section deals with the methodologies and the principles of supervised learning and the significance of using the data along with the label and the model is predicted with the help of ground truth value.

In social phobia, the basic step is to use feature selection and engineering, various techniques, and methods. It is used in the assessment of clinical parameters, observation of behaviour, and the neurological imaging of data, and also in the accuracy prediction [27].

```
# Initialize parameters
N = number_of_particles
max_iterations = maximum_number_of_iterations
w = inertia_weight
c1 = cognitive_coefficient
c2 = social_coefficient

# Initialize particles
particles = initialize_particles(N)
velocities = initialize_velocities(N)
personal_best_positions = particles
personal_best_fitness = evaluate_fitness(particles)
global_best_position = find_global_best(personal_best_positions)
global_best_fitness = evaluate_fitness(global_best_position)

# PSO main loop
for iteration in range(max_iterations):
    for i in range(N):
        # Update velocity
        r1, r2 = random(), random()
        velocities[i] = (w * velocities[i] +
                        c1 * r1 * (personal_best_positions[i] - particles[i]) +
                        c2 * r2 * (global_best_position - particles[i]))

        # Update position
        particles[i] = particles[i] + velocities[i]

        # Evaluate fitness
        current_fitness = evaluate_fitness(particles[i])

        # Update personal best
        if current_fitness > personal_best_fitness[i]:
            personal_best_positions[i] = particles[i]
            personal_best_fitness[i] = current_fitness

        # Update global best
        if current_fitness > global_best_fitness:
            global_best_position = particles[i]
            global_best_fitness = current_fitness

        # Check for termination criteria
        if check_termination(global_best_fitness):
            break

# Output the optimal therapy plan
optimal_therapy_plan = global_best_position
return optimal_therapy_plan
```

Fig. 1   Particle Swarm Optimization (PSO) Algorithm for Adaptive Therapy Planning in Social Phobia Treatment.

3.1.3   Model Training and Evaluation

This model is used in model training, pre-processing of data, best model selection, hyperparameter tuning, and the cross-validation technique for improving the performance prediction and for generalizing the ability [28].

3.1.4   Interpretability and Explainability

The evaluation of data interpretability and explain the ability of data metrics to determine the data transparency and reliability of data for the predictive models, and to ensure the clinicians interpret and comprehend the data from a clinical point of view. In this chapter, a lot of real-time use cases are discussed to predict the model outcome and the effective method in the treatment of social phobia [29].

The discussion focuses on challenges such as heterogeneity of data, sample size limitations, and the interoperability model. It also deals with the future gaps and the directions, including the data from multiple sources and its integration, its longitudinal analyses of and its collaborating efforts in the predictive model in the medical field [30].

3.2 Reinforcement Learning for Adaptive Treatment Strategies

Reinforcement learning (RL) plays an important role in improving treatment strategies for the development of social phobia therapy. It produces the data and the learning achievement from the environment and the feedback based on the data results which we have obtained. RL algorithms, such as data algorithms like Q-learning, data policy gradient methods, and the data actor-critic architectures are capable of changing the data dynamically and modifying treatment parameters, data reinforcement schedules, and the protocols for intervention to optimize the effect longitudinally. RL deals with the important parameter of the environment, the agent interaction, the reward system for the interaction, and to make the decision about the clinical parameter effectively [31].

3.2.1 Adaptive Treatment Planning

The treatment of social phobia therapy and its applications using RL algorithms is focused. The optimization goal is to schedule the reinforcement, intensity exposure, and interventions for therapeutic, and it is based on the trajectory response and the feedback of the patient [32].

The exploration-exploitation mechanism and the trade-off in reinforcement learning involve finding a new technique and a novel treatment for giving the rewards and the trade-off options.

The potential of RL is analysed with the help of wearable sensors digitally and for the preferences of the patients. The applications and the benefits of RL are shown in the treatment planning and for the eradication of social phobia therapy, the RL outcome, outcome of the treatment, patient engagement enhancement, and therapy adherence [33].

3.2.2 Challenges and Future Directions

Let's talk about the stuff we need to sort out, like making better use of samples, figuring out incentives, and considering ethics. We're also looking ahead at future studies, such as creating personalized learning algorithms, using wearable tech, and testing things out in real clinical settings [34].

3.3 Clinical Decision Support Systems: Integrating Predictive Models

Clinical decision support systems (CDSS) are used to provide predictive analytics and metrics and give therapy, especially for social phobia based on machine learning. With the help of predictive models and different data training, CDSS can give the young doctors personalized reports if needed, data in real-time recommendations, assessing the risks, and plans for the treatment based on the need [35].

3.3.1 Overview of Clinical Decision Support Systems

CDSS illustrate the basic data and the professional healthcare providers the information to make decisions, and also for giving evidence-based advice, and the insights received from them.

Predictive models' integration into the CDSS set the goal on incorporating new predictive models training for the decision systems clinically. The main motto is to predict treatment and the outcomes accurately, to identify the prognostic factors, and the patient classification based on the categorization and the treatment response.

3.3.2 Clinical Workflow Integration

The main goal of the existing study is to analyse the clinical workflows, and the data gathering in electronic health records, treatment of medical platform, and for the planning of data, data monitoring, and the patient follow-up considered. The recommendations of the data are analysed and gathered systemically and used to predict it clinically along with the techniques of machine learning [36].

4. Deep Learning Architectures for Treatment Adherence and Engagement

4.1 Utilizing Convolutional Neural Networks for the Analysis of Multimodal Data

Convolutional Neural Networks (CNNs) have a potential role in various techniques like data multimodality, including the different data text, images as data, audio data, and physiological data signals. Social phobia treatment is used in different domains [37]:

- Analyse the different data
- Identify the features importantly
- Prediction of individuals adherence level and treatment engagement.

4.1.1. Convolutional Neural Networks (CNNs)

Three main components of CNNs [38]:

1. **Convolutional layers**: To extract the relevant data features input data is used in this layer.
2. **Pooling layers**: Features are dimensionality reduced in this layer followed by the feature extraction.

3. ***Fully connected layers***: Learning of complex relationships are created by connecting the previous layer to the next layer.

Hierarchical representations from raw data are learned automatically from CNNs.

4.1.2 Combining Different Data Sources with CNNs

Social phobia therapy is used to integrate data from multiple sources of data [39]:

1. Transcripts of therapy sessions textually.
2. Patient-therapist interactions in audio.
3. Wearable sensors and the psychological signals.

The goal is to create a unified representation that captures important information from each source and can be used to predict treatment adherence and engagement.

Improving Prediction Accuracy with CNNs

Investigation of various techniques for feature extraction and representation learning and to improve the effectiveness are enhanced with the CNN. The meaningful patterns and relationships are derived from various sources and within the data [40].

4.1.3 Training CNN Models for Treatment Adherence and Engagement

Steps for training the CNN Model

1. ***Data pre-processing***: Compatibility of the data is maintained and the essential features are retrieved on this page.
2. ***Hyperparameter tuning***: Model optimization and the performance are adjusted in this stage.
3. ***Optimization techniques***: Analysing and giving the best algorithms for the effectiveness and the treatment of data.

The ultimate goal is for the predictive power and CNN model's generalizability for the engagement and the adherence [41].

Interoperability and the Explainability of the data and the predictive details are using the CNN model for producing the result accurately. The recommendation levels are predicted by the healthcare professionals.

Methods for making it interoperable include:

- Identifying and influencing the model to visualize the feature maps for understanding the text or the image.
- Highlighting the attention mechanisms for identifying the sequence.
- Decisions and the rules are used to provide the explanation [42].

4.2 Recurrent Neural Networks for Temporal Modelling of Treatment Progress

Recurrent Neural Networks (RNNs) are best for representing the data in time series and for producing sequential data. This helps in monitoring the data about the patient, the social phobia therapy interventions, and the progress of treatment over time in social phobia therapy. RNNs can examine the data longitudinally obtained from the overall therapy sessions, outcomes of the patient-report, and the assessment of behaviour. The course of the data is forecasted and the interventions and the crucial moments are pinpointed [43].

4.2.1 Recurrent Neural Networks (RNNs)

RNNs consist of recurrent layers and different memory cells. RNNs are used in processing the sequential data for capturing the temporal data [44].

4.2.2 Temporal Modelling of Treatment Progress

RNN progression and the treatment progress are known over the period by using the time-series model. It utilizes the longitudinal data using the different therapy sessions, data of the patient diaries, and data from the wearable in predicting the similarity, data functional impairment, and the response of the treatment.

The Long Short-Term Memory (LSTM) and Gated Recurrent Unit (GRU) are the new two types of advanced variants in RNNs. They are used for designing the gradient problem and capturing dependencies in the long term for the data sequentially. To improve the progress, the data are used dynamically.

Integration of RNNs with feedback mechanism and the real-time monitoring systems is a must for the clinicians to give the insights timely and to show the progress of the treatment. The interventions and the ability of the data are known in advance in the system [45].

RNNs case studies and the applications are useful and helpful for knowing the treatment progress in social phobia therapy and to identify the follow-up session. The strategies for getting the data and the personalized interventions are known in advance with the help of RNN.

4.2.3 Challenges and Future Directions

Some of the challenges faced by the RNN are the quality of the data, interoperability model, and data scalability. There is the possibility of developing this model by merging the model with the new techniques and methods like machine learning, digital health, and the new hybrid model by combining all the existing methods and techniques. The data and the longitudinal validation are known with the new digital health platforms [46, 47].

4.3 Using Virtual Agents and Wearable Sensors to Enhance Treatment Delivery

Wearable sensors and virtual agents offer new innovative ways to improve the data delivery and data monitoring in the treatment of social phobia therapy. A new Virtual agent, powered by the trending artificial intelligence (AI) and the sub-

Bio-inspired Algorithms in Machine Learning and Deep Learning for Disease Detection

branch of AI Natural Language Processing (NLP), can be given tailored therapy sessions, resources of educational data, and the information about the interactive interventions customized to each patient's unique needs and the data preferences. Wearable sensors, such as smartwatches and biosensors, collect physiological data from the biological data like heart rate, skin conductance, and the pattern of movement for monitoring the patient and the data related to health and the real-time assessment of the data [48].

4.3.1 Virtual Agents for Therapy Delivery

The virtual agents and the delivery of the therapy and the latest new techniques are elaborated in this section, as new conversational AI technologies, the ability of the personalized therapy sessions, interventions, and the implementation of cognitive-behavioural provide emotional support to individuals with social phobia. It also shows the method of how the techniques are used in analysing the characteristics of the students along with the social phobia, the sentiment of the data, and speech patterns in real time, emotion recognition is noted, perform sentiment analysis, and psychotherapeutic dialogues analysis [49].

A new exploration in wearable sensors and the new techniques like biosensors to detect physiological signals related to the person's anxiety, stress level, and emotional data arousal allows for the measurement of new and different treatment progress and the development of personalized strategies for the interventions [50].

4.3.2 Integration with Treatment Platforms

The current part of the chapter deals with how the virtual agents and a different wearable sensor help integrate into current treatment platforms, telemedicine services, and applications in digital health to improve treatment of data delivery, data engagement, and data adherence. It presents the new clinical applications and case studies showing the virtual agents and wearable sensors in the treatment of social phobia therapy, treatment, and effectiveness are discussed in this section [51].

The new techniques also deal with the challenges like privacy concerns, data user acceptance, and the data technical limitations, and the new future research directions which include the development of data related to context-aware virtual agents, clinical trials validation, and real-world scalability healthcare settings [52].

5. Challenges and Future Directions

5.1 Analysis of the Interpretability and Explainability of Algorithmic Predictions

Interpretability and explainability are the new two critical factors to consider when designing algorithmic predictions for social phobia treatment. The new innovative techniques like machine learning and deep learning models are useful in demonstrating exceptional predictive accuracy, internal mechanisms are now opaque, that makes the clinicians to understand and trust the predictions. Comprehensibility and clarity of algorithmic predictions are important in facilitating transparent decision-making, clinicians trust, and the building of methodologies in a clinical practice [53].

The Significance of Interpretability: Interpretability and the importance of algorithmic forecasts for social phobia treatment, underline the clinicians' trust knowledge to predict the new models for further recommendations [54].

Explainability Techniques: The factors and the explainability of the data and the algorithmic predictions offer the clinicians insights, which includes the feature importance analysis, method of model-agnostics techniques like SHAP and LIME, and the decision tree in post-hoc.

Examining the impact of data interpretability and explainability of data on the clinical relevance and utility of algorithmic predictions is important, as it allows clinicians to effectively include the predictive models in the decision-making treatment and customize interventions for the specific need of the patient [55].

Challenges and Limitations: Some of the challenges faced by this technique are trade-offs between data accuracy and data interpretability, using the model complexity, and the opaque deep learning architectures need.

5.2 *Ethical Considerations in Personalizing Algorithmic Treatment*

Ethical considerations play an important role in the algorithm customizing and the treatment of social phobia. Methods are very important in the clinical practice, addressing the issues ethically and the related work like data privacy, algorithmic bias, data transparency, accountability of data, and patient autonomy. Prioritizing ethical treatment personalization in the practices is essential in the patient's safeguard, maintaining the trust in healthcare systems, and upholding professional care standards.

Data personalizing algorithmic treatment, and safeguarding data privacy and confidentiality are very crucial and is significantly paramount. This makes the systems like data anonymization, data encryption, and secure data storage to protect patient privacy.

This chapter focuses on the issue of algorithmic bias and data fairness in predictive modelling in the treatment of social phobia. It underscores the prediction's bias for the healthcare access and outcome disparities. The study also addresses the biases of the data in the preprocessing, data incorporating fairness metrics in algorithms, and implementing transparency measures [56].

Ensuring the important informed consent and data transparency in algorithmic treatment personalization involves getting the patients' consent and the data providing clear explanations about how the model is a predictive one. It is important for the patient in algorithmic predictions and also to understand the data.

194 Bio-inspired Algorithms in Machine Learning and Deep Learning for Disease Detection

The chapter and the studies also concentrate on the importance of patient autonomy and data shared decision-making in the algorithmic treatment of data personalization. It highlights the necessity of the patient in the decision-making process, respecting their data preferences and data values, and empowering them to make data well-informed decisions about their treatment options.

5.3 Incorporation of Computational Methodologies into Clinical Practice

The integration of data computational methods into clinical practice has its own way of treating social phobia. Promising techniques like machine learning and deep learning techniques increases the improvement in the treatment outcomes and resource allocation, their real-world implementation focuses on the workflow integration, data clinician training, data usability, and regulatory of data compliance. Successfully incorporating the computational methods into the data clinical practice calls for the new collaboration across disciplines, data in active stakeholder involvement, and a commitment to evidence-based, patient-centred care [57].

Workflow Integration: This article showcases the new strategies for integrating computational methods into new clinical workflows, collection of electronic health record systems, and data telemedicine platforms to ensure seamless exchange of data and usability data for healthcare providers.

Clinician Training and Education: It's crucial and very important to provide clinicians with training in data and education in computational methods through workshops, continuing data medical education programmes, and the integration of interdisciplinary collaborations to enhance the ability to utilize predictive models for treatment decisions.

Usability and User Experience: Designing and data-implementing computational tools for the treatment of social phobia treatment in the user-friendly, need of the data, and the preferences.

Regulatory Compliance and Quality Assurance: Examining the regulatory requirements and data quality assurance measures for computational methods in the data clinical practice, ensuring compliance with regulation of protection, ethical guidelines, and the data best practices for model validation, data verification, and the data monitoring.

Scalability and Generalization: Ensuring data scalability and generalization of data of predictive models is crucial for effectively treating of social phobia. Challenges in the data scalability and generalization of data requires rigorous model validation, cross-validation techniques, data external validation studies, and the collaboration among different research institutions, data healthcare organizations, and the data regulatory agencies.

Model Validation Techniques: Discuss the data model validation techniques, data performance metrics, and cross-validation data strategies used to assess the scalability and generalization of predictive models across various patient populations, clinical contexts, and healthcare settings.

External Validation Studies: These studies aim to ensure that predictive models consistently perform well across different demographic groups, geographic regions, and healthcare systems in real-world implementation trials.

Collaborative Research and Data Sharing: Exploring collaborative research projects, data-sharing platforms, and the data consortia for combining different datasets in comparing predictive models and in establishing best practices for algorithmic personalization for social phobia.

Deployment and Implementation Challenges: Implementing and obtaining the predictive models in clinical practice for the infrastructure needs, issues in interoperability, data clinician acceptance, and data sustainability concerns.

To make progress in the future, interdisciplinary collaboration, stakeholder involvement, and a focus on ethical and evidence-based practices are essential for fully utilizing computational methods in treating social phobia and improving outcomes for individuals affected by this condition.

6. Analysis of Specific Instances and Practical Observations

In examining specific instances, one cannot overlook practical observations that complement theoretical frameworks. These observations provide tangible context for abstract concepts. Consider, for example, phenomenon of social loafing. This concept, extensively discussed in academic literature finds validation through everyday experiences. Individuals tend to exert less effort when working in groups. This is in contrast to working alone. Numerous studies have documented this tendency [58].

For instance, a research conducted by Latane Williams and Harkins (1979) involved participants clapping and shouting alone and in groups. They found that individual output decreased as the group size increased. This finding aligns with Diffusion of Responsibility theory. It posits that people feel less accountable when they are part of larger group. Consequently, individual contributions diminish.

Another example is related to decision-making processes within organizations. Studies indicate that consensus-based approaches often lead to better outcomes. A 2018 study on corporate board decisions found was significant correlation between diversity of perspectives and the quality of decisions. Such findings underscore the importance of inclusivity in group settings.

Practical observations further extend to the realm of marketing. Consumer behaviour research shows that product placement significantly influences purchasing decisions. For instance, products placed at eye-level shelves tend to sell more. This insight is utilized by retailers to optimize product arrangements. Maximizing sales is the primary goal.

In education, practical applications of theoretical principles also manifest clearly. Constructivist approaches in pedagogy that emphasize active student engagement have been shown to enhance learning outcomes. A 2020 study compared classrooms that employed active learning techniques with those that did not. Results indicated that students in active learning environments performed better academically.

Thus, specific instances and practical observations offer invaluable insights. They ground theoretical knowledge in concrete examples. This approach not only enriches academic discourse but also importantly enhances real-world applications. Through these instances and observations one can better understand complexities of abstract concepts. And their practical ramifications.

Case Studies and Practical Insights

6.1 Utilization of Bio-Inspired Algorithms in Clinical Environments

Bio-inspired algorithms provide novel approaches to optimize treatment parameters. They tailor interventions in the therapy of social phobia. Bio-inspired algorithms have been proven effective in improving treatment outcomes. They promote patient well-being in real-world clinical applications. Examining case studies that showcase effective applications of bio-inspired algorithms offers valuable insights. These insights reveal practical usefulness. They also reveal potential influence. This potential is on the delivery of treatments [59].

This case study demonstrates the use of genetic algorithms to optimize treatment parameters that include constructing exposure hierarchies and determining medication dosages. The goal is to maximize the effectiveness of therapy. It also aims to minimize the burden of treatment for individuals suffering from social phobia.

This case study showcases the application of swarm intelligence algorithms. Specifically, it looks at PSO and ant colony optimization. These algorithms enable real-time modifications to treatment protocols. They achieve this by incorporating patient feedback and response trajectories.

This case study demonstrates the integration of hybrid optimization algorithms. These algorithms combine evolutionary computation swarm intelligence and local search methods. They optimize treatment parameters. They improve treatment personalization in social phobia therapy.

6.2 Application of Machine Learning Models in Real-World Scenarios

Machine learning models are essential in forecasting treatment results. They help track treatment advancement. Additionally, they guide clinical decision-making in social phobia therapy. Real-world applications of machine learning models showcase their practicality and the ability to handle large-scale data. Their efficacy in clinical settings is clear. Case studies demonstrate successful implementations of machine learning models. They offer practical insights regarding integration into regular healthcare workflows.

Predictive Models for Treatment Outcome Prediction: This case study emphasizes the incorporation of supervised learning models. This includes logistic regression support vector machines and decision trees in CDSS. These models predict treatment outcomes. They guide treatment planning in social phobia therapy.

This case study showcases the application of reinforcement learning algorithms, specifically, Q-learning and policy gradient methods. These algorithms enable personalized interventions. They optimize treatment adherence and engagement. They also facilitate the development of adaptive treatment strategies [60].

This study demonstrates the use of RNNs and CNNs in temporal modelling. They are used for tracking treatment progress. They also monitor patient well-being in social phobia therapy.

6.3 Methods of Tailoring Treatment to Individual Patients

Treatment personalization in patient-centred approaches prioritizes specific needs preferences and values of individuals suffering from social phobia. Patient-centred care fosters engagement and empowerment. Satisfaction by actively involving patients in treatment decision-making. It customizes interventions to their characteristics and goals. Case studies demonstrate patient-centred approaches to customizing treatment. These provide practical insights. They show how to improve collaboration between patients and healthcare providers. They also enhance treatment outcomes [61].

This case study emphasizes the significance of shared decision-making. Tailoring treatment to individual needs enables patients to actively engage in planning treatment. They set goals and select interventions according to their own preferences and values.

Personalized Treatment Planning: This case study demonstrates the creation of customized treatment plans. These are designed to address unique requirements and abilities and difficulties of patients with social phobia. These plans incorporate patient-reported outcomes treatment preferences and expertise of clinicians [62].

This case study showcases utilization of digital health technologies including mobile applications, wearable sensors, and virtual agents. These tools continuously monitor the progress of treatment. They provide immediate feedback to both patients and clinicians. This approach enhances treatment adherence. It also boosts engagement and accountability [63].

By integrating patient-centred methodologies into therapy for social phobia, clinicians can enhance the efficacy of treatment. This also enhances patient contentment, promotes sustained recovery and resilience in individuals grappling with this demanding mental health condition [64–65].

7. Conclusion

The incorporation of computational methodologies such as bio-inspired algorithms and machine learning models into social phobia therapy signifies notable progress in tailored mental healthcare. Through utilization of data-driven insights, predictive analytics, and adaptive interventions, clinicians have the ability to customize treatments based on specific needs of each patient. They can maximize the effectiveness of therapy. This approach improves overall well-being of patient. Implementing individualized strategies in mental healthcare shows potential. It enhances treatment effectiveness, and can lessen treatment demands. It fosters resilience and recuperation in individuals with social phobia and other mental health disorders.

Customized mental healthcare provides chances for cultivating resilience and aiding recovery in individuals who have social phobia. Personalizsed interventions effectively address specific needs and challenges of individual patients. This leads to promotion of adaptive coping strategies. It also aids development of self-efficacy. Improvement of social functioning follows by employing a comprehensive strategy. This strategy combines psychological, pharmacological, and technological methods. Healthcare professionals enable patients, help them manage social difficulties and attain significant enhancements. in their quality of life. Personalized mental healthcare empowers individuals to develop resilience and facilitate their recovery. This allows them to lead fulfilling lives and excel in personal pursuits. It is crucial to close the divide between research and practice to advance personalized mental healthcare for social phobia. Collaboration among clinicians, researchers, policymakers, and industry stakeholders is essential. This is for translating scientific advancements into practical applications and implementing practices supported by evidence, as well as encouraging widespread use of personalized interventions. To effectively integrate computational methodologies into clinical practice, it is necessary to invest in interdisciplinary research. Data infrastructure and training programmes that provide clinicians with necessary knowledge, skills, and resources is essential for promoting cooperation and creativity within the healthcare system. We can utilize revolutionary capabilities of tailored mental healthcare to enhance results for individuals suffering from social phobia and propel advancement of mental health treatment as a whole.

References

[1] Heimberg, R.G. (Ed.). (1995). *Social Phobia: Diagnosis, Assessment, and Treatment*. Guilford Press.

[2] Wittchen, H.U. and Beloch, E. (1996). The impact of social phobia on quality of life. *International Clinical Psychopharmacology, 11*, 15–23.

[3] Wittchen, H.U. and Beloch, E. (1996). The impact of social phobia on quality of life. *International Clinical Psychopharmacology, 11*, 15–23.

[4] Amies, P.L., Gelder, M.G. and Shaw, P.M. (1983). Social phobia: A comparative clinical study. *The British Journal of Psychiatry, 142*(2), 174–79.

Bio-Inspired Algorithms using Machine Learning and Deep Learning for Social Phobia Treatment | 199

[5] Clark, D.M. and McManus, F. (2002). Information processing in social phobia. *Biological Psychiatry*, *51*(1), 92–100.

[6] Sheldon, B. (2011). *Cognitive-behavioural Therapy: Research and Practice in Health and Social Care*. Routledge.

[7] Cuijpers, P., Berking, M., Andersson, G., Quigley, L., Kleiboer, A. and Dobson, K.S. (2013). A meta-analysis of cognitive-behavioural therapy for adult depression, alone and in comparison with other treatments. *The Canadian Journal of Psychiatry*, *58*(7), 376–85.

[8] Song, F., Freemantle, N., Sheldon, T.A., House, A., Watson, P., Long, A. and Mason, J. (1993). Selective serotonin reuptake inhibitors: Meta-analysis of efficacy and acceptability. *British Medical Journal*, *306*(6879), 683–87.

[9] Sangkuhl, K., Klein, T.E. and Altman, R.B. (2009). Selective serotonin reuptake inhibitors pathway. *Pharmacogenetics and Genomics*, *19*(11), 907–909.

[10] Heimberg, R.G. (2001). Current status of psychotherapeutic interventions for social phobia. *Journal of Clinical Psychiatry*, *62*, 36–42.

[11] Ponniah, K. and Hollon, S.D. (2008). Empirically supported psychological interventions for social phobia in adults: A qualitative review of randomized controlled trials. *Psychological Medicine*, *38*(1), 3–14.

[12] Ponniah, K. and Hollon, S.D. (Jan. 2008). Empirically supported psychological interventions for social phobia in adults: A qualitative review of randomized controlled trials. *Psychological Medicine*, *38*(1), 3–14.

[13] Kessler, R.C. (2003). The impairments caused by social phobia in the general population: Implications for intervention. *Acta Psychiatrica Scandinavica*, *108*, 19–27.

[14] Taylor, S. (1996). Meta-analysis of cognitive-behavioural treatments for social phobia. *Journal of Behavior Therapy and Experimental Psychiatry*, *27*(1), 1–9.

[15] Eng, W., Heimberg, R.G., Coles, M.E., Schneier, F.R. and Liebowitz, M.R. (2000). An empirical approach to subtype identification in individuals with social phobia. *Psychological Medicine*, *30*(6), 1345–57.

[16] Huppert, J.D., Roth, D.A. and Foa, E.B. (2003). Cognitive-behavioural treatment of social phobia: New advances. *Current Psychiatry Reports*, *5*(4), 289–96.

[17] Jayasiri, D., Asanka, D., Udara, I. and Jayasiri, T. (Feb. 2024). Personalized Treatment Approaches for Social Phobia: An ML-based Decision Support System. *In: 2024 4th International Conference on Advanced Research in Computing (ICARC)* (pp. 43–48). IEEE.

[18] Mosing, M.A., Gordon, S.D., Medland, S.E., Statham, D.J., Nelson, E.C., Heath, A.C., ... and Wray, N.R. (2009). Genetic and environmental influences on the co-morbidity between depression, panic disorder, agoraphobia, and social phobia: A twin study. *Depression and Anxiety*, *26*(11), 1004–11.

[19] Irle, E., Ruhleder, M., Lange, C., Seidler-Brandler, U., Salzer, S., Dechent, P., ... and Leichsenring, F. (2010). Reduced amygdalar and hippocampal size in adults with generalized social phobia. *Journal of Psychiatry and Neuroscience*, *35*(2), 126–31.

[20] Husain, W., Yng, S.H., Rashid, N.A.A. and Jothi, N. (2017). Prediction of generalized anxiety disorder using particle swarm optimization. *In: Advances in Information and Communication Technology: Proceedings of the International Conference, ICTA 2016* (pp. 480–89). Springer International Publishing.

[21] Alghawli, A.S. and Taloba, A.I. (2022). An enhanced ant colony optimization mechanism for the classification of depressive disorders. *Computational Intelligence and Neuroscience*, *2022*, 1332664.

[22] Pang, X., Chen, C., Tong, X., Shi, L. and Liu, X. (2023, August). Application of Improved Genetic Algorithm and Ant Colony Algorithm in Multi-objective Path Planning. *In: Journal of Physics: Conference Series*, *2562*(1), 012011. IOP Publishing.

[23] Li, C., Xu, B., Chen, Z., Huang, X., He, J. and Xie, X. (2024). A Stacking Model-Based Classification Algorithm is Used to Predict Social Phobia. *Applied Sciences, 14*(1), 433.

[24] D'monte, S. and Panchal, D. (2015, May). Data-mining approach for diagnoses of anxiety disorder. *In: International Conference on Computing, Communication & Automation* (pp. 124–27). IEEE.

[25] Ebenfeld, L., Lehr, D., Ebert, D.D., Kleine Stegemann, S., Riper, H., Funk, B. and Berking, M. (2021). Evaluating a hybrid web-based training program for panic disorder and agoraphobia: Randomized controlled trial. *Journal of Medical Internet Research, 23*(3), e20829.

[26] Scholing, A. and Emmelkamp, P.M. (1999). Prediction of treatment outcome in social phobia: A cross-validation. *Behaviour Research and Therapy, 37*(7), 659–70.

[27] Mörtberg, E. and Andersson, G. (2014). Predictors of response to individual and group cognitive behaviour therapy of social phobia. *Psychology and Psychotherapy: Theory, Research and Practice, 87*(1), 32–43.

[28] Borge, F.M., Hoffart, A. and Sexton, H. (2010). Predictors of outcome in residential cognitive and interpersonal treatment for social phobia: Do cognitive and social dysfunction moderate treatment outcome? *Journal of Behavior Therapy and Experimental Psychiatry, 41*(3), 212–19.

[29] Amir, N., Taylor, C.T. and Donohue, M.C. (2011). Predictors of response to an attention modification program in generalized social phobia. *Journal of Consulting and Clinical Psychology, 79*(4), 533.

[30] Kimbrel, N.A. (2008). A model of the development and maintenance of generalized social phobia. *Clinical Psychology Review, 28*(4), 592–612.

[31] Beltzer, M.L., Daniel, K.E., Daros, A.R. and Teachman, B.A. (2023). Examining social reinforcement learning in social anxiety. *Journal of Behavior Therapy and Experimental Psychiatry, 80*, 101810.

[32] Ørskov, P.T., Lichtenstein, M.B., Ernst, M.T., Fasterholdt, I., Matthiesen, A.F., Scirea, M., ... and Andersen, T.E. (2022). Cognitive-behavioural therapy with adaptive virtual reality exposure vs. cognitive behavioural therapy with *in vivo* exposure in the treatment of social anxiety disorder: A study protocol for a randomized controlled trial. *Frontiers in Psychiatry, 13*, 991755.

[33] Spence, S.H., Donovan, C. and Brechman-Toussaint, M. (2000). The treatment of childhood social phobia: The effectiveness of a social skills training-based, cognitive-behavioural intervention, with and without parental involvement. *The Journal of Child Psychology and Psychiatry and Allied Disciplines, 41*(6), 713–26.

[34] Rahmani, A.M., Yousefpoor, E., Yousefpoor, M.S., Mehmood, Z., Haider, A., Hosseinzadeh, M. and Ali Naqvi, R. (2021). Machine learning (ML) in medicine: Review, applications, and challenges. *Mathematics, 9*(22), 2970.

[35] Fathi, S., Ahmadi, M., Birashk, B. and Dehnad, A. (2020). Development and use of a clinical decision support system for the diagnosis of social anxiety disorder. *Computer Methods and Programs in Biomedicine, 190*, 105354.

[36] Dunn, E.J., Aldao, A. and De Los Reyes, A. (2015). Implementing physiology in clinical assessments of adult social anxiety: A method for graphically representing physiological arousal to facilitate clinical decision-making. *Journal of Psychopathology and Behavioral Assessment, 37*, 587–96.

[37] Xie, W., Wang, C., Lin, Z., Luo, X., Chen, W., Xu, M., ... and Cheng, M. (2022). Multimodal fusion diagnosis of depression and anxiety based on CNN-LSTM model. *Computerized Medical Imaging and Graphics, 102*, 102128.

[38] Mo, H., Hui, S.C., Liao, X., Li, Y., Zhang, W. and Ding, S. (2024). A multimodal data-driven framework for anxiety screening. *IEEE Transactions on Instrumentation and Measurement, PP*(99), 1–13.

Bio-Inspired Algorithms using Machine Learning and Deep Learning for Social Phobia Treatment | 201

[39] Kumari, K., Singh, J.P., Dwivedi, Y.K. and Rana, N.P. (2021). Multimodal aggression identification using convolutional neural network and binary particle swarm optimization. *Future Generation Computer Systems, 118*, 187–97.

[40] Guo, T., Zhao, W., Alrashoud, M., Tolba, A., Firmin, S. and Xia, F. (2022). Multimodal educational data fusion for students' mental health detection. *IEEE Access, 10*, 70370–70382.

[41] Meshram, P. and Rambola, R.K. (2023). Diagnosis of depression level using multimodal approaches using deep learning techniques with multiple selective features. *Expert Systems, 40*(4), e12933.

[42] Rai, B.K., Jain, I., Tiwari, B. and Saxena, A. (2024). Multimodal mental state analysis. *Health Services and Outcomes Research Methodology*, 1–28. Springer.

[43] Bouarara, H.A. (2021). Recurrent neural network (RNN) to analyse mental behaviour in social media. *International Journal of Software Science and Computational Intelligence (IJSSCI), 13*(3), 1–11.

[44] Al-Ezzi, A., Kamel, N., Faye, I. and Gunaseli, E. (2020). Review of EEG, ERP, and brain connectivity estimators as predictive biomarkers of social anxiety disorder. *Frontiers in Psychology, 11*, 517065.

[45] Noori, F.M., Kahlon, S., Lindner, P., Nordgreen, T., Torresen, J. and Riegler, M. (Sept. 2019). Heart rate prediction from head movement during virtual reality treatment for social anxiety. *In: 2019 International Conference on Content-Based Multimedia Indexing (CBMI)* (pp. 1–5). IEEE.

[46] Al-Ezzi, A., Kamel, N., Faye, I. and Gunaseli, E. (2021). Analysis of default mode network in social anxiety disorder: EEG resting-state effective connectivity study. *Sensors, 21*(12), 4098.

[47] Salehi, E., Mehrabi, M., Fatehi, F. and Salehi, A. (2020). Virtual reality therapy for social phobia: A scoping review. *In: Medical Informatics in Europe Conference (MIE) 2020* (pp. 713–717). IOS Press.

[48] Herbelin, B. (2005). *Virtual Reality Exposure Therapy for Social Phobia* (No. 3351). EPFL.

[49] Anderson, P.L., Price, M., Edwards, S.M., Obasaju, M.A., Schmertz, S.K., Zimand, E. and Calamaras, M.R. (2013). Virtual reality exposure therapy for social anxiety disorder: A randomized controlled trial. *Journal of Consulting and Clinical Psychology, 81*(5), 751.

[50] Kampmann, I.L., Emmelkamp, P.M., Hartanto, D., Brinkman, W.P., Zijlstra, B.J. and Morina, N. (2016). Exposure to virtual social interactions in the treatment of social anxiety disorder: A randomized controlled trial. *Behaviour Research and Therapy, 77*, 147–56.

[51] Price, M., Mehta, N., Tone, E.B. and Anderson, P.L. (2011). Does engagement with exposure yield better outcomes? Components of presence as a predictor of treatment response for virtual reality exposure therapy for social phobia. *Journal of Anxiety Disorders, 25*(6), 763–70.

[52] Price, M., Mehta, N., Tone, E.B. and Anderson, P.L. (2011). Does engagement with exposure yield better outcomes? Components of presence as a predictor of treatment response for virtual reality exposure therapy for social phobia. *Journal of Anxiety Disorders, 25*(6), 763–70.

[53] Peng, Z. and Wan, Y. (2024). Human vs. AI: Exploring students' preferences between human and AI TA and the effect of social anxiety and problem complexity. *Education and Information Technologies, 29*(1), 1217–46.

[54] Nazar, M., Alam, M.M., Yafi, E. and Su'ud, M.M. (2021). A systematic review of human–computer interaction and explainable artificial intelligence in healthcare with artificial intelligence techniques. *IEEE Access, 9*, 153316–153348.

[55] Joyce, D.W., Kormilitzin, A., Smith, K.A. and Cipriani, A. (2023). Explainable artificial intelligence for mental health through transparency and interpretability for understandability. *NPJ Digital Medicine, 6*(1), 6.

[56] Altis, K.L., Elwood, L.S. and Olatunji, B.O. (2015). Ethical issues and ethical therapy associated with anxiety disorders. *Ethical Issues in Behavioral Neuroscience*, 265–78.

[57] Jayasiri, D., Asanka, D., Udara, I. and Jayasiri, T. (Feb. 2024). Personalized Treatment Approaches for Social Phobia: An ML-Based Decision Support System. *In: 2024 4th International Conference on Advanced Research in Computing (ICARC)* (pp. 43–48). IEEE.

[58] Rowa, K., McCabe, R.E. and Antony, M. (2008). Specific phobia and social phobia. *A Guide to Assessments That Work, 207,* 228.

[59] Butler, G. (1989). Issues in the application of cognitive and behavioural strategies to the treatment of social phobia. *Clinical Psychology Review, 9*(1), 91–106.

[60] Rowa, K. and Antony, M.M. (2005). Psychological treatments for social phobia. *The Canadian Journal of Psychiatry, 50*(6), 308–316.

[61] Jayasiri, D., Asanka, D., Udara, I. and Jayasiri, T. (2024, February). Personalized Treatment Approaches for Social Phobia: An ML-Based Decision Support System. *In: 2024 4th International Conference on Advanced Research in Computing (ICARC)* (pp. 43–48). IEEE.

[62] Balasubramaniam, S. and Kumar, K.S. (2022). Fractional Feedback Political Optimizer with Prioritization-based Charge Scheduling in Cloud-Assisted Electric Vehicular Network. *Ad Hoc and Sensor Wireless Networks, 52*(3–4), 173–98.

[63] Balasubramaniam, S., Syed, M.H., More, N.S. and Polepally, V. (2023). Deep learning-based power prediction aware charge scheduling approach in cloud-based electric vehicular network. *Engineering Applications of Artificial Intelligence, 121,* 105869.

[64] Pelissolo, A., Abou Kassm, S. and Delhay, L. (2019). Therapeutic strategies for social anxiety disorder: Where are we now? *Expert Review of Neurotherapeutics, 19*(12), 1179–89.

[65] Perna, G., Alciati, A., Sangiorgio, E., Caldirola, D. and Nemeroff, C.B. (2020). Personalized clinical approaches to anxiety disorders. *Anxiety Disorders: Rethinking and Understanding Recent Discoveries,* 489–521.

11 | Bio-Inspired Algorithms Based Machine Learning Models for Neural Disorders Prediction
A Focus on Depression Detection

Tekulapally Shriya Reddy,[1*] Kishor Kumar Reddy C.,[2]
Manoj Kumar Reddy D.[3] and Srinath Doss[4]

Depression and neurological disorders together can have a very negative effect on a person's life. The good news is that there is a workable solution in the form of bio-inspired algorithms and machine-learning models. To more accurately diagnose depression and other neurological disorders, scientists combine data from behavioural hints, linguistic patterns, and physiological indicators with information from biological systems like brain networks and genetic algorithms. Utilizing machine learning models like Decision Trees, KNN (K-Nearest Neighbors), and Naive Bayes can lead to a thorough detection and understanding of mental health concerns. With the use of these state-of-the-art techniques, neurological disease patients can receive a more personalized and comprehensive approach to diagnosis and management. It offers an early diagnostic and treatment approach for neurological illnesses based on data-centric prediction, which can improve patient outcomes and raise living standards for millions of people globally. This strategy is useful in recognizing early symptoms of depression and allowing for intervention before the disease develops, as demonstrated by empirical study and validation. A major advancement in neuroscience has been made possible by combining machine learning methods and bio-inspired algorithms, which opens new avenues for the early detection and treatment of neurological conditions. With individualized care, improved results, and a higher standard of living for people with neurological illnesses, we can all work together to build a more positive and health-conscious society.

1. Introduction to Neural Disorders

Neural diseases refer to all the variants of diseases that affect people's nervous system in one way or the other. The latter includes the brain, spinal cord, and the

---

[1,2] Department of Computer Science & Engineering, Stanley College of Engineering and Technology for Women, India.

[3] Department of Electrical and Electronics Engineering, Vardhaman College of Engineering, Hyderabad, India.

[4] Faculty of Engineering & Technology, Botho University, Botswana.

* Corresponding author: tekulapallyshriyaram1104@gmail.com

peripheral nerves. These diseases cause substantial amount of disability in physical, cognitive, and even psychological compartment of an individual. It is important to emphasize that neural developmental issues can be lifelong, and their effects are restraining a person's ability to have a fulfilling life, also, they pose a serious threat to healthcare initiatives [11]. Neural disorders may be classified in many indices based on the zone of the nervous system they are impacting or based on the sort of condition. Neurological disorders can be grouped in different categories according to the system involved or the process involved. Some neurodegenerative diseases include Alzheimer, Parkinson, Huntington diseases; they slow down the neuron destruction and substantially disorient clients in their thinking and movement capability [1]. They are mostly chronic illnesses and a large percentage of them do not have a known cure at the current times; this makes them a priority in medical research.

The major neurodevelopmental disorders include intelligence disability, attention deficit hyperactivity disorders, and autism spectrum disorders which are usually because of improper formation of the brain and their signs are conspicuous in the young stages of development. It leads to alterations in behaviour, social relationships, and learning abilities and so should be diagnosed before the school-going age because they would require inter professional approaches in their management [3]-[4]. Ischemic cerebral injuries, also referred to as cerebrovascular accidents, can be classified into stroke and transient ischemic attack which is defined by focal cerebral infarction due to obstruction of a cerebral artery. These conditions call for professional care for the patient to avoid further harm as they progress later in life. Neuropathic infections are conditions that affect the nervous system and can be treated; they include meningitis and encephalitis that result from bacterial, viral, or ret fungi. Like any other diseases, these diseases have the tendencies of causing acute and chronic neurological complications and hence require vaccination and early treatment and management to be provided [5]-[6].

Traumatic brain injury (TBI) is the result of a physical injury that occurs to the head when an external force, great enough to cause damage to the brain, is applied to the skull and may result in either permanent or temporary loss of the normal use of the brain. It may result from a fall, car accident, sports, and even violence where a person may develop alteration in his physiologic, cognitive, and psychologic competence. It appears that what patients need most after the episode are physical and occupational therapy, and other forms of care, which aim at trying to help people get back to their normal lives. Seizure disorders and epilepsy are unique due to the tendency to recur and are characterized by the failure of the human being to control the electric seizures that occur in the brain [7]-[8]. Epilepsy is a neurological disease that is associated with disorders of brain cells with intermittent electric impulse irregularities requiring both short- and long-term management with the help of drugs, special diet regimens, and sometimes neurosurgery.

Crucially, neural networks can detect diseases at the early stages that can lead to optimal treatment outcomes and patient prognosis. Additionally, they are

Bio-Inspired Algorithms Based Machine Learning Models for Neural Disorders Prediction | 205

adaptive, allowing ongoing education from new cases so as to be updated with what is happening in medicine all the time. Besides that, neural networks can incorporate a wide range of medical information types like medical images, genetic information as well as clinical records which help in providing comprehensive diagnostic insights for medical cases. Enhancement of diagnostics reliability through elimination of human faults and provision of consistent and objective analysis is among their values. In addition to this, these systems over time save costs by reducing unnecessary tests or lesser known diagnoses, thus cutting down on overhead costs while ensuring quality diagnostics availability even in remote or undeserved areas thus scaling up medical practices. Therefore, neural networks are such a game-changing technology for diseases identification which guarantees better healthcare deliveries.

1.1 Understanding Depression: Causes, Symptoms, and Diagnosis

Out of all the neurological disorders, depression is one of the most prevalent, causing concerns depending on the extent of the occurrences and their effects on society and the lives of the victims. Depression is commonly recognized as a broad clinical mood disorder with effects on the patient's emotions, thinking patterns, and behaviours [9]-[10]. The factors causing depression are not clearly understood although the development of depression is thought to be attributed to a combination of hormonal, genetic, and environmental factors as well as psychological factors. Some of these include: Gender, as women are at a higher risk than men due to hormonal changes and other factors; genetic factors and heredity, as people who have a family history of depression or any of the mood disorders are at a higher risk. What this indicates is that the genetic factor could contribute to the tendency of a person to develop a depression gene [11]. Apart from lifestyle factors, certain biological causes also play a significant role in depression and include structural and functional changes in the brain; hormonal dysregulation, and differences in neurochemistry.

For instance, disruptions in some neurotransmitters as serotonin, norepinephrine, and dopamine have been linked to depressive disorders [12]-[13]. These biological components indicate that medical and pharmacological approaches should play a role in dealing with depression. Environmental indicators are also another factor that needs to be considered. Among the identified factors that might cause or worsen depressive episodes, various life changes can be recognized, including financial difficulties, loss of a close person, traumatic experiences, or long-term stress. This highlights the need for supportive environment and stress intervention measures in managing depression. Other available data show that it is also linked to anxiety disorders, and other psychological factors affect the risk of depression. Self-destructive thoughts and behaviours as well as low self-esteem or excessively critical attitudes make a person even more susceptible to depression. It is essential to recognize these psychological aspects to create therapeutic modalities that engage and treat both the cognitive and the affective domains of clients' personalities [14].

The following are some of the mild to severe symptoms of depression:

- Depressive mood can therefore be described as a constant state of hopelessness or feeling of having no control over whatever is going to happen, or at worst, a complete lack of hope [15]-[17].
- Inert, not a lot of fun doing things that were once enjoyable or interesting the patient has no interest in most of the things that previously used to fascinate him/her [18].
- Difficulty in swallowing and alterations in hunger (increased appetite/food craving or total loss of appetite).
- One can turn into a night creature, or an afternoon slumbered; or they may be an insomniac or a person who sleeps much in the daytime [19]. This is a condition that makes a student to develop a difficulty in concentrating, solving a problem, or in remembering.
- Exhausted, either mentally or physically, because of being conquered by the feeling of guilt or feeling that one does not deserve anything [20].
- Desire to commit suicide and ideas associated with it.
- Diagnostic symptoms that cannot be viewed as having a medical root, which is that people experience everyday distress, flu-like discomfort, and restlessness that are often chronic [21].

Anxiety medical diagnosis needs an extensive assessment by an accredited healthcare company, typically a psychotherapist or psychoanalyst. The American Psychiatric Association's Diagnostic and Statistical Manual of Mental Disorders (DSM-5) has the analysis standards for clinical depression. These demands consist of problems in social work or various other crucial domain names of working, along with the presence of certain signs and symptoms such as anhedonia or clinical depression that take place for the most part of the day practically each day for a minimum of 2 weeks.

Healthcare specialists might do a complete psychological analysis, a summary of case history, a health examination, and research laboratory screening along with analysing signs to eliminate hidden clinical troubles that might appear like clinical depression signs and symptoms. To evaluate the extent of anxiety and track the performance of therapy testing tools like the Beck Depression Inventory (BDI) coupled with Patient Health Questionnaire (PHQ-9) might be made use of. To properly deal with and sustain those influenced by this prevalent psychological problem, comprehending clinical depression needs a holistic strategy that takes into consideration the complex communications in between organic, mental, plus ecological variables along with exact signs and symptom acknowledgment and medical diagnosis.

1.2 Importance of Early Detection and Intervention

Timely diagnosis and treatment are major factors that are applicable to most several diseases and medical conditions in the healthcare sector. This approach focuses on the assessment of visible symptoms when they are most apparent and probably even before they have developed into extreme conditions. Better diagnosis and diagnosis at an early stage is very effective in improving patients' prognosis and reduction of the prevalence of diseases, mortality among patients, as well as reducing costs for the healthcare sector. This is so because the nature of diseases differs and some are easy to diagnose and treat, when identified early. There are those that may be too complex in their nature for early diagnoses and treatment. For instance, cancer, cardiovascular illnesses, and the human immunodeficiency virus/ acquired immune deficiency syndrome can be better managed once diagnosed in the earlier stages [22]. It also allows healthcare practice to diagnose illnesses in its early stage and early treatment, risk reduction, change in lifestyles, and the evidence-based practices to reduce further advancement of the diseases and to increase the healthy life of the patients.

Moreover, since children are involved, then the strategies must strongly emphasize early identification and treatment. Early diagnosis of the Developmental delays, genetic disorders, and congenital malformations ensure that children can be offered timely therapies, medications, and proper care and this fairs well for the development of children. Altogether, the significance of screening and assessment are extremely important and cannot be underestimated in any sector, including healthcare. In essence, about disease control and treatment, population health promotion and management, it provides a foundation for these goals that can enhance health outcomes and therefore the quantity and quality of life across the human life span.

As shown in the Figure 1, the prevalence of depression is high in teenagers who are sensitive of matter. Therefore, decreasing preconception related to psychological wellness, broadening accessibility to very early testing and treatment solutions, and

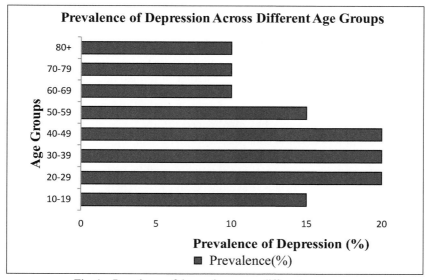

Fig. 1 Prevalence of depression across different age groups.

208 | Bio-inspired Algorithms in Machine Learning and Deep Learning for Disease Detection

raising public understanding are all necessary components of alternative healthcare programmes. As a whole, very early recognition and treatment are important to promoting psychological wellness. The development of mental wellness problems improving the top quality of therapy plus decreasing the general toll that mental disease has on people coupled with culture.

2. Machine Learning Techniques in Healthcare

2.1 Evolution of Machine Learning in Healthcare

Featuring major milestones in the advancement of artificial intelligence (AI) and machine learning (ML) in the context of healthcare, the technology has found its feet in a field characterized by strong evidence of its applicability and tremendous potential for shaping the future of healthcare services delivery. The idea of using ML in healthcare was pioneered by the expertise systems and rule-based algorithms in the 1970s and 1980s; MYCIN is an example of the latest discovery which was used to diagnose bacteria. New methods also entered the scene in the 1990s with the use of new statistical procedures such as Decision tree and Logistic regression for better forecasting.

There was the beginning of the ideas of data mining and of the concept of big data in the early 2000s because the fields of healthcare generated large amounts of electronic health records (EHRs), genetic study, and uses of imaging. The past decade in the 2010s started a new epoch with the progression of ML and deep learning algorithms especially the convolutional neural networks (CNNs) and the recurrent neural networks (RNNs) that showcased possibilities in the medical image analysis and the natural language processing of the medical notes. There was further development in the concept of personalized medicine and predative analytics using ML algorithms that studies in-depth genetic, clinical, and lifestyle data with a view to enhance the physician's approach in developing the best treatment plan that would yield positive patient results.

The combination of ML with IoT (internet of things) and wearable devices facilitated constant health check and chronic ailment management for users to adhere to a constant stream of information on their health and potential illnesses. Research within recent years has also placed efforts for explication into more explanation and an ethical agenda like data privacy or algorithmic bias. Future developments are expected in an even greater extent with regards to multimodal data fusion as well as new, sound, and autonomous ethical AI solutions within the medical field where physicians, developers, and researchers are working hand-in-hand.

As shown in the Table 1, significant advancements in the application of ML techniques within the healthcare sector over the past few decades is outlined. Each year represents a milestone where ML technologies have contributed to various aspects of healthcare, from medical image processing to personalized medicine and telemedicine. These advancements have revolutionized patient- care, diagnosis accuracy, medication research, and healthcare delivery systems. By examining these key advancements, one can gain insights into the transformative impact of ML on healthcare practices and the continuous evolution of AI-driven solutions to address healthcare challenges.

Table 1 Evolution of Machine Learning advancements in healthcare.

Year	Key Advancements in Machine Learning for Healthcare
1980	The application of machine learning techniques to the processing of medical images has advanced computer-aided diagnosis.
1995	Creation of clinical decision support systems that use machine learning algorithms to assess patient data and recommend courses of action.
2000	Use of machine learning in personalized medicine and genomics, which makes it possible to analyse vast amounts of genetic data for the purpose of optimizing treatment and predicting disease.
2005	Machine learning integration with electronic health records (EHRs) enables data-driven insights into patient health outcomes, trends, and population health management at scale.
2010	Development of deep learning algorithms for the interpretation of medical images, which has improved the accuracy of diagnosis for diseases including cancer and neurological problems.
2015	Increased use of machine learning in medication research and discovery, leading to quicker identification of new therapeutic targets and potential uses for repurposing drugs.
2020	Machine learning-driven telemedicine and remote patient monitoring are on the rise, allowing for proactive patient care and real-time patient health metrics monitoring.
2024	Constant improvements in AI-powered healthcare delivery systems, with a stronger emphasis on precision medicine, predictive analytics, and AI-assisted screening and diagnosis.

3. Bio-Inspired Algorithms for Neural Disorders Prediction

3.1 Introduction to Bio-Inspired Algorithms

Bio-inspired formulas which are based upon all-natural procedures and organic systems have shown substantial capacity for projecting neurological conditions. These formulas utilize sensations like development, crowd habits, and neural task to tackle hard medical care issues, especially in the forecast of neurological conditions such as clinical depression, Alzheimer's and Parkinson's condition. Benefits of each are defined thoroughly listed below:

Hereditary Algorithms

- *Principle*: These algorithms simulate a choice by creating, establishing, and enhancing a populace of remedies throughout succeeding generations.
- *Application*: In a neurological condition forecast, hereditary algorithms are made use of to choose along with enhance functions. It boosts the version,

anticipating precision by choosing one of the most pertinent attributes from large datasets (such as hereditary information and mind imaging). As an example, they can aid in recognizing hereditary pens connected to a raised threat of clinical depression or Alzheimer's illness [23].

Particle Swarm Optimization (PSO)

- *Principle*: PSO is designed after the social habits of birds gathering or fish education. It enhances an issue by permitting a populace (group) of prospective remedies (bits) to move around in the search area making use of fundamental mathematical ideas based upon their very own and their next-door neighbours' experiences.
- *Application*: PSO is utilized to maximize the specifications of AI versions that anticipate neurological illness. It can effectively look for the ideal criteria in intricate versions, leading to boosted efficiency in jobs like spotting Parkinson's condition based upon movement signs plus mind-imaging information [24].

Artificial Neural Networks (ANN) and Deep Learning

- *Principle*: Artificial neural networks (ANNs) are computer system designs motivated by the human mind that include adjoined devices (nerve cells) that refine information in layers. Deep discovering, a kind of synthetic neural network contains countless layers that enable the understanding of complex patterns.
- *Application*: Deep discovering versions, RNNs are commonly utilized to evaluate neuroimaging information (e.g., MRI, fMRI) to spot very early signs of neurological issues. They can spot complicated patterns in imaging information that might show problems such as clinical depression also prior to medical signs show up.

Ant Colony Optimization (ACO)

- *Principle*: ACO was motivated by ants' foraging habits and capacity to find the quickest courses to food resources. Chemical routes are utilized as an indirect interaction technique to locate suitable services.
- *Application*: In conditions of neurological problems, ACO can be utilized to enhance paths in mind link networks. As an example, it can aid in recognizing exactly how neural circuits are changed in problems such as schizophrenia by enhancing the look for irregular patterns in mind link information.

Transformative Techniques and Differential Evaluation

- *Principle*: These techniques are all-natural evolution-inspired optimization methods that look for ideal options by focusing on the flexibility and advancement of people within a populace.
- *Application*: These formulas are utilized to enhance advanced versions that project neurological illness. For instance, they can make use of longitudinal individual information to enhance the criteria and framework of neural network versions that anticipate the programme of illness like numerous scleroses.

Swarm Intelligence (SI)

- **Principle**: SI formulas are motivated by the cumulative habits of decentralized, self-organized systems, such as pests or birds.
- **Application**: SI techniques are made use of, to gather and classify large datasets pertinent to neurological diseases. As an example, they can team clients based upon resemblances in their mind task patterns or hereditary accounts which can aid recognize subtypes of anxiety or various other neural ailments.

As shown in Table 2, Bio-inspired algorithms leverage mechanisms and principles observed in natural systems to address complex computational problems. These algorithms draw inspiration from biological processes, adapting them into computational strategies to find optimal solutions in various domains. Here is a brief overview of several bio-inspired algorithms, their foundational inspirations, and common applications, particularly in medical fields such as depression, epilepsy, Parkinson's, schizophrenia, and Alzheimer's disease.

Table 2 Overview of Bio-inspired algorithms for neural disorder prediction.

Bio-Inspired Algorithms	Description	Sector-Inspired Algorithmic Innovation	Common Application
Genetic Algorithm (GA)	Uses principles of natural selection and genetics to find optimal solutions.	Natural selection and genetics	Depression, Epilepsy
Particle Swarm Optimization (PSO)	Models the social behaviour of birds flocking or fish schooling to find optimal solutions.	Swarm behaviour of birds/fish	Parkinson's, Depression
Artificial Neural Networks (ANN)	Simulates the neural structure of the human brain to learn from data and recognize patterns.	Human brain structure	Depression, Schizophrenia
Ant Colony Optimization (ACO)	Mimics the behaviour of ants finding paths to food sources to solve optimization problems.	Foraging behaviour of ants	Alzheimer's, Depression
Evolutionary Strategies (ES)	Encompasses various algorithms inspired by natural evolutionary processes to solve complex optimization tasks.	Darwinian evolution principles	Depression, Schizophrenia
Differential Evaluation (DE)	Uses mechanisms of natural evolution such as mutation, crossover, and selection for optimization problems.	Evolutionary strategies	Depression, Epilepsy
Swarm Intelligence (SI)	Utilizes the collective behaviour of decentralized, self-organized systems like ant colonies or bird flocks.	Collective behaviour of social organisms	Parkinson's, Depression

As shown in Figure 2, a comparative overview of several bio-inspired algorithms is depicted, along with a CNN for depression identification. The algorithms used are GA, PSO, ACO, Swarm Algorithm (SA), DE, and CNN. The performance criteria evaluated include accuracy, precision, specificity, and efficiency, as measured by execution time. This comparison emphasizes the pros and disadvantages of each strategy, allowing you to choose the best algorithm depending on your individual accuracy, precision, and computational efficiency needs.

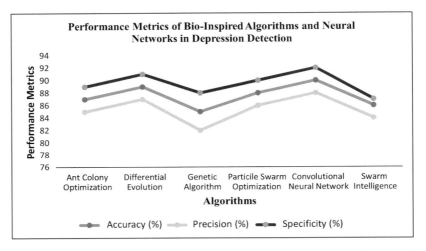

Fig. 2 Performance metrics of Bio-Inspired Algorithms and neural networks in depression detection.

3.2 Principles and Applications of Bio-Inspired ML Models in Mental Health

The use of bio-inspired artificial intelligence (ML) versions in psychological wellness is rapidly broadening incorporating the concepts of all-natural and organic systems to resolve the intricacies of psychological health and wellness conditions. These versions, influenced by transformative procedures, swarm knowledge plus neural networks supply unique strategies to the forecast, medical diagnosis along with administration of psychological health and wellness conditions [25]. Listed below is a thorough introduction of their applications:

Recognition and Forecasting of Depression
- To determine and projection of clinical depression, a selection of information resources consisting of wearable sensing units, digital wellness documents, coupled with patient-reported results are examined making use of bio-inspired AI formulas.
- GAs improve the accuracy of clinical depression forecast designs by helping in the recognition of hereditary pens and the option of one of the most significant elements from big datasets.

- Deep Learning techniques like fabricated neural networks (ANNs) evaluate detailed patterns in behaviour together with neuroimaging information to detect very early advising signals of clinical depression and track the efficiency of therapy.

Tracking Stress along with Anxiety

- Mobile wellness applications that assess information from heart price irregularity, galvanic skin reaction coupled with various other physical indicators to supply real-time responses and therapies are implemented by PSO formulas.
- SI formulas collection coupled with categorize stress-related information to find patterns along with projection stress and anxiety episodes.

Medical Diagnosis of Schizophrenia

- Neural network-inspired deep understanding designs specifically, are vital for detecting schizophrenia because they can recognize both architectural and practical irregularities in the mind by reviewing neuroimaging information.
- CNNs evaluate fMRI together with MRI information to spot distinctive mind patterns connected to mental illness, helping with very early medical diagnosis and surveillance the training course of the ailment.
- ACO, which makes best use of mind network connection courses, can be used to recognize constant disruptions related to mental illness.

Administration of Bipolar Disorder

- Making use of a selection of information resources such as state of mind journals plus sensing unit information, bio-inspired AI designs projection state of mind swings in individuals with bipolar affective disorder.
- Sequential information might be refined well by RNNs and Long Short-Term Memory (LSTM) networks to prepare for manic together with depressive episodes. This enables punctual treatments and individualized therapy programmes.

Autism Spectrum Disorders and ADHD

- To determine and deal with attention deficit hyperactivity disorder (ADHD), autism spectrum disorders (ASD) bioinspired formulas analyse behaviour and neuroimaging information [26].
- DE and Evolutionary Strategies (ES) maximize designs to discover hereditary together with mind link patterns symptomatic of ASD and ADHD.
- ANNs and deep understanding designs review neuroimaging information and behaviour assessments to discover very early biomarkers and sustain tailored treatment strategies.

Post Traumatic Stress Disorder (PTSD)

- Device finding out formulas utilize information from army soldiers, injury survivors along with various other at-risk teams to forecast the start along with development of PTSD.

- GAs and PSO maximize designs that analyse physical information historic information, and emotional analyses to determine individuals that might go to threat of establishing PTSD and to personalize therapy in action.

Real-Time Surveillance and Supervision
- Utilizing details from wearable innovation plus mobile wellness applications, bio-inspired AI designs permit real-time monitoring together with therapy of a series of psychological health and wellness concerns.
- ANNs and deep learning versions keep an eye on rest patterns task degrees together with physical actions by evaluating constant streams of information from wearable sensing units.
- SI approaches make it much easier to develop flexible systems that respond to changes in an individual's mind state and give customized, real-time aid.

Information Integration Using Multiple Modes
- To improve the forecast and medical diagnosis of psychological wellness health problems GAs and ACOs maximize the option and assimilation of multimodal information (e.g., hereditary, neuroimaging, professional, coupled with behaviour information).
- Diverse datasets are refined and assessed by deep understanding designs which expose fancy affiliations and patterns that might not show up with standard evaluation.

As shown in Table 3, details of numerous usages of bio-inspired formulas in medical care are listed. These formulas, influenced by organic systems are being used throughout various domain names to change condition, medical diagnosis, medication exploration individualized medication, positive modelling wellness surveillance, clinical robotics, and automation. By taking advantage of the power of bio-inspired formulas, medical care experts can improve client treatment, boost therapy results, and simplify healthcare procedures. Table 3 offers a thorough summary of just how these formulas are being used to attend to varied healthcare obstacles.

Table 3 Applications of Bio-inspired algorithm in healthcare.

Application	Description
Disease Diagnosis	Bio-inspired algorithms are used to assess medical imaging data (e.g., MRI, CT scans) to identify irregularities that may indicate cancer or tumours.
Drug Discovery	Bio-inspired algorithms facilitate virtual screening of chemical compounds to identify prospective medication candidates and optimize molecular structures for increased efficacy.
Personalized Medicine	Bio-inspired algorithms examine genomic data to find genetic markers related to illness susceptibility, therapeutic response, and treatment outcomes in specific patients.

Contd.

Prognostic Modeling	Bio-inspired algorithms anticipate disease progression and patient outcomes based on clinical data, biomarkers, and physiological signals, which aid in treatment planning and management.
Health Monitoring and Wearables	Bio-inspired algorithms evaluate data from wearable devices (e.g., smartwatches, fitness trackers) to monitor vital signs, detect anomalies, and give consumers with real-time health insights.
Medical Robotics and Automation	Bio-inspired algorithms drive robotic devices to perform minimally invasive surgeries, aid in rehabilitation exercises, and automate healthcare chores such as medicine administration.

3.3 Evaluating the Advantages and Limitations of Bio-Inspired Approaches

- *Strength and Versatility*: Bioinspired approaches are fundamentally durable and adaptable, making use of ideas discovered in all-natural systems to adjust to ever-changing and challenging circumstances.
- *International Optimization*: Bio-inspired formulas such as PSO coupled with hereditary formulas can undergo huge option rooms together with recognizing around the world optimum response to testing optimization concerns. These formulas can properly look for the maximum options without ending up being entrapped in regional optima by imitating the procedures of all-natural option together with advancement [26].
- *Parallelism plus Scalability*: A great deal of bio-inspired formulas is normally identical coupled with scalable which allows them to successfully make use of calculation sources and address complicated jobs. These techniques can manage large information troubles and increase convergence by being parallelized over various CPUs or dispersed computer systems.
- *Interpretability and Explainability*: A variety of bio-inspired designs supply reasonable descriptions for their decision-making treatments and options, such as genetic formulas and ant swarm optimization. This explainability enhances client expertise and self-confidence particularly in essential sectors like financing and healthcare where responsibility and visibility are important.
- *Imagination and Innovation*: By contrasting numerous organic systems and all-natural occasions, bioinspired techniques often produce initial remedies to testing problems. These techniques advertise initial idea and the examination of unique methods with interdisciplinary teamwork which causes imaginative explorations coupled with breakthroughs in scientific research along with innovation.

Despite its capacity, bio-inspired approaches additionally deal with numerous difficulties.

- *Level of Sensitivity and Specification Adjusting*: Bio-inspired formulas generally consist of a collection of criteria that need to be effectively readjusted to run at their finest. These formulas can be tough to set up because of their level of sensitivity to specification options; in order to get superb outcomes a lot of trial and error and subject experience are needed.

- *Computational Complexity*: Large-scale optimization troubles call for computationally costly together with taxing bio-inspired formulas specifically those that depend on move knowledge or transformative calculation.
- *Early Convergence and Stagnation*: Search procedures in bio-inspired formulas might experience untimely convergence or stagnancy which avoids them from completely analysing the entire option area or from ending up being stuck in less-than-ideal solutions. Poor populace range, wrong criterion setups, or misleading physical fitness landscapes can all add to this trouble.
- *Restricted Transferability*: The specific concern domain name and the residential or commercial properties of the underlying information are regularly important consider the success of bio-inspired methods. Although some techniques could operate well in some scenarios their transferability and larger efficiency might be restricted if they do not do continually throughout datasets or generalize well to various other locations.

As shown in Table 4, Bio-inspired approaches leverage natural processes to solve complex problems in computer science, engineering, and applied mathematics. These methods offer numerous advantages, such as robustness to noisy environments and adaptability, but also come with limitations like high computational complexity and sensitivity to parameters. Table 4 provides a concise overview of the key advantages and limitations of bio-inspired approaches, aiding in the assessment of their suitability for various applications.

Table 4   Evaluating the advantages and limitations of Bio-inspired approaches.

Advantages	Limitations
Robustness to noisy or uncertain environments	High computational complexity
Adaptability to changing conditions	Sensitivity to parameter settings
Ability to handle complex, nonlinear problems	Difficulty in interpreting and explaining model behaviours
Parallel processing capabilities	Lack of scalability for large-scale problems
Exploration of novel and innovative solutions	Overfitting or underfitting of models
Flexibility in problem-solving	Limited understanding of convergence and optimization dynamics
Inspiration for interdisciplinary research	Vulnerability to local optima
Potential for mimicking natural processes	Challenges in integrating with existing systems and methodologies
Efficient global search strategies	Dependency on domain-specific knowledge and expertise
Ability to find near-optimal solutions	Ethical considerations regarding the use of living organisms or natural processes

4. Integration of Bio-Inspired Algorithms with Machine Learning

4.1 Understanding the Synergies between Bio-Inspired Algorithms and Traditional ML Techniques

Bio-inspired formulas give unique methods to problem-solving by taking motivation from organic systems and all-natural sensations. On the various other hand, typical AI strategies are based upon mathematical formulas and analytical concepts. Even though these two techniques can show up various, they both intend to make use of information to find out to projection or choose. The complementing top qualities of bio-inspired formulas and traditional device discovering strategies are where they function best with each other. Solutions with organic motivation, such hereditary formulas, bit guidebook optimization and ant swarm optimization, are very competent in maximizing and checking out complex search locations. They are durable, adaptable, and with the ability of taking care of transforming and uncertain problems.

Nevertheless, much more traditional AI techniques such as neural networks, decision trees and SVMs use efficient devices for anticipating modelling, pattern recognition, and information evaluation. They are extensively made use of in various applications since they supply scalability, performance and interpretability. The benefits of both strategies can be used by scientists and specialists via the combination of bio-inspired formulas with traditional maker finding out methods. Genes for example, can be put on semantic network hyperparameter optimization and attribute option. For category troubles, assistance vector makers can do far better when enhanced with bit guidebook optimization. Ant swarm optimization can boost information collections decision tree strategies.

4.2 Benefits of Integrating Bio-Inspired Algorithms with Machine Learning

ML designs that make use of bioinspired concepts should very carefully incorporate these principles with present formulas and strategies. Here's a summary of just how to attain this assimilation perfectly:

- *Hybridization of Algorithms*: One technique includes standard artificial intelligence approaches with bio-inspired formulas. This strategy uses the benefits of both standards to create even more resistant and effective designs. As an example, transformative formulas can be paired with neural networks to choose functions or maximize design criteria.
- *Hyperparameter Adjusting and Optimization*: Bio-inspired optimization strategies, such as bit throng optimization along with substitute annealing can be utilized to play hyperparameters and enhance design efficiency. By swiftly discovering the search room and determining ideal options for these formulas replicate all-natural procedures such as throng actions or thermal annealing.

218 | Bio-inspired Algorithms in Machine Learning and Deep Learning for Disease Detection

- *Neuromorphic Computing*: This cutting-edge technique of ML design layout is based upon the style together with procedures of the mind. Contrasted to standard computer designs, neuromorphic systems have the ability to execute jobs quicker and adaptably since they mimic the identical handling coupled with connection of nerve cells.
- *Self-Organizing Maps (SOM)*: SOMs apply for without supervision discovering and organizing troubles as they are influenced by the framework of neural networks in the mind. These designs keep the topological partnerships in between information factors by arranging the inbound information in a low-dimensional area. In device-discovering application, this approach container assistance with information visualization and pattern acknowledgment.
- *Developmentary Strategies and Formulas*: Developmentary strategies and formulas, like genetic formulas simulate the procedures of all-natural option in order to discover the most effective options or enhance version criteria. In time these formulas enhance version efficiency by over and over choosing, interbreeding coupled with changing a populace of possible options.

4.3 Case Studies Demonstrating Successful Integration Approaches in Depression Detection

Studies showcasing reliable assimilation methods in anxiety discovery give instances of exactly how AI strategies and bio-inspired formulas have been effectively incorporated to boost the accuracy, efficiency, and stability of clinical depression discovery designs. Right here are some instances to assist you recognize:

- *Assistance Vector Device and Hybrid Hereditary Formula Design*: In this study, researchers integrated making use of assistance vector makers (SVM) and hereditary formulas (GA) to produce a crossbreed design that utilizes electroencephalography (EEG) information to detect clinical depression [6]. By selecting one of the most making clear EEG functions connected with clinical depression, the hereditary formula was used to enhance the function option treatment. In order to compare individuals that were dispirited and those that weren't based upon their EEG patterns the picked functions were ultimately fed right into the SVM classifier.
- *PSO for Neural Network Feature Selection*: In this study, multimodal information was made use of to refine the function option treatment in neural network-based anxiety discovery versions with making use of bit movement optimization (PSO). PSO was used to discover the very best part of functions from a range of information resources, such as demographics, neuroimaging information, and scientific assessments. After that, a neural network classifier was educated with the selected functions to forecast anxiety state from the amount of the information. The incorporated version went beyond versions without attribute option regarding category precision and generalization efficiency by making use of PSO for function option. This suggests that bio-inspired optimization strategies can be efficiently made use of to boost clinical depression discovery designs.

- ***Ant Swarm Optimization for Signs Pattern Collection Evaluation***: Ant swarm optimization was utilized in this situation research to classify individuals according to their signs accounts and determine certain subgroups within a populace. Ant Swarm Optimization was utilized to team individuals right into collections according to common signs patterns as established by medical meetings or self-reported surveys. This highlights the worth of bio-inspired formulas in revealing concealed patterns and substructures in anxiety information.

As shown in Table 5, lifetime frequency prices of different DSM conditions classified by sex is depicted. These occurrence prices supply understandings right into the regularity of incident of various mental wellness problems amongst women and men. Recognizing the occurrence prices of these conditions is vital for doctors, policymakers, and scientists to establish efficient treatment techniques along with designate sources properly to deal with psychological wellness difficulties within various market teams.

Table 5 Comparative case study of DSM disorders.

DSM Disorder	*Lifetime Prevalence Rates*		
	Females	*Males*	*Total*
Major Depressive Disorder	20	12.8	17.4
Drug Abuse	5	12.3	7.6
Social Anxiety Disorder	12.7	11.9	12.4
Post-Traumatic Stress Disorder	9.8	4	7
Panic Disorder	6.9	2.9	4.9
Specific Phobia	16	9	12.5
Dysthymia	2.7	2	2.5
Alcohol Abuse	7.5	19.9	12.8

5. Application of Bio-Inspired Algorithms in Depression Detection

5.1 Overview of Studies Utilizing Bio-Inspired Algorithms for Depression Prediction

The application of bio-inspired algorithms in developing anxiety is an example towards very simple applicative development, towards improving the precision and the performance of any existing models. Together with the capability to perform feature selection and thus improve the interpretability of a model and avoid overfitting, tools of GA for important features selection from different data sources. This makes the resulting prediction models to be realistic and can be of practical use. In this case, PSO aids in improving in relation to hyperparameters of the model and the general effectiveness and flexibility of the model. These

Bio-inspired Algorithms in Machine Learning and Deep Learning for Disease Detection

approaches are helpful in anticipating even specifics and aspects of anxiety that are attached to a calculus.

Ensemble learning in ACO is worthwhile in the following way since it makes input to the improvement of the Generalized Predictive Accuracy since it comprises of several models with weights set depending in their efficiency. This ties up rather strong set of models that assists to reduce the overfitting issue. Integration of swarm-based heuristics like ant colony and PSO results in a model, which was earlier learned, that can adapt to the changing anxiety manifestation to make interventions earlier. Techniques such as genetic programming, in explicit terms, provide a superior level of interpretability and accuracy than normal model analysis and help in enhancing the usage of a superior therapeutic model for treatment as well as making better decisions for practicing.

5.2 Comparative Analysis of Bio-Inspired Algorithms against Traditional Methods

Standard and buffed formulas are compared to one another, and it is described what advantages and disadvantages accompany working with each of them, and how they comport themselves in practical implementation. Strategies such as logistic regression, SVM, decision tree have been used in the past to carry out the depression prediction. Such methods are based input metrics like demographics, clinical lab results, and self-reported symptoms to categorize a person as being depressed or not. Several criteria are considered when comparing these approaches. Analysing flexibility, it can be mentioned that bio-inspired formulations are more flexible and adjustable than the classic approach. It is for this reason that they are generally better suited for interaction and higher order terms such as quadratic and cubic, which in essence are nonlinear relationships, and they capture more of the details of the data than linear models. Unlike deterministic algorithms, stochastic bio-inspired algorithms can travel over the space of solutions and recognize more consistent patterns even if they are located within a noisy environment.

This factor assumes significance as the sizes and volume of the data encounter in scenarios continue to expand. Optimization methods inspired by nature and by some principles such as evolution or SI capabilities are higher than those of traditional methods may face difficulty at large datasets. One is the difficulty in providing interpretations of bio-inspired solutions because these are usually looked at as black boxes, which hinders people's ability to understand why decisions were made in a certain way. On the other hand, approaches that have been previously used more often provide obvious interpretability with clear rules or model coefficients that can signal the importance of characteristics. Lastly, it is essential to evaluate how well an induction performance or the predictive model to learn from previous inputs to predict inputs not used in the learning process which is fundamental to the applicability of computer learning in real-world applications. The generalization performance of both traditional statistical techniques and bio-inspired algorithms must be compared on different datasets for the task to analyse success.

Table 6 depicts the comparative performance measures for traditional and bio-inspired algorithms in healthcare applications. Traditional methods, such as logistic regression and decision trees, go up against bio-inspired algorithms like as GAs, PSO, and ACO. Each algorithm's accuracy, sensitivity, and specificity are highlighted, providing information about its usefulness in many different types of healthcare jobs. By comparing these results, healthcare professionals can make more informed decisions about algorithm selection for various healthcare applications.

Table 6 Comparative evaluation of Bio-inspired algorithms with conventional approaches.

Algorithm	Traditional Method	Accuracy (%)	Sensitivity (%)	Specificity (%)
Genetic Algorithm	Logistic Regression	87	80	91
Particle Swarm Optimization	Support Vector Machine	84	78	90
Ant Colony Optimization	Decision Trees	88	81	92

5.3 Comparison of Different Algorithms in Terms of Accuracy and Efficiency

This research clarifies the concessions in between design efficiency together with source usage in the context of anxiety forecast where both accuracy and computational sources are substantial elements. In this contrast, the efficiency of numerous formulas may be as compared with:

Logistic Regression

- *Accuracy*: Although extremely uncomplicated and user-friendly, logistic regression might have difficulty determining elaborate connections in the information. Specifically, when the relationships in between forecasters and anxiety are nonlinear its efficiency in anxiety forecast might be modest.
- *Efficiency*: Large-scale applications and real-time forecast jobs can gain from logistic regression's reduced training together with induction source needs and calculating performance.

Support Vector Devices

- *Accuracy*: When incorporated with appropriate bit features assistance vector makers (SVMs) can accomplish high precision in anxiety forecast jobs and excel in recognizing nonlinear choice limits. Nevertheless, the bit plus hyperparameter choice might have an influence on exactly how well they work.
- *Efficiency*: SVMs could need a great deal of sources particularly when taking care of substantial datasets or function areas that have many measurements.

Bio-inspired Algorithms in Machine Learning and Deep Learning for Disease Detection

SVM training can take longer and make use of even more calculating power than educating even more simple designs like logistic regression.

Decision Trees

- *Accuracy*: Decision trees function well for anxiety forecast issues with nonlinear connections since they can properly catch intricate communications in between variables plus results. However, choice trees are at risk to overfitting which might jeopardize their capacity to generalize.
- *Efficiency*: Decision trees, specifically throughout induction, are reliable in regard to computer system sources. Nonetheless, choice tree training can be computationally costly especially if huge trees are made use of if set strategies such as arbitrary woodlands are used.

Random Forests

- *Accuracy*: By integrating forecasts from numerous trees arbitrary woodlands enhance generalization efficiency by solving the overfitting trouble with choice trees. Also, amidst complicated activities and sound they typically do well on anxiety forecast examinations.
- *Efficiency*: Because arbitrary woodlands need educating several trees all at once, they might be computationally more pricey than specific choice trees. When contrasted to a few other set methods, such as slope improving, they are still reliable, nonetheless.

Neural Networks

- *Accuracy*: In a selection of maker finding out jobs consisting of anxiety forecast, neural networks and particularly deep understanding designs, have revealed state-of-the-art efficiency. From unprocessed information they can recognize innovative patterns plus adapt to complex partnerships.
- *Effectiveness*: Deep semantic network training can be computationally stressful especially for huge datasets plus detailed frameworks. However, renovations in innovation (such as GPUs [graphic processing units] plus TPUs [tensor processing units]) together with optimization approaches have enhanced their efficiency making sensible use them in real-world applications feasible.

Easier designs like logistic regression or choice trees could provide a reasonable give-and-take in between precision and effectiveness specifically in resource-constrained contexts even though much more advanced formulas like neural networks might use greater precision.

6. Future Directions and Challenges in Bio-Inspired ML Models for Depression Detection

Using bio-inspired artificial intelligence designs to anxiousness discovery encounters a number of considerable difficulties. The top quality as well as accessibility of information are significant obstacles, as clinical depression information originated from varied resources like genes, neuroimaging plus patient-reported results, making complex reliable assimilation. In addition, the interpretability of intricate designs, such as hereditary formulas along with neural networks is frequently restricted preventing their approval in medical setups. Overfitting stays an essential problem, where versions succeed on training information however stop working to generalize to brand-new information. Making certain strength as well as dependability throughout various populaces and also atmospheres is necessary. Computational intricacy is an additional difficulty, as bio-inspired formulas typically need substantial sources for training as well as release. In addition, ethical factors to consider consisting of information personal privacy together with possible predispositions in ML designs, require cautious administration to make sure reasonable along with fair usage. Attending to these difficulties is important for the effective application of bio-inspired ML designs in clinical depression discovery.

Bio-inspired formulas as well as artificial intelligence (ML) in medical care are swiftly developing driven by technical breakthroughs plus raising information schedule. An essential fad is incorporating multimodal information, incorporating hereditary, neuroimaging, medical and also behaviour information for even more precise anticipating designs. Scientists are likewise concentrating on creating interpretable ML designs that equilibrium precision with openness, making them extra trustworthy for medical professionals. Transfer finding out is getting grip enabling designs educated on one information to be adjusted for usage in an additional, maximizing restricted information sources. Real-time information incorporation from wearable tools and also mobile wellness applications is boosting vibrant tracking plus forecast of mental wellness problems. Improvements in computational power as well as formulas are making it possible for the release of innovative bio-inspired ML versions at range. These fads jointly assurance to enhance individual end results as well as expand the effect of ML in medical care. There will be a major leap in the future for detecting depression with advancements driven by technology, better data integration and in-depth knowledge of mental health issues. These new systems are likely to combine multiple data sources such as social media activity, wearable device metrics, voice analysis, or facial recognition to give a comprehensive and accurate understanding of one's mental well-being. Furthermore, there should be new applications for ML and AI that would allow personalized diagnostics and customized treatment recommendations free from other considerations like unique genetic make-up, environmental factors or behavioural issues. There will be improved algorithms for early detection and prediction of depressive episodes leading to timely interventions among patients affected by this condition.

Figure 3 demonstrates the new developments, how bio-inspired algorithms coupled with machine learning pose the capability of profoundly revolutionizing the practice of medicine in every aspect from drug design and precision diagnosis and targeted therapy to health management by remote monitoring and AI-based clinical decision support. These strategies are creating the path for a positive change in the existing healthcare system one that is better optimized, improved, and enhanced from focusing on the patient-centred computing intelligence and integrated insights.

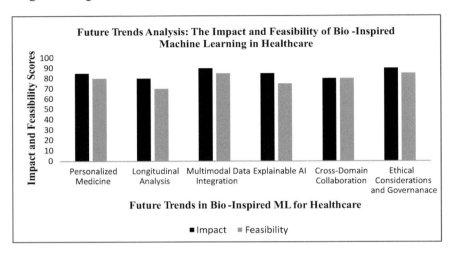

Fig. 3 Upcoming developments in Bio-Inspired Machine Learning for healthcare.

7. Ethical Considerations and Implications

7.1 Ethical Considerations in Using Bio-Inspired ML Models for Healthcare

Applying Bio-inspired ML in healthcare settings involves facing several ethical because it indirectly deals with the patient's safety and identity, while at the same time interfering with patients' liberty. The sombre concern arising out of this is the security and privacy of data. Secure access to and transmission of personal patient data including genetic data, EHRs, and diagnostic images is imperative. Possible solutions, such as strong security and encryption, access control mechanisms, and anonymization approaches should be applied to counter threats to privacy and ensure patients' data protection from illicit use and leakage. Respect for patient's self-determination and right to receive adequate information are basic ethical pillars in research and practice of medicine. It has also found that patients must be fully informed of the goals, potential harm or risks which are involved, and possible benefits when using bio-inspired ML models in research, diagnosis, or therapy. Describing how patient data will be used, by whom, and what consequences it may lead to educating the patient and allowing them to deliberate on whether they are willing to be involved in the utilization of ML in their healthcare.

One major aspect of ML that must be handled carefully is the questions of fairness and avoiding bias when feeding the algorithm and in its outcomes. It is noteworthy that the same set of training data that is used to develop predictive

Bio-Inspired Algorithms Based Machine Learning Models for Neural Disorders Prediction | 225

models may contain pre-existing inequalities in terms of healthcare access, treatment, or demography; this makes these models detrimental to patients as they serve to prolong such prejudices and disparities. To optimize the fairness and justice in the healthcare system, the use of fairness-sensitive algorithms, different training datasets, as well as bias-detection tools, will allow minimizing the problem and developing the equitable healthcare policies. Accountability, collaboration, and trust are essential in the current and future healthcare setting, and compelling understanding and explication of this are expected to guide clinical informatics research and practice by emphasizing explainability and transparency. It is not sufficient for patients, physicians and other actors in the healthcare environment just to get a prediction from the ML algorithm; they have to know about the factors that comprise this prediction and about potential weaknesses and vagueness of the prediction. It has been pointed out that framing logical explanations, training and reports, figures and tables promote meaningful communication and informed consent in clinical management.

Sufficiency, accountability, and liability issues are crucial when incorporating bio-inspired ML models in the healthcare domain. It is essential also to determine who bears the responsibility for the accuracy, reliability, and consequences of the predictions, diagnosis, or proposed treatment arrived at through the use of the ML applications in the varied healthcare setting, including ML developers, practitioners in the field of healthcare, regulatory bodies, and healthcare institutions. Using risk management processes, legal responsibility models, and complaint mechanisms may further reduce the ethical and legal implications which affect the application of ML in the healthcare system. Therefore, providing right resources for fair distribution and access to the healthcare products and aides empowered by ML is critical in availing healthcare delivery equity. By considering these ethical factors, healthcare stakeholders can sufficiently unlock the possible positive impact of bio-inspired ML models on patient experiences, patient treatment and care, clinicians' decisions, and public health and achieve the ethical goals and principles of adequately handling patients' data, promoting their rights, and rewarding justice in healthcare systems.

7.2 Implications of Bio-Inspired ML Models in Depression Diagnosis and Treatment

Modern AI and bio-inspired ML approaches are improving clinical decision-making in diagnosis and management of depression great outcomes and changing the entire landscape of mental healthcare. Due to these models, the behavioural patterns such as the actions and interactions can be observed, monitored and early signs of depression detected using the physiological signs, the neuroimages so that the treatment is enhanced, and the misery of the untreated mental disorders advances reduced. The fourth element relates to individualized treatment plans as an advantage. Through the focus on patient characteristics, the results achieved by treatments, and heritable markers, bio-inspired ML prescribes customized depression therapies respecting patients' needs and preferences. These models combine multiple parameters, including clinical risk indicants, genetic data, characterization of patient's medication past with the goal to boost the compliance and effectiveness of the therapy.

Risk assessment and prognostic markers are also promoted with these models that identify the path of the disease, relapse, and therapy effectiveness. This enables recognition of the vulnerable persons, theologians, decedent providential track, and fundamentals, hence enhancing the organizational efficiency and patient well-being. Clinicians and researchers need ML-based decision support systems as they help clinicians diagnose depression, select relevant treatments, and track the progression of the disease. These tools help in gathering real-time information, scientific information, and alerts to help in improving treatment plans and overall quality of care that is offered. Telemonitoring and telepsychiatry solutions use all strategies that mimic bio systems to evaluate signs as well as the response to treatment and other management plans. Sensors, applications installed in mobile devices, and telehealth sessions offer ways to provide constant tracking of the mental state of patients, predict relapses, and respond to them, increasing patient participation in the recovery process and improving access to the necessary healthcare services [27-28].

Moreover, self-evolving ML algorithms foster advancement in knowledge on the one hand by processing data regarding the depressive disorder and its treatment and, on the other hand, the prospects of using bio-inspired algorithms create a new generation of analytic instruments. This enhances the discovery of both diagnostic biomarkers and prospective indicators, in addition to therapies geared towards specific patient subpopulations. Altogether, the bio-inspired ML models contribute to offering patient-specific care to mental diagnosis and treatment, increasing the patients' benefits, decreasing the inequalities, and substantially contributing to improving the role and efficacy of depression treatment interventions, thus likely to promote the welfare of those struggling with depression.

Conclusion

To conclude the applications of bio-inspired AI versions stand for an appealing frontier in psychological wellness. Attracting motivation from all-natural and organic systems these versions use cutting-edge options for anticipating, identifying, plus taking care of a vast array of psychological health and wellness problems. Using strategies such as hereditary formulas, bit can swarm optimization, and man-made neural networks, scientists and doctors have the ability to utilize large quantities of information to get much deeper understandings right into the hidden systems of psychological problems.

By incorporating multimodal information resources consisting of hereditary, neuroimaging, professional along with behaviour details, these designs give a holistic strategy to recognizing psychological health and wellness and customizing therapy techniques. Furthermore, the real-time tracking plus treatment abilities of bio-inspired ML versions provides the prospective to reinvent psychological medical distribution making it possible for prompt treatments, and boosting individual results. Nonetheless, obstacles such as information personal privacy, version interpretability plus honest factors to consider should be very carefully attended to guarantee the liable release of these modem technologies.

Continuing the development of collaboration in terms of the initiatives of scientists, medical practitioners, policymakers, and industries is important to enhance the use of bio-inspired AI models for mental healthcare and deterioration of patients' lives due to mental disorders. Such collaborations can help to cease developing bio-inspired AI by making sure that the major findings put into practice to serve the core issues in mental health. This allows one to avoid the siloed mentality that is present in some professions, and different views, being incorporated into a project, will lead to it becoming more well-rounded and efficient. Also, incorporating ethical issues as an early area of concern will assist to ward off possible risks attached to these technologies. This includes preventing abuses in the development and use of AI solutions to respect the users' rights to privacy, equity, and clarity. Semantically complex and often multifactorial, mental health problems can benefit from the permanent progress of bio-inspired ML models as more accurate diagnostic aids, treatment plans, or long-term monitoring solutions.

While these models are continuously refined and developed, it remains critical to ensure their transparency, the responsibility of its developers, and its adherence to patients' best interest. The implementation of transparency in AI model development and operation provides an opportunity for explaining to the stakeholders how the decision is made and helps in easier integration of AI into clinical practice. Accountability involves holding the developers and the consumers of the applicable technology to heed for the consequences, which helps in the avoidance of misuse of the technology and rectifying the impact from its wrong use. Patient-centred care puts the individual, their needs and preferences, first; guaranteeing that progressive innovations in the field directly and positively impacts those with mental health afflictions. Through the application of state of the art technology alongside clinical and empirical knowledge, a new and progressive idea can be presented regarding the provision of mental healthcare to people in the future. Moreover, it improves the quality of care provided to the patients as well as positioning the technologies that are planned to be implemented to fit better into the patient's interests in terms of their mental state and, as a result, a better quality of life.

Progressing collective initiatives in between scientists, medical professionals, policymakers plus sector stakeholders will certainly be vital to take advantage of the complete capacity of bio-inspired AI designs in changing psychological medical and boosting the lives of people affected by mental disease. By promoting interdisciplinary partnerships and focusing on honest factors to consider can optimize the influence of these modern technologies while lessening possible threats. The recurring development of bio-inspired ML designs holds assurance for resolving the complicated and complex nature of psychological wellness problems. As remained to modify and create these versions it is essential to focus on openness, responsibility, and also patient-centred treatment. By integrating cutting-edge modern technology with understanding and evidence-based methods, can lead the way for a future where psychological medical is a lot more available, reliable, and fair for all people.

References

[1] Teng, S., Chai, S., Liu, J., Tateyama, T., Lin, L. and Chen, Y.W. (Jan. 2024). Multi-Modal and Multi-Task Depression Detection with Sentiment Assistance. *In: 2024 IEEE International Conference on Consumer Electronics (ICCE)* (pp. 1–5). IEEE.

[2] Sini, P.J. and Sherfy, K.K. (Mar. 2023). Early Detection of Anxiety, Depression, and Stress among Potential Patients using Machine Learning and Deep Learning Models. *2023 2nd International Conference on Computational Systems and Communication (ICCSC)*, Thiruvananthapuram, India. Research Gate.

[3] Digumarthi, J., Gayathri, V.M. and Pitchai, R. (Apr. 2022). Early Prediction of Cardiac Arrhythmia using Novel Bio-inspired Algorithms. *In: 2022 8th International Conference on Smart Structures and Systems (ICSSS)* (pp. 01–04). IEEE.

[4] Dixit, S., Gaikwad, A., Vyas, V., Shindikar, M. and Kamble, K. (Aug. 2022). United Neurological study of disorders: Alzheimer's disease, Parkinson's disease detection, Anxiety detection, and Stress detection using various Machine Learning Algorithms. *In: 2022 International Conference on Signal and Information Processing (IConSIP)* (pp. 1–6). IEEE.

[5] Reddy, C.K.K., Pullannagari, S.R., Doss, S. and Anisha, P.R. (2024). Dactylology Prediction using Convolution Neural Networks. *In: Fostering Cross-Industry Sustainability with Intelligent Technologies* (pp. 61–72). IGI Global.

[6] Loh, H.W., Ooi, C.P., Aydemir, E., Tuncer, T., Dogan, S. and Acharya, U.R. (2022). Decision support system for major depression detection using spectrogram and convolution neural network with EEG signals. *Expert Systems*, 39(3), e12773.

[7] Shah, K., Patel, U. and Kumar, Y. (Jan. 2024). Machine Learning-based Approaches for Early Prediction of Depression. *In: 2024 International Conference on Intelligent and Innovative Technologies in Computing, Electrical, and Electronics (IITCEE)* (pp. 1–7). IEEE.

[8] Shusharina, N., Yukhnenko, D., Botman, S., Sapunov, V., Savinov, V., Kamyshov, G., ... and Voznyuk, I. (2023). Modern methods of diagnostics and treatment of neurodegenerative diseases and depression. *Diagnostics*, 13(3), 573.

[9] Yang, J., Li, X., Mao, L., Dong, J., Fan, R. and Zhang, L. (2023). Path analysis of influencing factors of depression in middle-aged and elderly patients with diabetes. *Patient Preference and Adherence*, 273–80.

[10] Lin, H., Zhou, W., Tian, X. and Wang, F. (2024). Detection rates of mental health problems among sexual minorities in mainland China: A meta-analysis. *Journal of Homosexuality*, 71(8), 1991–2009.

[11] Zhang, J., Yu, Y., Barra, V., Ruan, X., Chen, Y. and Cai, B. (2023). Feasibility study on using house-tree-person drawings for automatic analysis of depression. *Computer Methods in Biomechanics and Biomedical Engineering*, 1–12.

[12] Kim, K., Ryu, J.I., Lee, B.J., Na, E., Xiang, Y.T., Kanba, S., ... and Park, S.C. (2022). A machine-learning-algorithm-based prediction model for psychotic symptoms in patients with depressive disorder. *Journal of Personalized Medicine*, 12(8), 1218.

[13] Kaseb, A., Galal, O. and Elreedy, D. (Oct. 2022). Analysis on Tweets Towards COVID-19 Pandemic: An Application of Text-Based Depression Detection. *In: 2022 4th Novel Intelligent and Leading Emerging Sciences Conference (NILES)* (pp. 131–36). IEEE.

[14] Nadeem, M., Rashid, J., Moon, H. and Dosset, A. (Jun. 2023). Machine Learning for Mental Health: A Systematic Study of Seven Approaches for Detecting Mental Disorders. *In: 2023 International Technical Conference on Circuits/Systems, Computers, and Communications (ITC-CSCC)* (pp. 1–6). IEEE.

[15] Kuchibhotla, S., Dogga, S.S., Thota, N.G.V., Puli, G., Niranjan, M.S.R. and Vankayalapati, H.D. (May, 2023). Depression detection from speech emotions using MFCC-based recurrent neural network. *In: 2023 2nd International Conference on Vision Towards Emerging Trends in Communication and Networking Technologies (ViTECoN)* (pp. 1–5). IEEE.

[16] Anisha, P.R., Reddy, C.K.K., Nguyen, N.G., Bhushan, M., Kumar, A. and Hanafiah, M.M. (Eds.). (2022). *Intelligent Systems and Machine Learning for Industry: Advancements, Challenges, and Practices.* CRC Press.

[17] Shen, Y., Yang, H. and Lin, L. (May, 2022). Automatic depression detection: An emotional audio-textual corpus and a GRU/BiLSTM-based model. *In: 2022IEEE International Conference on Acoustics, Speech, and Signal Processing (ICASSP)* (pp. 6247–51). IEEE.

[18] Wang, Q. and Liu, N. (Dec. 2022). Speech detection of depression based on multi-mlp. *In: 2022 IEEE International Conference on Bioinformatics and Biomedicine (BIBM)* (pp. 3896–98). IEEE.

[19] Yu, W., Kang, H., Sun, G., Liang, S. and Li, J. (2022). Bio-inspired feature selection in brain disease detection via an improved sparrow search algorithm. *IEEE Transactions on Instrumentation and Measurement, 72,* 1–15.

[20] Zhang, J., Xu, B. and Yin, H. (2023). Depression screening using hybrid neural network. *Multimedia Tools and Applications, 82*(17), 26955–26970.

[21] Acharya, R. and Dash, S.P. (Jul. 2022). Automatic depression detection based on merged convolutional neural networks using facial features.. *In: 2022 IEEE International Conference on Signal Processing and Communications (SPCOM)* (pp. 1–5). IEEE.

[22] Dev, A., Roy, N., Islam, M.K., Biswas, C., Ahmed, H.U., Amin, M.A., ... and Mamun, K.A. (2022). Exploration of EEG-based depression biomarkers identification techniques and their applications: A systematic review. *IEEE Access, 10,* 16756–16781.

[23] Reddy, C.K.K. (May, 2023). An Efficient Healthcare Monitoring System for Cardiovascular Diseases using Deep Modified Neural Networks. Research Gate.

[24] Awotunde, J.B., Ajagbe, S.A. and Florez, H. (Oct. 2023). A Bio-Inspired-Based Salp Swarm Algorithm Enabled with Deep Learning for Alzheimer's Classification. *In: International Conference on Applied Informatics* (pp. 157–70). Cham: Springer Nature Switzerland.

[25] Gollagi, S.G. and Balasubramaniam, S. (2023). Hybrid model with optimization tactics for software defect prediction. *International Journal of Modeling, Simulation, and Scientific Computing, 14*(02), 2350031.

[26] Balasubramaniam, S. and Kumar, K.S. (2022). Fractional Feedback Political Optimizer with Prioritization-based Charge Scheduling in Cloud-Assisted Electric Vehicular Network. *Ad Hoc & Sensor Wireless Networks, 52*(3–4), 173–98.

[27] Park, D., Lee, G., Kim, S., Seo, T., Oh, H. and Kim, S.J. (2024). Probability-based multi-label classification considering correlation between labels–focusing on DSM-5 depressive disorder diagnostic criteria. *IEEE Access.*

[28] Pham, T.H. and Raahemi, B. (2023). Bio-inspired feature selection algorithms with their applications: A systematic literature review. *IEEE Access, 11,* 43733–43758.

12 | Research Directions and Challenges in Bio-Inspired Algorithms for Machine Learning and Deep Learning Models in Healthcare

Mani Deepak Choudhry,[1*] Sundarrajan M,[2] Akshya Jothi[3] and Seifedine Kadry[4]

In the recent past, there has been growing interest in bio-inspired algorithms for their potential to enhance machine learning and deep learning models, especially for applications in healthcare. This chapter covers the nascent domain of bio-inspired algorithms applied in healthcare, discussing research directions and challenges. This chapter discusses several bio-inspired techniques: genetic algorithms, artificial neural networks, evolutionary strategies, swarm intelligence, and ant colony optimization—underpinning their flexibility and efficiency in optimizing complex healthcare systems. The chapter also describes how these algorithms have been combined in machine learning and deep learning frameworks that exhibit the ability for feature selection challenges, parameter optimization, and model explainability on healthcare datasets. Moreover, the chapter looks into the state-of-the-art application of bio-inspired algorithms in healthcare, including disease diagnosis, medical image analysis, drug discovery, and recommendation systems for personalized treatment. While there have been promising developments, several challenges persist, involving algorithm scalability, computational complexity, robustness to noise and uncertainty, ethical consideration, and regulatory compliance. The chapter suggests potential research directions that could overcome those challenges, emphasizing an interdisciplinary approach among computer scientists, healthcare professionals, and domain experts.

1. Introduction to Bio-Inspired Algorithms in Healthcare

Although the application of computers to biology is relatively recent, the increased use of computers means that the application of computers to healthcare is also

---

[1] Department of Computing Technologies, SRM Institute of Science and Technology, Kattankalathur, Chengalpattu, Tamil Nadu, India.
[2] Department of Networking and Communications, SRM Institute of Science and Technology, Kattankalathur, Chengalpattu, Tamil Nadu, India.
[3] Department of Computational Intelligence, SRM Institute of Science and Technology, Kattankalathur, Chengalpattu, Tamil Nadu, India.
[4] Department of Applied Data Science, Noroff University College, Norway.
  Email: sundarrm1@srmist.edu.in; akshyaj@srmist.edu.in; seifedine.kadry@noroff.no
* Corresponding author: manideec@srmist.edu.in

almost as old as computing itself. In the past few years, one of the most promising in developing more advanced decision-making systems in healthcare is applying algorithms inspired by natural processes and evolutionary principles [1]. These algorithms simulate the adaptive and optimization mechanisms of biological systems for novel solutions to complex problems in medical diagnosis, treatment optimization, and healthcare management.

A long tradition of computational biology and evolutionary computing has inspired the development of bio-inspired algorithms in healthcare [2]. These ideas have motivated scientists to construct algorithms based on the fundamentals that Charles Darwin set for natural selection, genetic mutation, and survival of the fittest in optimization problems. The obvious ones are genetic algorithms (GAs), evolutionary strategies (ES), and ant colony optimization (ACO), all of which base their working models on the principles of natural selection in the sense of iteratively improving solutions by adapting to changes in the environment. In so doing, bio-inspired algorithms capture the essence of evolution to provide a flexible and powerful means of optimizing healthcare processes and decision-making [3].

The development of big data and machine learning (ML) has opened doors for bio-inspired algorithms to be applied to more areas, one of which is healthcare analytics and predictive modeling. Data generated in healthcare assumes an exponentially large proportion, and, in general, traditional computational methods are usually not able to address the complexity and variability of medical datasets [4]. On the other hand, bio-inspired algorithms naturally perform extremely well when optimizing over large-scale, high-dimensional data, making them suitable candidates for feature selection, parameter optimization, and pattern recognition tasks in healthcare [5]. From there, scientists can merge bio-inspired techniques with ML and deep learning (DL) models in health systems to make them more accurate, effective, and interpretable for better patient outcomes.

Combining bio-inspired algorithms with ML and DL models in healthcare analytics is changing the game. GAs, particle swarm optimization (PSO), and artificial bee colonies are examples of bio-inspired algorithms that mimic some natural processes' evolution, swarming, and foraging and delivering solutions for complex optimization problems. They perform very well in the context of large-scale, high-dimensional data spaces that emerge with the numerous and complex data sources that characterize healthcare today. For example, GAs have previously been used for feature selection, where they extract the most relevant features from patient data that contribute to disease prediction or diagnosis. It reduces data dimensionality while at the same time enhancing model performance and interpretability because it will highlight the most important variables in the modeling process. On the other side of the coin, the integration of PSO for hyperparameter tuning within ML models has yielded improved accuracy with reduced computational costs.

Using bio-inspired algorithms to supplement the model of ML and DL creates robustness and adaptability. Quite often, the data associated with healthcare tends to be very noisy, heterogeneous, and incomplete, which poses a big challenge for classical computational methods [6]. Such complexities make bio-inspired algorithms flexible and adaptive, hence coming up with robust solutions that are supplied even in an uncertain environment. For example, ACO has been utilized in improving the medical resources' routing and scheduling to optimize the system for healthcare services. Moreover, bio-inspired techniques can be integrated with neural networks to form hybrid models, which possess the benefits of both approaches. Such hybrid models can learn automatically from data while optimizing their structure and parameter values through bio-inspired processes and produce better performance for disease progression modeling and prediction of treatment outcomes [7].

Another critical aspect of the application of bio-inspired algorithms could be interpretability in healthcare models. ML models, especially DL, are predominantly considered "black boxes", due to the complex and non-transparent mode of making decisions [8]. Bio-inspired algorithms would increase interpretability in a way that insights toward feature importance and decision rules are derived from data. For instance, evolutionary algorithms can result in easy-to-understand and trustable rule-based systems, which would be understandable for clinicians [9]. Systems will be able to explain why a certain decision was made, thereby improving transparency and ensuring better clinical decision-making. At the same time, bio-inspired algorithms can be further fused with ML to give way to the development of personalized medicine in which treatment and intervention are tailored to individual patients based on their unique data profiles. Such synergy brings a further improvement in the accuracy and effectiveness of healthcare delivery while maintaining the interpretability and trustworthiness of the models, and so leads to further enhancement in patient outcomes [10].

In addition, beyond its promise for bio-inspired algorithms, such widespread adoption in healthcare will also come with challenges in terms of collaboration that would be required from the computer scientists, healthcare professionals, and domain experts; concerns on scalability and computational efficiency of the algorithms; ethical concerns; and so on. These create combined research efforts of the researchers, policymakers, and industry toward the development of robust, ethical, and clinically validated bio-inspired solutions. The current chapter has focused on applying bio-inspired algorithms within healthcare and discussing how such works are strong and have their limitations in transforming the face of medical practice and research.

2. Overview of Machine Learning and Deep Learning Models in Healthcare

The health sector has been revolutionized to become data-driven by insights and decisions, which emanate from ML and DL, with a resultant trickle-down effect of better care to the patients and improved diagnoses and treatments. ML is the broad application of artificial intelligence (AI) for training the algorithm with large datasets to recognize patterns or make predictions or decisions about the outcomes of the processes under consideration, without being explicitly programmed. In healthcare, ML involves everything from predicting outbreaks to personalizing treatment plans and advancing diagnoses. It learns models from historical data, including electronic health records (EHRs), medical images, genomic sequences, and much more, to dig out trends and correlations that are unknown to human clinicians. DL is a more advanced subset of ML that employs deep artificial neural networks for the analysis of many-layered data: in the medical field, images, audio recordings, and text. DL has resulted in very impressive improvements with the models based on convonutional neural networks (CNNs) and recurrent neural networks (RNNs) in applications related to image and speech recognition. Specifically, for healthcare, CNNs are widely used in the interpretation of medical imaging, such as X-rays, MRIs, and CTs, with accuracy almost always equivalent to or even better than that of human experts. RNNs, further extended to models such as long short-term memory (LSTM) networks, are good at learning sequential data and are therefore an excellent fit for predicting patient outcomes using time-series data from wearables or continuous monitoring systems.

Integrating ML and DL into healthcare portends great advances in personalized medicine, early disease detection, and operation efficiencies. For example, ML models can analyze genetic information and subsequently tailor individual treatments for optimal benefits to an individual in personalized medicine. For example, the early diagnosis of diseases, such as cancers and diabetic retinopathy, is greatly enhanced by DL models that spot changes in medical images effortlessly traversable by the human eye. Besides, ML models can optimize health operations by planning resources, admissions of patients, and streamlining administrative procedures. Continuous development of these technologies is likely to reshape healthcare delivery to be more predictive, preventive, and precise. Various ML and DL algorithms involved in healthcare are depicted in Figure 1 followed by subsequent subsections describing ML and DL models in detail.

2.1 ML Models for Healthcare

ML is the wide range of statistical learning and study that allows computer systems to learn from experience and hence improve their way of operation without being programmed for specific activities. This learning involves modifying the way the machine behaves. For instance, an ML system may be capable of learning how to recognize faces by combing over a set of images. The two main subdivisions of ML are unsupervised learning and supervised learning. One of the sectors poised to gain tremendously from such a move is healthcare [11, 12, 13]. Over the last century, the development of technology has played a large role in pushing the average human lifespan higher. Even the slightest details of operations can be optimized today because of the power of computing. AI and ML, with growing technology, are set to drastically change healthcare. Currently, ML is playing a role in the sector; the scope for future implementation remains unlimited [14, 15]. The healthcare industry has embraced the cutting edge of modern technologies,

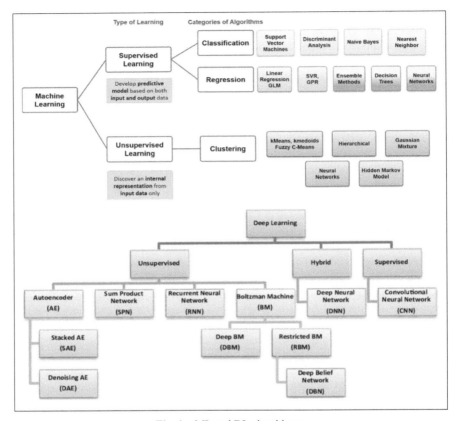

Fig. 1 ML and DL algorithms.

and AI and ML are no exceptions. It has many applications in health, just like the way it plays roles in business and e-commerce. ML is changing the healthcare industry through new, innovative applications combined with Big Data tools, such as Electronic Medical Records, for advanced data analytics. ML tools have the potential to upgrade automation and intelligent decision-making for patient care and public health systems, thus improving the quality of life for billions across the globe [16,17,18].

2.1.1 Revolutionizing Healthcare by ML

ML can analyze and interpret complex medical data more efficiently and accurately than traditional methods. The possibilities that could be opened in the process of improving patient care are diverse. Here are some key ways in which ML is revolutionizing the healthcare industry:

- ML algorithms are very competent at detecting patterns and even minute correlations in huge datasets. The result in healthcare will be improved by early disease detection and timely diagnosis. ML algorithms are now applied in revealing early indicators of diseases missed by the human doctor through patient data—medical histories, genetic profiles, and imaging. This can be tantamount to prompt intervention, saving lives, and improving patient outcomes.

- Different people have distinct natures and may respond differently to varied treatments. ML algorithms could look through the characteristics of patients, their medical history, and the results of the treatment provided to define an individualized treatment plan. Considering all factors, from genetic markers and lifestyle to environmental factors, ML can help healthcare providers personalize the treatment of patients in such a way as to maximize the possibility of their successful recovery.
- ML algorithms learn from historical data of patient cases to predict disease course and high-risk potential for certain conditions. Analyzing trends and factors of risk, such models provide healthcare professionals with important insights for proactive intervention. For example, in chronic conditions, such as diabetes or hypertension, ML can predict when a patient's condition might get worse, enabling physicians to take precautionary measures and avoid complications.

2.1.2 Benefits of using ML in Healthcare

- Improvement in accuracy and efficiency.
- Personalized Treatment.
- Real-Time Monitoring.
- Data-Driven Insight.

2.1.3. Challenges of using ML in Healthcare

- **Data Quality and Availability**
  - Fragmented and inconsistent data across different systems.
  - Difficulty in aggregating and preprocessing data.
    Sensitivity and privacy concerns regarding patient data.
    Compliance with regulations like HIPAA.
- **Model Interpretability**
  - Advanced ML models, particularly DL, often act as "black boxes".
  - Lack of transparency in model decision-making processes.
  - Need for clear explanations for clinical validation and trust.
  - Physicians require interpretable outputs to integrate ML into patient care.
- **Generalizability**
  - ML models may not generalize across different patient populations or clinical settings.
  - Variability in demographics, genetics, and healthcare practices.
  - Extensive need for validation and retraining with diverse datasets.

236 | Bio-inspired Algorithms in Machine Learning and Deep Learning for Disease Detection

- Challenges of integration into existing clinical workflow.
- Ensuring that the models augment, rather than interfere with, the decision-making processes.

2.2 DL Models for Healthcare

AI, including ML and DL, is one of the latest technologies transforming healthcare today. It involves the training of artificial neural networks in a tremendous amount of data to learn complicated patterns and predict with great precision. Healthcare is a unique sector that has benefited, for the last couple of years, from DL models in medical imaging and diagnostics, personalized treatment planning, and drug discovery [19]. These models are most relevant in healthcare data because of their ability to handle and analyze large datasets with a huge number of variables. The most popular application of DL in healthcare has been within the domain of medical imaging. CNNs are important types of DL models that specialize in image recognition and classification tasks. Such models have been applied to the task of detecting and diagnosing diseases from medical images like X-rays, MRIs, and CT scans. For example, CNNs can detect tumors, fractures, and other abnormalities more accurately, if not better, than human radiologists. This not only results in an improvement in the accuracy of diagnoses but also in faster diagnosing, hence enabling early intervention in the treatment process. Apart from diagnostics, DL models transform personalized medicine. By studying the patient's genetic data, EHRs, and other data, these models can predict the risk of acquiring some diseases and provide personalized treatment plans. The best models for this function are RNNs and LSTMs, as they can handle sequential data and recognize temporal patterns. This is pretty important for estimating the disease course and delivering patient-tailored treatment plans, not only to improve the patient's state but also to reduce the cost of healthcare.

DL also forms significant contributions to the discovery of drugs and their subsequent development. The traditional approaches toward drug discovery are time-consuming and expensive, but DL models predict how different molecules will interact with biological targets and, hence, dramatically speed up this process. Generative adversarial networks (GANs) and other DL techniques can generate fresh drug candidates and simulate the potential effects these drugs are likely to elicit. This has the impact of significantly reducing the development timeline. These models could also reveal existing drugs that could be repurposed to treat other conditions, thereby offering new hope for diseases with few options. However, implementation comes with a lot of challenges [20]. Data privacy and security are key aspects since data within healthcare are sensitive. It is very important to ensure that the models are trained on representative quality data to avoid biases, which then lead to inaccurate predictions and care disparities. Another area of concern is the interpretability of DL models since these models normally operate as a "black box" with decision-making processes not easily understandable by a human. These challenges need continual collaboration between AI researchers, healthcare professionals, and regulatory bodies to ensure the technologies of DL are safe, effective, and fair to patients in general.

2.2.1. DL in Medical Imaging

DL techniques in medical imaging enhance the image acquisition and pathology identification process. They improve the quality of images from different modalities and enable effective detection of pathological markers. As an illustration, CNN improves the resolution of MRI images to visualize possible pathologies [21]. In addition to increasing resolution, CNNs are great for processing acquired images to detect features that point to specific pathologies [22]. That is, this technology has a dual ability to enhance acquisition while supporting pathology identification. The high-dimensional structure of data and the imbalance between positive and negative samples make many diseases, especially tumors, relatively rare, posing a great challenge for the model-training task in these problems. DL has brought profound changes to medical imaging in the last few years in addressing the classification, segmentation, and detection tasks in MRI, CT, and PET modalities [23, 24, 25]. It is notoriously true that training DL algorithms is data-thirsty in the low-sample scenario. Data augmentation comes as a solution by providing the artificial generation of new samples, a paramount procedure in DL fields characterized by sparse rich datasets. This is also useful for missing modalities in multimodal image segmentation, hence generalizing the model and reducing overfitting. PyTorch supports data augmentation on the fly, which makes the process efficient without needing a physically larger dataset. The basic augmentation operations are rotations, crops, flips, and noise injection, but these are often not sufficient for complex medical images. Advanced techniques and domain-specific augmentation strategies are necessary to effectively enhance the training process for DL models in medical imaging.

2.2.2 Challenges faced by DL models

DL models in healthcare, particularly in medical imaging, face several challenges, including:

- **Data Privacy and Security:** Ensuring the protection of sensitive patient data and complying with regulations like HIPAA and GDPR.
- **Limited Training Data:** The scarcity of annotated medical data, especially for rare diseases, hampers the effective training of DL models.
- **Data Quality and Variability:** Variations in imaging protocols, equipment, and patient populations can lead to inconsistencies in data quality.
- **Interpretability:** The "black box" nature of DL models makes it difficult to understand and explain their decision-making processes.
- **Bias and Fairness:** Models trained on unrepresentative datasets may exhibit biases, leading to disparities in diagnosis and treatment.
- **Computational Resources:** High computational power and memory are required to train and deploy DL models, which can be costly and resource-intensive.

- *Integration with Clinical Workflows*: Incorporating DL solutions into existing clinical workflows and ensuring user acceptance among healthcare professionals.
- *Regulatory Approval*: Meeting stringent regulatory standards for medical device approval and demonstrating clinical efficacy and safety.
- *Generalization*: Ensuring that models generalize well across different populations, healthcare settings, and imaging modalities.
- *Ethical Concerns*: Addressing ethical issues related to AI in healthcare, including informed consent, accountability, and the impact on healthcare jobs. Table 1 defines various models involved in DL with their uniqueness.

Table 1   Different DL models with their uniqueness.

S. No.	DL Models	Uniqueness
		Various DL Models
1.	CNN	• Excellent at image recognition and classification. • Capable of automatic feature extraction.
2.	RNN	• Effective in handling sequential data. • Suitable for time-series analysis and predicting disease progression.
3.	LSTM	• Maintains long-term dependencies in data. • Ideal for patient monitoring and EHR analysis.
4.	GAN	• Generates synthetic data to augment training datasets. • Useful in drug discovery and personalized medicine.
5.	Autoencoders	• Effective in unsupervised learning and dimensionality reduction. • Useful for anomaly detection in medical images.
6.	Deep Belief Networks	• Combines multiple layers of stochastic latent variables. • Useful for pre-training and initializing deep networks.
7.	Restricted Boltzmann Machines	• Efficient in learning a probability distribution over its input. • Can be used for collaborative filtering in medical recommendations.
8.	Transformers	• Highly efficient in processing large-scale data. • Excellent for natural language processing tasks like medical text analysis.

3. Bio-Inspired Optimization Techniques for Healthcare Data

Bio-inspired optimization techniques, drawing inspiration from natural processes and biological systems, offer innovative solutions to complex problems in various fields, including healthcare [26–30]. These techniques emulate the efficiency, adaptability, and resilience of biological systems to optimize decision-making processes. In healthcare, where data is vast, complex, and often uncertain, bio-inspired algorithms can enhance data analysis, predictive modeling, and resource management. They provide robust frameworks to tackle challenges such as disease diagnosis, treatment planning, and patient management. Figures 2 and 3 provide an overview and describe the various bio-inspired techniques.

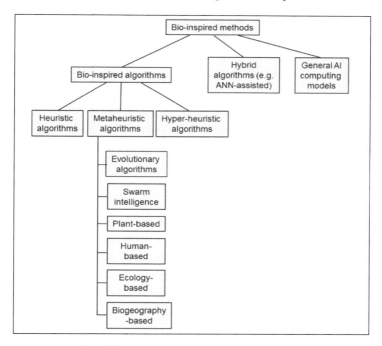

Fig. 2 Different classifications of Bio-inspired methods.

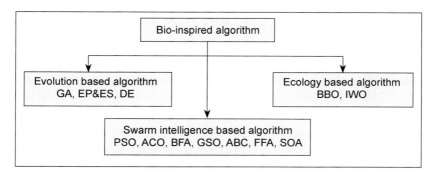

Fig. 3 Taxonomy of Bio-inspired algorithms.

One of the most prominent bio-inspired techniques is GAs, which, inspired by natural selection by selection, crossover, and mutation, aim to solve the optimization problem [31, 32]. Healthcare applications of GAs include staff schedule optimization, resource allocation in hospitals, and personal treatment planning, all to arrive at workable, high-quality decisions that will improve patient outcomes and operational efficiency. Another popular technique is the PSO, inspired by the social behavior of birds and fish. It employs numerous particles, which refer to potential solutions, moving throughout the search space and guided by their own and neighbors' experiences searching for an optimal solution [32]. In healthcare, PSO optimizes medical imaging, such as enhancing MRI and CT scans, and bioinformatics tasks, like gene selection for disease classification. The coordination of PSO toward achieving a common goal makes it powerful in solving high-dimensional optimization problems common in healthcare data.

ACO, inspired by the foraging behavior of ants, is another bio-inspired technique used in healthcare. ACO algorithms simulate the pheromone-laying and following behavior of ants to find optimal paths through graphs, making them suitable for network optimization problems [32, 33]. ACO is also used in healthcare to optimize the routing of emergency vehicles, design efficient patient referral networks, and improve the logistics of drug delivery systems. This is justifiable because the algorithm can come up with near-optimal solutions, even with complex and dynamic environments, making it appropriate for real-time decision-making in healthcare logistics.

Another field that follows the human immune system learning and memory approach is that of Artificial Immune Systems (AIS). AIS will contribute to anomaly detection and diagnostics since they are able to recognize patterns, remember interactions, and adapt to new challenges. For instance, in medicine, this technology is used in the detection of disease outbreaks, personalized medicine, and adaptive control systems in medical devices. These abilities make AIS a powerful tool for improving healthcare monitoring and response systems. These bio-inspired optimization techniques are applied to ML and predictive modeling in healthcare. Techniques such as Differential Evolution and Bee Colony Optimization can be used to improve ML techniques with optimized hyperparameters and feature selection processes during training. These methods improve the accuracy and efficiency of predictive models to be used for disease prognosis, patient risk assessment, and treatment outcome prediction. These bio-inspired algorithms allow the model development by healthcare data scientists to be more reliable and interpretable because of their adaptive and exploratory nature.

4. Applications of Bio-Inspired Algorithms in Healthcare

The next frontier where bio-inspired algorithms have found applications in health is by revolutionizing the field of health care [34–38]. Bio-inspired algorithms have come as a result of the phenomena in nature, and they offer solutions to various complex problems. Noteworthy applications of bio-inspired algorithms in health are outlined below:

- ***Disease Diagnosis and Prognosis***: In disease diagnosis and prognosis, bio-inspired algorithms, such as GAs and AIS, are used. Such algorithms look at

Research Directions and Challenges in BIA for ML, DL Models in Healthcare | 241

patient data—that is, history of sickness, symptoms, and results of diagnosis tests—so that doctors can diagnose the disease at an early stage and predict the course of the disease.

- **Personalized Medicine**: Personalized medicine is the use of therapeutics by taking into account patient molecular characteristics along with lifestyle and environmental influences. In this regard, bio-inspired algorithms might offer a way to adequately explore the huge space of genomic and clinical databases to devise optimal treatment strategies for a target patient population. The use of techniques for optimization of treatment plans, dosage regimens, and combinations of drugs includes PSO and ACO to make the outcomes of the patients better and to alleviate their adverse effects.
- **Medical Imaging**: Bio-inspired algorithm applications have been found in several medical imaging problems, where quality and efficiency both are increased in the diagnostic imaging techniques. These techniques are mostly based on MRI, CT, and PET scans. Examples are swarm-inspired algorithms, PSO, and ACO that help in processes of image reconstruction and noise reduction, as well as helping in optimization for feature extraction, processes that lead to clearer and more informative images in the medical field. These improved imaging techniques help radiologists to diagnose accurately and to plan the right course for treatment.
- **Healthcare Resource Allocation**: One of the important components of timely and effective patient care is the efficient allocation of resources in healthcare, in terms of medical staff, equipment, and facilities. Several bio-inspired algorithms have been researched in the optimization of resource allocation processes within health systems, including GAs and ACOs. The algorithms take into account parameters like demand, resource availability, and operating constraints in areas of scheduling, staffing, and facility layout. In this way, the best healthcare delivery is rendered and made most cost-effective.
- **Drug Discovery and Development**: Bio-inspired algorithms are increasingly being used in the processes of drug discovery and development to speed up the identification of potential drug candidates and optimum drug designs. Techniques like (GAs), PSO, and Evolutionary Strategies (ES) are put to work for tasks in virtual screening, molecular docking, and pharmacophore modeling toward the identification of new drug-target interactions and lead compound identification.
- **Healthcare Logistics and Supply Chain Management**: Effective healthcare logistics and supply chain management is the key to the timely supply of medical supplies, medicines, and equipment to healthcare providers. Bio-inspired algorithms like ACO and PSO are used in this process of optimization of routing, scheduling, and inventory management processes in healthcare logistics.
- **Healthcare Data Analytics and Decision Support**: Healthcare data analytics and building decision support systems is one of the applications where bio-inspired algorithms are very popular. They develop predictive models,

risk stratification algorithms, and treatment recommendation systems with techniques like GAs, artificial neural networks, and evolutionary computation. These algorithms pave the way toward the adaptability and self-learning of healthcare organizations to increase their analytics capabilities to improve patient care outcomes.

5. Challenges in Implementing Bio-Inspired Algorithms

Application of bio-inspired algorithms can be a very difficult task due to their complexity and the nature of the biological systems they are based on [39–45]. The following are typical challenges:

- *Complexity of Biological Systems*: Biological systems are usually of very high complexity and dynamism, which is why representing them in an algorithmic form turns out to be very difficult. Translating such systems' complexity into computationally tractable algorithms requires deep domain and computation understanding to be effective.
- *Parameter Tuning*: Most bio-inspired algorithms have one or more parameters that have to be tuned very carefully for well-performing assignments. Getting good parameter configurations is not easy because it is highly experimental, and, in most cases, this necessitates a large amount of previous experience and domain knowledge on the subject.
- *Scalability*: The bio-inspired techniques are pretty good at most small-scale problems. However, the problem of scaling large problems or those involving large datasets or complex problems with bio-inspired algorithms can be quite formidable. The increase in scale of a problem naturally increases the computational complexity and memory requirements.
- *Premature Convergence*: This is a problem from which bio-inspired algorithms, notably evolutionary algorithms, unfortunately, suffer. A suboptimal solution usually arises from early stagnation before reaching a global optimum.
- *Selection of Algorithms*: There are so many different bio-inspired algorithms that work best for different types of problems. Designing the most appropriate one for a particular problem requires a sound understanding both of the strengths and weaknesses of each algorithm and the problem domain.
- *Interpretability*: Some bio-inspired algorithms, like artificial neural networks, can be difficult to interpret and understand. This makes interpretability a barrier to their adoption, especially in applications where the rationale behind the decision is important.
- *Computational Resources*: Bio-inspired algorithms are sometimes very computationally intensive and require many computational resources for effective running. This may be limiting, especially in the case of those applications where time and resource constraints have to be adhered to strictly.
- *Validation and Benchmarking*: Performance evaluation of bio-inspired algorithms against other techniques is hard. One has to devise appropriate validation methodologies and benchmarking datasets that are effective, and this is very important but nontrivial.

- ***Robustness and Adaptability***: The biological systems often depict these characteristics in robustness and adaptability to variations in environments. In robustness and adaptability to variations in environments, the biological systems often depict these characteristics. Designing algorithms that have these properties is tough, especially in environments that are dynamic and uncertain.
- ***Ethical and Social Implications***: The more influential and pervasive bio-inspired algorithms become, the more important the ethical and social implications. From algorithmic bias to fairness and transparency, problems will need to be properly tackled to ensure that such algorithms will be used responsibly.

Addressing these challenges requires a multidisciplinary approach, combining insights from biology, computer science, mathematics, and other fields. It is impossible to make progress in this exciting and rapidly developing field without cooperation between researchers of different specializations.

6. Future Research Directions and Innovations

Future research and innovation in bio-inspired algorithms are expected to focus on current challenges and push the envelope of feasibility [46–47]. Some potential areas of interest include:

1. ***Hybridization and Integration***: The combination of several bio-inspired algorithms, or simply integration, may lead to the development of stronger and more versatile optimization methods when combined with other optimization techniques. A hybrid approach would make it feasible to capture the strong points of different algorithms while alleviating the weaknesses of individual members.
2. ***Explainability and Interpretability***: Bio-inspired algorithms, particularly ML, for instance, neural networks, require an additional level of interpretation to be interpretable and explainable in the application domain under considerations where transparency and accountability is a concern. Future research might contribute to the development of techniques that make the reasoning of such algorithms interpretable to humans.
3. ***Adaptive, Self-learning Systems***: Bio-inspired algorithms that adapt and self-learn in the face of a changing environment—very much like biological organisms—are a very attractive subject in research. Robust self-learners, capable of improving their functioning without human interaction, could be explosively applied in the fields of robotics, autonomous driving, and care applications.
4. ***Ethical and Fairness Considerations***: The broader the deployment of bioinspired algorithms, the more urgency the ethical and fairness issues impart. So, an expected area of important research in this facet would be the development of methodologies that can be helpful in the mitigation of

244 | Bio-inspired Algorithms in Machine Learning and Deep Learning for Disease Detection

issues related to algorithmic bias, promotion of fairness and transparency, and injecting ethical consideration into design and deployment.

5. ***Biologically Plausible Computing***: The research in the direction of bio-inspired algorithms should give immense jumps to the next plane in the fields of AI and cognitive sciences. Computing of this kind, inspired by the structure and working of the brain, does enable the understanding of biological intelligence, and it also makes much more efficient and robust AI systems.

6. ***Robustness and Resilience***: Designing bio-inspired algorithms to be robust and resilient against adversarial attacks, noise, and uncertainty are some of the foremost research areas. It is important to design algorithms capable of handling unpredictable perturbations and maintaining the performance of the system under difficult conditions for real-world application.

7. ***Multi-objective and Multimodal Optimization***: It is important to continue the process of extension of bio-inspired algorithms to deal with multi-objective optimization problems where multiple objectives may conflict with each other. Similarly, the development of algorithms that will effectively explore and exploit multiple search spaces (multimodal optimization) might yield more effective and efficient optimization techniques.

8. ***Applications in Emerging Technologies***: It also opens the doors to exploring applications for such bio-inspired algorithms in emerging technologies, be it quantum computing, nanotechnology, or biotechnology, that might open up avenues for out-of-the-box innovation. The algorithms can be put to use in solving complicated optimization problems in these domains and in aiding to break barriers in the spheres of drug discovery, material science, and renewable energy.

Furthermore, future research on bio-inspired algorithms will be inspired by interdisciplinarity collaboration, pushing the limits of what can be done and solving, with innovative solutions inspired by nature, true real-world problems.

Conclusion

In this chapter, we have taken an interesting exploration through bio-inspired algorithms and their application in health. It begins with the very basics of bio-inspired algorithms and the importance of these algorithms to the health sector. It then goes further in-depth regarding ML and DL models, considering their huge influence on medical diagnosis, patient treatment, and care. Then, we saw the world of optimization, particularly health data optimization, and brought to light how the techniques developed for optimization are capable of effectively handling the complex optimization challenges emanating from health analytics. We then consider diverse applications of bio-inspired algorithms in health, ranging from medical image analysis and disease diagnosis to personalized treatment planning and healthcare resource management. On one hand, the potential for these algorithms seems vast; yet, challenges always come hand-in-hand. Starting from the complexities of biological systems to algorithm selection and scaling issues, we review some of the issues researchers and practitioners have to face to make the most out of these novel methodologies. Looking toward the future, we outline some very exciting research avenues and advancements that could revolutionize the challenges faced now and have the potential to take bio-inspired algorithms in health to new heights. From hybridization to explainability and ethical considerations to emerging technologies, the landscape is rife with the opportunity to drive forward the frontiers of healthcare analytics with interdisciplinary collaboration and creative exploration.

References

[1] Pham, T.H. and Raahemi, B. (2023). Bio-inspired feature selection algorithms with their applications: A systematic literature review. *IEEE Access*.

[2] Siddiqui, M.F., Alam, A., Kalmatov, R., Mouna, A., Villela, R., Mitalipova, A., ... and Parween, Z. (2022). Leveraging healthcare system with nature-inspired computing techniques: An overview and future perspective. *Nature-Inspired Intelligent Computing Techniques in Bioinformatics*, 19–42.

[3] Amiri, Z., Heidari, A., Zavvar, M., Navimipour, N.J. and Esmaeilpour, M. (2024). The applications of nature-inspired algorithms in Internet of Things-based healthcare service: A systematic literature review. *Transactions on Emerging Telecommunications Technologies*, 35(6), e4969.

[4] Kumari, N. and Acharjya, D.P. (2023). Data classification using rough set and bio-inspired computing in healthcare applications: An extensive review. *Multimedia Tools and Applications*, 82(9), 13479–13505.

[5] Sripriyanka, G. and Mahendran, A. (2022). Bio-inspired computing techniques for data security challenges and controls. *SN Computer Science*, 3(6), 427.

[6] Pandiyan, N. and Narayan, S. (2023). A Survey on Deep Learning Models Embed Bio-Inspired Algorithms in Cardiac Disease Classification. *The Open Biomedical Engineering Journal*, 17(1).

[7] Munish Khanna, Singh, L.K. and Garg, H. (2024). A novel approach for human diseases prediction using nature inspired computing and machine learning approach. *Multimedia Tools and Applications*, 83(6), 17773–17809.

[8] Mujawar, S. and Gupta, J. (Mar. 2022). A Statistical Perspective for Empirical Analysis of Bio-Inspired Algorithms for Medical Disease Detection. *In: 2022 International Conference on Emerging Smart Computing and Informatics (ESCI)* (pp. 1–7). IEEE.

[9] Baburaj, E. (2022). Comparative analysis of bio-inspired optimization algorithms in neural network-based data mining classification. *International Journal of Swarm Intelligence Research (IJSIR)*, 13(1), 1–25.

[10] Schirner, M., Deco, G. and Ritter, P. (2023). Learning how network structure shapes decision-making for bio-inspired computing. *Nature Communications*, 14(1), 2963.

[11] Abdelaziz, A., Elhoseny, M., Salama, A.S. and Riad, A.M. (2018). A machine learning model for improving healthcare services on cloud computing environment. *Measurement*, 119, 117–28.

[12] Char, D.S., Abràmoff, M.D. and Feudtner, C. (2020). Identifying ethical considerations for machine learning healthcare applications. *The American Journal of Bioethics*, 20(11), 7–17.

[13] Ahmad, M.A., Eckert, C. and Teredesai, A. (Aug. 2018). Interpretable machine learning in healthcare. *In: Proceedings of the 2018 ACM International Conference on Bioinformatics, Computational Biology, and Health Informatics* (pp. 559–60). IEEE.

[14] Kaur, P., Sharma, M. and Mittal, M. (2018). Big data and machine learning based secure healthcare framework. *Procedia Computer Science*, 132, 1049–59.

[15] Sarwar, M.A., Kamal, N., Hamid, W. and Shah, M.A. (Sept. 2018). Prediction of diabetes using machine learning algorithms in healthcare. *In: 2018 24th International Conference on Automation and Computing (ICAC)* (pp. 1–6). IEEE.

[16] Sendak, M.P., D'Arcy, J., Kashyap, S., Gao, M., Nichols, M., Corey, K., ... and Balu, S. (2020). A path for translation of machine learning products into healthcare delivery. *EMJ Innov., 10*, 19–00172.

[17] Gupta, A. and Katarya, R. (2020). Social media-based surveillance systems for healthcare using machine learning: A systematic review. *Journal of Biomedical Informatics, 108*, 103500.

[18] Tucker, A., Wang, Z., Rotalinti, Y. and Myles, P. (2020). Generating high-fidelity synthetic patient data for assessing machine learning healthcare software. *NPJ Digital Medicine, 3*(1), 1–13.

[19] Purushotham, S., Meng, C., Che, Z. and Liu, Y. (2018). Benchmarking deep learning models on large healthcare datasets. *Journal of Biomedical Informatics, 83*, 112–34.

[20] Miotto, R., Wang, F., Wang, S., Jiang, X. and Dudley, J.T. (2018). Deep learning for healthcare: Review, opportunities, and challenges. *Briefings in Bioinformatics, 19*(6), 1236–46.

[21] He, K., Zhang, X., Ren, S. and Sun, J. (2016). Deep residual learning for image recognition. *In: Proceedings of the IEEE Conference on Computer Vision and Pattern Recognition* (pp. 770–78). IEEE.

[22] Ghorbanali, A. and Sohrabi, M.K. (2023). A comprehensive survey on deep learning-based approaches for multimodal sentiment analysis. *Artificial Intelligence Review, 56*(Suppl 1), 1479–1512.

[23] Amyar, A., Modzelewski, R., Vera, P., Morard, V. and Ruan, S. (2022). Weakly supervised tumor detection in PET using class response for treatment outcome prediction. *Journal of Imaging, 8*(5), 130.

[24] Brochet, T., Lapuyade-Lahorgue, J., Huat, A., Thureau, S., Pasquier, D., Gardin, I., ... and Ruan, S. (2022). A quantitative comparison between Shannon and Tsallis–Havrda–Charvat entropies applied to cancer outcome prediction. *Entropy, 24*(4), 436.

[25] Lundervold, A.S. and Lundervold, A. (2019). An overview of deep learning in medical imaging focusing on MRI. *Zeitschrift für Medizinische Physik, 29*(2), 102–27.

[26] Gill, S.S. and Buyya, R. (2019). Bio-inspired algorithms for big data analytics: A survey, taxonomy, and open challenges. *In: Big Data Analytics for Intelligent Healthcare Management* (pp. 1–17). Academic Press.

[27] Torre-Bastida, A.I., Díaz-de-Arcaya, J., Osaba, E., Muhammad, K., Camacho, D., and Del Ser, J. (2021). Bio-inspired computation for big data fusion, storage, processing, learning and visualization: State-of-the-art and future directions. *Neural Computing and Applications*, 1–31.

[28] Kar, A.K. (2016). Bio-inspired computing: A review of algorithms and scope of applications. *Expert Systems with Applications, 59*, 20–32.

[29] Jabbar, S., Iram, R., Minhas, A.A., Shafi, I., Khalid, S. and Ahmad, M. (2013). Intelligent optimization of wireless sensor networks through bio-inspired computing: Survey and future directions. *International Journal of Distributed Sensor Networks, 9*(2), 421084.

[30] Alabdulatif, A. and Thilakarathne, N.N. (2023). Bio-inspired internet of things: Current status, benefits, challenges, and future directions. *Biomimetics, 8*(4), 373.

[31] Gonçalves, C.B., Souza, J.R. and Fernandes, H. (2022). CNN architecture optimization using bio-inspired algorithms for breast cancer detection in infrared images. *Computers in Biology and Medicine, 142*, 105205.

[32] Swain, A., Swain, K.P., Palai, G. and Nayak, S.R. (2021). Optimization of wireless sensor networks using bio-inspired algorithm. *In: Smart Sensor Networks Using AI for Industry 4.0* (pp. 1–24). CRC Press.

[33] Khan, F.A., Ullah, K., ur Rahman, A. and Anwar, S. (2023). Energy optimization in smart urban buildings using bio-inspired ant colony optimization. *Soft Computing, 27*(2), 973–89.

Research Directions and Challenges in BIA for ML, DL Models in Healthcare | 247

[34] Aldossri, R. and Hafizur Rahman, M.M. (2023). A Systematic Literature Review on Cybersecurity Issues in Healthcare. *Computational Vision and Bio-Inspired Computing: Proceedings of ICCVBIC 2022*, 813–23.

[35] Paneerselvam, S. (2020). Role of AI and Bio-Inspired Computing in Decision Making. *Internet of Things for Industry 4.0: Design, Challenges, and Solutions*, 115–36.

[36] Ma, Y., Xiao, X., Ren, H. and Meng, M.Q.H. (2022). A review of bio-inspired needle for percutaneous interventions. *Biomimetic Intelligence and Robotics*, 2(4), 100064.

[37] Eid, H.F. (2023). Bio-Inspired Algorithms for Wireless Network Optimization: Recent Trends and Applications. *Applications of Artificial Intelligence in Wireless Communication Systems* (pp. 13–35). IGI Global.

[38] Larabi-Marie-Sainte, S., Alskireen, R. and Alhalawani, S. (2021). Emerging applications of bio-inspired algorithms in image segmentation. *Electronics*, 10(24), 3116.

[39] Poudel, S., Arafat, M.Y. and Moh, S. (2023). Bio-inspired optimization-based path planning algorithms in unmanned aerial vehicles: A survey. *Sensors*, 23(6), 3051.

[40] Chui, K.T., Liu, R.W., Zhao, M. and Zhang, X. (2024). Bio-inspired algorithms for cybersecurity: A review of the state-of-the-art and challenges. *International Journal of Bio-Inspired Computation*, 23(1), 1–15.

[41] Yadav, R., Sreedevi, I. and Gupta, D. (2022). Bio-inspired hybrid optimization algorithms for energy efficient wireless sensor networks: A comprehensive review. *Electronics*, 11(10), 1545.

[42] Johnvictor, A.C., Durgamahanthi, V., Pariti Venkata, R.M. and Jethi, N. (2022). Critical review of bio-inspired optimization techniques. *Wiley Interdisciplinary Reviews: Computational Statistics*, 14(1), e1528.

[43] Thankaraj Ambujam, S. (2024). Power quality enhancement in the wind energy distribution system using HHO algorithm-based UPFC. *Journal of the Chinese Institute of Engineers*, 1–21.

[44] Balasubramaniam, S., Prasanth, A., Kumar, K.S. and Kavitha, V. (2024). Medical Image Analysis Based on Deep Learning Approach for Early Diagnosis of Diseases. *In: Deep Learning for Smart Healthcare* (pp. 54–75). Auerbach Publications.

[45] Ali, A., Hafeez, Y., Hussainn, S.M. and Nazir, M.U. (Jan. 2020). Bio-inspired communication: A review on solution of complex problems for highly configurable systems. *In: 2020 3rd International Conference on Computing, Mathematics, and Engineering Technologies (iCoMET)* (pp. 1–6). IEEE.

[46] Bale, A.S., Tiwari, S., Khatokar, A., Vinay, N. and Mohan, K. (2021). Bio-Inspired Computing: A Dive into Critical Problems, Potential Architecture, and Techniques. *Trends in Sciences*, 18(23), 1–14.

[47] Balasaraswathi, M., Sivasankaran, V., Akshaya, N., Baskar, R. and Suganya, E. (2020). Internet of things (IoT) based bio-inspired artificial intelligent technique to combat cybercrimes: A review. *Internet of Things in Smart Technologies for Sustainable Urban Development*, 141–55.

Index

A

Alex-Net 143, 144

Algorithm 1, 2, 6, 7, 10, 16, 17, 23, 25, 29, 31, 48-60, 62, 63, 66, 85, 88, 92, 95, 98, 100, 101, 107, 109, 111, 113, 116, 123, 125, 130, 132, 137, 141, 147, 151, 160, 161, 166, 185, 203, 209, 211, 217, 219, 221, 230, 234, 240, 241, 245

Artificial Neural Networks 4, 27, 48, 78, 89, 112, 113, 133, 159, 210, 211, 230, 233, 236, 242

Autism Spectrum Disorder 158, 173, 204, 213

B

Bio-inspired 1-5, 7, 10, 11, 17-19, 23, 24, 34, 37, 39, 41, 48, 50-53, 66, 70, 79, 80, 88, 89, 94, 97, 99, 100, 107, 109, 122, 123, 130, 141, 147, 148, 149, 151-154, 158-168, 173, 175, 177, 180, 209, 211, 214, 215, 220, 224, 230, 232, 242, 245

Bio-inspired Algorithms (BIAs) 1-5, 7, 9-11, 17-19, 23, 26, 88, 93, 94, 101, 102, 107-110, 113, 114, 116, 117, 183, 185, 196, 198, 203, 209, 211, 212, 214, 215, 217, 219, 220, 221, 223, 226, 230, 231, 239-243

Bio-inspired Intelligence 122, 123

Bio-inspired Optimization 34, 41, 49-52, 59, 108, 117, 130, 134, 165, 166, 168, 180, 183, 217, 238, 240

C

Cancer Diagnosis 50, 82, 92, 122, 123, 129-138

Cardiac Health Monitoring 88, 91-95, 97-99, 101, 104

Comparative Analysis 80, 220

Computational intelligence 1, 33, 102, 135, 183

Convolutional Network 5, 42, 52, 71, 76, 116, 142, 159, 189, 208

COVID-19 107, 109, 114-118, 122, 166

D

Data-Centric Prediction 203

Decision Trees 27, 53, 56, 128, 136, 186, 197, 203, 217, 221, 222

Deep Learning 1, 2, 23, 29, 34-36, 39, 41, 44, 45, 48, 52, 54, 71, 78, 80, 84, 89, 90, 91, 97, 102, 107, 108, 112, 116, 141, 143, 147-155, 158, 159, 164, 183, 189, 192-194, 230-232

Depression 203, 205-207, 209-213, 218-220, 222, 223, 225, 226

Diabetic diagnosis 141-147, 156

Diagnosis 5, 10, 23, 34, 41-43, 51, 52, 70-72, 107, 108, 113, 114, 116, 118, 122, 123, 127, 128, 130, 131, 134, 135, 137, 141, 142, 145, 147, 156, 158, 159, 163, 165, 179, 180, 203, 205, 207, 208, 212, 213, 223, 225, 231, 233, 239, 240, 244

Disease Detection 41, 42, 44, 45, 83, 100, 159, 164, 166, 233, 235

DL-based Accuracy 64-66

E

Early Diagnosis 10, 42, 72, 88, 117, 166, 167, 180, 207, 233

Electronic Health Records 73, 189, 208, 233

Ethical Decisions 73

Evolutionary Algorithms (EAs) 7, 10, 11, 23, 24, 26, 28, 52, 77, 78, 92, 123, 125, 232, 242

Explainable AI 38, 39, 83, 84, 224

F

Feature Selection 25, 27, 32, 34, 38, 41, 42, 51, 53, 77, 78, 81, 92-95, 97, 99, 101, 123, 124, 134, 136, 146, 158, 165, 166, 170, 173, 175, 177, 178, 180, 218, 230

Fuzzy DL 53

Contents

G

Genetic Algorithms 1, 2, 9, 11, 23, 24, 29, 48, 54, 70, 90, 93, 100, 125, 133, 161, 185, 196, 203, 230, 231

Genetic Programming 15, 24, 30, 51, 77, 125, 133, 220

GridSearch Optimization 158

H

Healthcare 2, 4, 7, 10, 18, 38, 39, 41, 48-50, 52, 61, 80, 83, 84, 89, 100, 103, 104, 137, 145, 162, 166, 167, 175, 177, 189, 190, 192, 193, 195, 197, 198, 204-208, 214, 215, 221, 224, 225, 227, 230, 232, 233, 235, 236-238, 240-242, 245

K

KNN (K-Nearest Neighbors) 203

L

Learning 1, 2, 5, 8, 10, 12, 23, 25, 27, 33, 34, 36, 39, 49, 53, 71, 73, 75, 77, 78, 80, 83, 85, 102, 107, 108, 111, 123, 128, 135, 143, 147, 155, 158, 168, 183, 186, 188, 191, 196, 203, 208, 220, 230, 233, 240, 243

M

Machine Learning 1, 2 23, 25, 27, 28, 35, 37, 39, 43, 48, 50, 107, 108, 111, 113, 122, 123, 128, 130, 136, 141, 145, 150, 158, 159, 170, 183, 185, 186, 189, 191, 192, 196-198, 203, 208, 209, 217, 223, 224, 230-231

Medical Diagnosis 34, 71, 78, 79, 206, 212, 214, 231, 244

Mental Health 183, 197, 198, 203, 212, 223, 225, 227

ML-based Accuracy 62, 63

N

Neural Network 1, 2, 4, 5, 9, 14, 27, 29, 34, 36, 42, 48, 52, 54, 71, 74, 76, 78, 83, 88, 90-92, 94, 97-99, 103, 107, 108, 112, 113, 116, 128, 130, 133-136, 141, 142, 145, 158, 159, 165, 189-191, 204, 205, 208, 210, 213, 217, 218, 222, 223, 226, 230, 232, 233, 236, 242, 243

Neurological Disorders 5, 73, 166, 203-205

O

Optimization 1, 2, 5-7, 9-11, 14, 16-19, 23-26, 28-30, 48-55, 60-63, 65, 66, 70, 71, 74, 78, 80, 88, 91-97, 99, 100, 104, 107, 108, 117, 125, 130, 131, 133, 134, 147, 158, 160-163, 168, 175-177, 183, 185, 188, 190, 210, 215, 217, 218, 222, 226, 230, 231, 238-241, 243, 244

Optimization Models 23

Optimization Techniques 19, 33, 43, 49, 50, 52, 53, 63, 66, 89, 92, 93, 97, 160, 180, 190, 238, 240, 243, 244

P

Particle-Swarm Optimization 1, 2, 6, 23, 24, 31, 32, 34, 48, 51, 71, 78, 89, 91, 94, 133, 158, 159, 161, 185, 186, 210, 231

R

Res-Net 143, 144

S

Social Anxiety 183, 184, 219

Social Phobia 183-186, 188, 189, 191-193, 196-198

SVM 53, 55, 62, 63, 66, 101, 107, 108, 113, 114, 118, 129, 130, 136, 143, 145, 146, 150-153, 155, 165, 166, 177, 180, 217, 218, 220, 221

Swarm intelligence 1, 2, 4, 11, 14, 15, 31, 38, 45, 48, 51, 77, 88, 91, 98-100, 103, 110, 122, 133, 134, 160-162, 185, 196, 211, 230

Swarm Intelligence Algorithms 11, 14, 45, 98, 99, 133, 134, 196

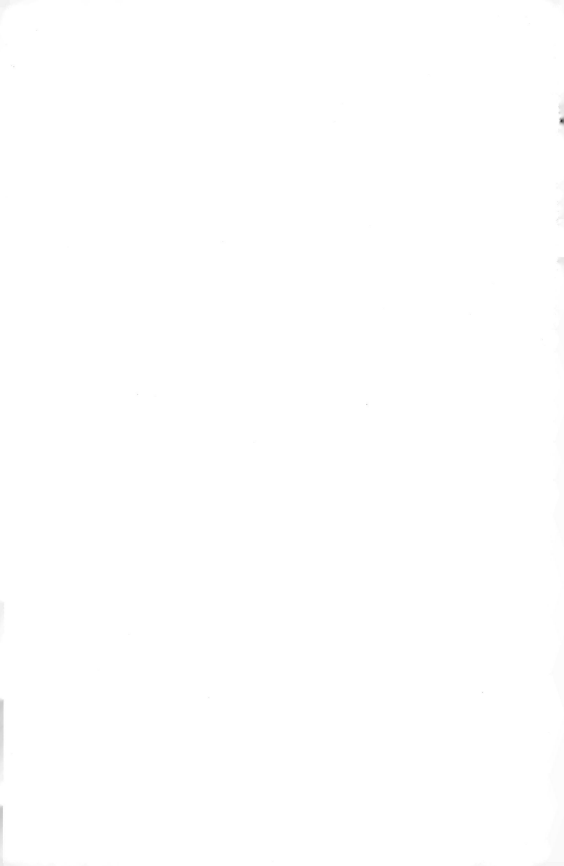